NUTRITION AND AGRICULTURAL DEVELOPMENT

Significance and Potential for the Tropics

BASIC LIFE SCIENCES

Alexander Hollaender, General Editor

Associated Universities, Inc.
Washington, D. C.
and The University of Tennessee
Knoxville

1973: Volume 1 • GENE EXPRESSION AND ITS REGULATION
Edited by F. T. Kenney, B. A. Hamkalo, G. Favelukes, and J. T. August

Volume 2 • GENES, ENZYMES, AND POPULATIONS
Edited by A. M. Srb

1974: Volume 3 • CONTROL OF TRANSCRIPTION
Edited by B. B. Biswas, R. K. Mandal, A. Stevens, and W. E. Cohn

Volume 4 • PHYSIOLOGY AND GENETICS OF REPRODUCTION (Parts A and B)
Edited by E. M. Coutinho and F. Fuchs

1975: Volume 5 • MOLECULAR MECHANISMS FOR REPAIR OF DNA (Parts A and B)
Edited by P. C. Hanawalt and R. B. Setlow

Volume 6 • ENZYME INDUCTION
Edited by D. V. Parke

1976: Volume 7 • NUTRITION AND AGRICULTURAL DEVELOPMENT
Edited by N. Scrimshaw and M. Béhar

NUTRITION AND AGRICULTURAL DEVELOPMENT

Significance and Potential for the Tropics

Edited by

Nevin S. Scrimshaw
Massachusetts Institute of Technology

and

Moisés Béhar
World Health Organization

PLENUM PRESS . NEW YORK AND LONDON

Library of Congress Cataloging in Publication Data

Symposium on Nutrition and Agricultural and Economic Development in the Tropics, Guatemala, 1974.
Nutrition and agricultural development.

(Basic life sciences; v. 7)
Held in celebration of the 25th anniversary of the Institute of Nutrition of Central America and Panama.
Includes bibliographical references and index.
1. Food supply—Tropics—Congresses. 2. Nutrition—Congresses. 3. Agriculture—Tropics—Congresses. I. Scrimshaw, Nevin S. II. Béhar, Moisés. III. Guatemala (City). Instituto de Nutrición de Centro América y Panamá. IV. Title.
HD9000.1.S96 1974 388.1'9'13 76-2043
ISBN 0-306-36507-3

Proceedings of the Fourteenth International Biological Symposium
held in Guatemala City, Guatemala, December 2-6, 1974

A Division of Plenum Publishing Corporation
227 West 17th Street, New York, N.Y. 10011

United Kingdom edition published by Plenum Press, London
A Division of Plenum Publishing Company, Ltd.
Davis House (4th Floor), 8 Scrubs Lane, Harlesden, London, NW10 6SE, England

Printed in the United States of America

Foreword

For the past thirteen years, symposia have been held either in South America or in Mexico on subjects of special interest to Latin American scientists. When the opportunity of holding the 14th International Biological Symposium in Guatemala was offered, it was most welcome, especially as the occasion was the celebration of the 25th Anniversary of the Institute of Nutrition of Central America and Panama (INCAP).

With the encouragement of members of the Ford Foundation staff and the National Academy of Sciences, the idea for a symposium on the broad approach to the problem of nutrition was developed by Dr. Moisés Béhar, the second director of INCAP, 1961–1974, Dr. Nevin Scrimshaw, first director of INCAP, 1949–1961, and members of the INCAP staff. Because the availability of food has become a serious international problem, a discussion of the underlying problems was most timely. INCAP, one of the pioneer and leading institutions in the area of nutrition, has a profound influence on nutrition in Latin America.

The meeting was attended by about 300 scientists from more than 20 countries. Because this was the first symposium in this series to be held in Central America, it provided an opportunity to get acquainted with scientists from many of the Central American republics. It was especially rewarding that so many students from the Central American universities attended this meeting.

We had excellent cooperation from our speakers and discussants, and the great hospitality of the members of INCAP was very much appreciated. Credit should also go to Plenum Press for bringing out the proceedings of this symposium so promptly.

A complete list of previous Latin American Symposia, with publication information on each, is given below.

1961

I. International Symposium on Tissue Transplantation–Santiago, Viña del Mar, and Valparaiso, Chile. Published in 1962 by the University of Chile Press, Santiago; edited by A. P. Cristoffanini and Gustavo Hoecker; 269 pp.

1962

II. International Symposium on Mammalian Cytogenetics and Related Problems in Radiobiology–Sao Paulo and Rio de Janeiro, Brazil. Published in 1964 by The Macmillan Company, New York, under arrangement with Pergamon Press, Ltd., Oxford; edited by C. Pavan, C. Chagas, O. Frota-Pessoa, and L. R. Caldas; 427 pp.

1963

III. International Symposium on Control of Cell Division and the Induction of Cancer–Lima, Peru, and Cali, Colombia. Published in 1964 by the U.S. Department of Health, Education, and Welfare as *National Cancer Institute Monograph 14;* edited by C. C. Congdon and Pablo Mori-Chavez; 403 pp.

1964

IV. International Symposium on Genes and Chromosomes, Structure and Function–Buenos Aires, Argentina. Published in 1965 by the U.S. Department of Health, Education, and Welfare as *National Cancer Institute Monograph 18;* edited by J. I. Valencia and Rhoda F. Grell, with the cooperation of Ruby Marie Valencia; 354 pp.

1965

V. International Symposium on the Nucleolus–Its Structure and Function–Montevideo, Uruguay. Published in 1966 by the U.S. Department of Health, Education, and Welfare as *National Cancer Institute Monograph 23;* edited by W. S. Vincent and O. L. Miller, Jr.; 610 pp.

1966

VI. International Symposium on Enzymatic Aspects of Metabolic Regulation–Mexico City, Mexico. Published in 1967 by the U.S. Department of Health, Education, and Welfare as *National Cancer Institute Monograph 27;* edited by M. P. Stulberg; 343 pp.

1967

VII. International Symposium on Basic Mechanisms in Photochemistry and Photobiology–Caracas, Venezuela. Published in 1968 by Pergamon Press as Volume 7, No. 6, *Photochemistry and Photobiology;* edited by J. W. Longworth; 326 pp.

1968

VIII. International Symposium on Nuclear Physiology and Differentiation–Belo Horizonte, Minas Gerais, Brazil. Published in 1969 by The Genetics Society of America as a supplement to *Genetics,* Volume 61, No. 1; edited by R. P. Wagner; 469 pp.

1969

IX. International Symposium on Fertility of the Sea–Sao Paulo, Brazil. Published in 1971 by Gordon and Breach Science Publishers, New York; edited by J. D. Costlow; 2 volumes, 622 pp.

1970

X. International Symposium on Visual Processes in Vertebrates–Santiago, Chile. Published in 1971 by Pergamon Press as Volume 11, Supplement No. 3, *Vision Research;* edited by Thorne Shipley and J. E. Dowling; 477 pp.

1971

XI. International Symposium on Gene Expression and Its Regulation–La Plata, Argentina. Published in 1973 by Plenum Publishing Corporation, New York, as *Vol. 1 Basic Life Sciences Series* (Alexander Hollaender, General Editor); edited by Francis T. Kenney, Barbara A. Hamkalo, Gabriel Favelukes, and J. Thomas August.

1972

XII. International Symposium on Genes, Enzymes, and Populations–Cali, Colombia. Published in 1973 by Plenum Publishing Corporation, New York, as *Vol. 2 Basic Life Sciences Series* (Alexander Hollaender, General Editor); edited by Adrian M. Srb; 359 pp.

1973

XIII. International Symposium on Physiologic and Genetic Aspects of Reproduction–Salvador da Bahia, Brazil. Published in 1974 by Plenum Publishing Corporation, New York, as *Vol. 4 (Parts A and B) Basic Life Sciences Series* (Alexander Hollaender, General Editor); edited by Elsimar M. Coutinho and Fritz Fuchs; 871 pp.

Alexander Hollaender

Preface

The articles in this volume were presented and discussed at the Symposium on Nutrition and Agricultural and Economic Development in the Tropics, held in Guatemala City December 2–6, 1974, to celebrate the XXVth Anniversary of the Institute of Nutrition of Central America and Panama (INCAP). This Institute was an early manifestation of the movement toward integration of the six countries of the Central American Isthmus. When a cooperative effort to study, and look for solutions to, the prevailing nutritional problems of the populations of these countries was first proposed in 1945, it seemed almost utopian. However, the Pan American Health Organization convened a meeting in Guatemala City in February, 1946, at which the idea was discussed and approved by the representatives of the Ministries of Health of all six countries.

The mission entrusted to INCAP was the achievement of three essential objectives: to study the nutrition problems of the member countries; to seek ways and means of solving them; and to provide member governments with advice and assistance in applying the measures best calculated to solve those problems. The following year, Guatemala, Honduras, and El Salvador ratified the agreement and began paying annual contributions of $8,500 each.

From the very beginning, the basic purpose was to develop the internal capabilities of the countries to determine and solve their own nutritional problems, with the Institute acting as a technical supporting agency. Activities were to be integrated. In 1948, recent graduates from the local universities of Guatemala, Honduras, and El Salvador were selected and trained for one year in the United States in clinical nutrition, food chemistry, and nutrition and dietetics, to form the initial nucleus of the scientific staff.

INCAP was inaugurated on September 15, 1949, with nine Central American professionals from three countries. It was a modest start in a tin-roofed adobe building in the Botanical Gardens, provided by the Government of Guatemala, but the group was young, enthusiastic, dedicated, and hardworking. The other three countries of Central America joined subsequently: Nicaragua in 1954, Costa Rica in 1955, and Panama in 1956. As each country joined, additional young professionals from each joined the INCAP staff or were sent to the United States for advanced training.

The W. K. Kellogg Foundation gave an initial grant of $15,000 per year for three years to PAHO to support its administrative participation in INCAP, provided fellowships for the necessary training of professionals, and donated $50,000 for equipment and supplies, supplemented by a generous grant to establish a library with the major current nutrition books and journals. These funds supplemented the $25,500 for the first year's budget derived from the country's quota.

The annual quotas per member country were increased to $12,500 in 1949, $17,500 in 1956, $25,000 in 1964, and $62,424 in 1967. It was soon realized that larger quarters would be needed, and the Government of Guatemala constructed a modern, three-story building on the outskirts of Guatemala City, which was inaugurated September 15, 1954. In the years since, a clinical research center has been added and an experimental farm for work with large animals was opened in 1961. A second, larger three-story building was completed in 1972, and a pilot plant for food technology was constructed in 1973.

In 1971, the contribution system of the member countries was adjusted to a total of $250,000, with a quota from each country proportional to its economic capabilities. With expiration of the initial grant from the W. K. Kellogg Foundation, the member countries asked PAHO to continue administering the Institute on their behalf, and PAHO contributions gradually increased to a present total of nearly $600,000 per year.

In cooperation with the national health departments, the first years were devoted to epidemiological studies of the nature and magnitude of the nutritional problems of the population and to completion of an analysis of the nutritional value of Central American foods. As local problems were revealed, efforts were initiated to find solutions within the resources and local characteristics of the countries. Progressively, new personnel were recruited locally and trained both at INCAP and in the United States. A strong program of research developed as the basis for training and advisory responsibilities to its member countries.

From the beginning, INCAP was heavily dependent on outside assistance for its research program. The first research grants came from the Nutrition Foundation and the Williams–Waterman Program of the Research Corporation. Subsequently, major research support was provided for various projects by the U.S. National Institutes of Health and many other sources. In its 25th year, INCAP received approximately $2,250,000 in research grants or contracts from different sources.

The *research programs* of the Institute were established to obtain a better understanding of the epidemiology and effects of the more important nutritional deficiencies found in the countries–protein-energy malnutrition, endemic goiter, vitamin A deficiency, and nutritional anemias–and to search for the means to correct them. From an initial emphasis on food analysis, food habits, and clinical nutritional status, the program expanded into agricultural sciences, food safety, social anthropology, and, more recently, economics, in order to understand better the complex food and nutrition problems needing correction.

The *training programs* of INCAP started with ad hoc or in-service training in Guatemala of the personnel working in the member countries, and developed progressively into short courses and workshops for field training to complement the background and experience of key personnel (physicians, nurses, teachers, agricultural extension workers, nutritionists). Finally, in agreement with the other Central American universities and in cooperation with the University of San Carlos, Guatemala, formal courses leading to academic degrees were developed.

At present, the following academic degree programs are offered at INCAP. A four-year undergraduate program for the training of nutritionists, and graduate-level courses leading to a master's degree in the following four areas: Public Health, with emphasis on nutrition and maternal and child health; Food Science and Technology; Food Science and Animal Nutrition; and Biochemistry and Human Nutrition. In addition, students are still received for ad hoc in-service training in the different areas of INCAP competence. An average of 150 students are enrolled every year in these training programs.

The *advisory services* started with technical cooperation from INCAP headquarters staff to the Ministries of Health of the member countries, in each of which a department of nutrition was created, largely utilizing personnel whose training was provided or arranged by INCAP. Progressively, this technical cooperation was expanded to other ministries of the member countries, especially those of agriculture and education, as well as to the universities and to private industry. More recently, it extended to the newly organized national planning commissions.

The objective has always been to help the countries develop their own technical capabilities, their own nutrition programs, and to assist in training the personnel needed for this purpose. In this way, INCAP has worked, not as an outside agency telling the countries what to do, but rather as a body that has collaborated with them in defining their problems, helping them to decide what could be done to correct them, and training their personnel to do it. Meanwhile, it has undertaken the technical work needed to support this purpose, with the cooperation, wherever appropriate and convenient, of other national or regional Central American institutions.

Among the specific accomplishments of INCAP are the following:

1. Complete and detailed studies of the nutritional status and dietary habits of the populations of the six member countries.

2. The completion of a composition table for the foods of Central America and Panama, which later formed the core of a Latin American Food Composition Table prepared by INCAP with consultant help.

3. Better understanding of (a) the effects of pre- and postnatal malnutrition on growth and development of children, including learning and behavior; (b) the interactions of nutrition and work performance of adults.

4. Better understanding of the epidemiology of protein-calorie malnutrition, including the role of infections.

5. Improved methods for the treatment and rehabilitation of malnourished children.

6. Development and practical application of the principle of combining different plant sources to make highly nutritious, low-cost foods such as Incaparina.

7. Development of original methods of food fortification, including the iodization of moist, unrefined salt with potassium iodate and the fortification of sugar with vitamin A.

8. Utilization of local products and development of improved management systems for animal feeding, including the use of cottonseed meal in monogastric animals, feeding systems for raising calves with little milk, and the use of available waste products and by-products for animal feeding.

9. Development of principles and materials for nutrition education and for the teaching of nutrition at various levels.

10. Development and application of new methods for assessment of the nutritional status of population groups.

Equally important, however, are the contributions of INCAP toward a better understanding of the food and nutritional problems of communities; to recognition of their public health and social importance; to knowledge of what can and should be done about them; and to creation of an awareness of and interest in these subjects on the part of national officials, university professors and other influential citizens, and the international community.

Although INCAP was created for, and maintains, a primary responsibility for the six member countries, it also helps the food and nutrition programs of other countries in the Latin American region and the world by its training and research programs and, through PAHO and WHO, by advisory services.

During its first 25 years, more than 1600 students have passed through INCAP's classrooms and laboratories, and its staff and students have contributed over 1500 scientific publications. Starting from a small number of workers in a limited number of disciplines, its staff now includes 60 specialists in agronomy, food science and technology, microbiology, physiology, biochemistry, general medicine, pediatrics, gastroenterology, dietetics, human and animal nutrition, social and physical anthropology, psychology, economics, education, statistics, systems analysis, communications, and library sciences.

At present, its annual budget is over $3 million, and it operates in modern and ample buildings on the outskirts of Guatemala City, with excellent laboratories of biochemistry, microbiology, virology, tissue culture, food chemistry, work physiology, and hematology, plus a pilot plant for food processing, a computer center, teaching laboratories and classrooms, an animal colony for small experimental animals, an excellent library with more than 30,000 volumes that also receives more than 500 journals, and a clinical center especially equipped for metabolic and clinical investigations. It has, in addition, an experimental farm for agronomic research and studies in large animals, as well as eight field stations located in different ecological areas for epidemiological and other studies in human populations.

INCAP has been a highly successful venture, developing in 25 years from a very modest attempt at international cooperation among six small countries, into a large and strong institution that has made significant contributions in the field of human nutrition, not only to its member countries, but to the world at large. The following factors that contributed to its development are particularly worth noting: well trained scientific personnel, mainly from its member countries, working with enthusiasm and dedication; the utilization of problem-solving research as the basis for its advisory services and training programs; and a multidisciplinary and multisectorial approach to the problems of food and nutrition. Of great significance also was the fact that it was able to utilize the best available knowledge and expertise from around the world by bringing experts to advise on its programs from a variety of fields, either as consultants or as members of its Technical Advisory Committee.

The technical, administrative, and financial support of the Pan American Health Organization Regional Office for the Americas of WHO has been fundamental, as well as has the support from many fund-granting institutions. The Institute is especially indebted to the W. K. Kellogg Foundation, The Nutrition Foundation, The Research Corporation, the Josiah Macy, Jr., Ford, Rockefeller, and Nestlé foundations, the U.S. National Institutes of Health, the International Committee on Nutrition for National Development, the U.S. Agency for International Development, the International Development Research Centre of Canada, UNICEF, and WHO.

With INCAP's help, the countries of Central America have made significant progress in the understanding of the nutritional problems of their populations and in the control or alleviation of some of them. Unfortunately, because of economic, social, and political factors in Central America, malnutrition is still a serious problem in the area, and present world conditions may aggravate the problem further. Clearly, the nutritional situation would have been far worse in a number of ways without INCAP-sponsored efforts, such as salt iodization, flour fortification with B vitamins and iron, the development of Incaparina and other weaning foods, and provision of nutrition education and incorporation of nutrition in public health programs.

In INCAP, the governments now have at their service a strong and able technical institution on which they can count for sound advice and help in dealing with food and nutrition problems. In addition, they have available well-trained personnel in the field, and the facilities of INCAP for the training of more as needed. The main limitations will continue to be of a socioeconomic and political nature, and INCAP is now devoting considerable effort to assisting countries to make improved nutrition one of the objectives of their social and economic development and to encourage them to include nutritional considerations in their national development planning.

The Central American area can produce the food it needs, and it has the human and material resources for accelerated social and economic development. We are confident that INCAP will play an increasing role in the efforts of its member countries to improve the nutritional and health status of their populations, and that its work will continue to be of value to Latin America as a whole and to other developing regions.

Dr. Nevin S. Scrimshaw
Director, 1949–1961

Dr. Moisés Béhar
Director 1961–1974

ACKNOWLEDGMENTS

We are indebted to the participants in the Symposium for so promptly supplying manuscripts and graciously accepting editorial changes. Most particularly, we acknowledge the effective and dedicated editorial assistance of Amalia G. de Ramírez of INCAP and Jane Dittrich of MIT.

We acknowledge the financial support for the meeting provided by the Pan American Health Organization, the Organization of American States, the Atomic Energy Commission, the Williams-Waterman Program of the Research Corporation, the Ford Foundation, and The Rockefeller Foundation.

Contributors

J. C. Abbott, Food and Agriculture Organization of the United Nations, Rome, Italy

M. W. Adams, Department of Crop and Soil Sciences, Michigan State University, East Lansing, Michigan

R. G. Anderson, International Maize and Wheat Improvement Center, Calle Londres No. 40, Mexico, D. F.

Hildebrando Araica A., Ministry of Health, Department of Population and Planning, Panama

Eduardo E. Arriaga, Data Evaluation Branch, International Statistical Programs Center, U.S. Bureau of the Census, Washington, D. C.

Guillermo Arroyave, Division of Physiological Chemistry, Institute of Nutrition of Central America and Panama, Guatemala City, Guatemala

Antonio Arteaga L., Nutrition Department, Catholic University, Santiago, Chile

Antonio Bacigalupo, Universidad Nacional Agraria, Lima, Peru

John E. Bardach, Hawaii Institute of Marine Biology, University of Hawaii at Manoa, Kaneohe, Hawaii

George H. Beaton, Department of Nutrition, School of Hygiene, University of Toronto, Toronto, Canada

Pedro Belli, Instituto Centroamericano de Administración de Empresas, Managua, Nicaragua

Georg Borgstrom, Department of Food Science and Human Nutrition, Michigan State University, East Lansing, Michigan

Ricardo Bressani, Division of Agricultural and Food Sciences, Institute of Nutrition of Central America and Panama, Guatemala City, Guatemala

Lester R. Brown, Worldwatch Institute, Washington, D. C.

William L. Brown, Pioneer Hi-Bred International, Inc., Des Moines, Iowa

Marco Tulio Cabezas, Division of Agricultural and Food Sciences, Institute of Nutrition of Central America and Panama, Guatemala City, Guatemala

Robert F. Chandler, Jr., The Asian Vegetable Research and Development Center, P. O. Box 42, Shanhua, Taiwan

Claudio F. Chicco, Centro de Investigaciones Agropecuarias, Ministerio de Agricultura y Cria, Maracay, Venezuela

C. M. Christensen, Department of Plant Pathology, University of Minnesota, St. Paul, Minnesota

Joaquin Cravioto, División de Investigación Scientífica, Institución Mexicana de Asistencia a la Niñez (IMAN), Mexico 20, D.F.

Tony J. Cunha, Department of Animal Science, University of Florida, Gainesville, Florida

William J. Darby, The Nutrition Foundation, Inc., New York and Washington, D.C.

Elsa R. DeLicardie, División de Investigacion Scientífica, Institución Mexiana de Asistencia a la Niñez (IMAN), Mexico 22, D.F.

Juan del Canto, Division of Applied Nutrition, Institute of Nutrition of Central America and Panama, Guatemala City, Guatemala

John Osgood Field, International Nutrition Planning Program, Massachusetts Institute of Technology, Cambridge, Massachusetts

Marina Flores, Division of Applied Nutrition, Institute of Nutrition of Central America and Panama, Guatemala City, Guatemala

Hernán Fonseca, University of Costa Rica, San José, Costa Rica

Manuel Cuca García, Colegio de Postgraduados, Escuela Nacional de Agricultura, Chapingo, Mexico

Ricardo Garza T., Instituto Nacional de Investigaciones Pecurias, Palo Alto, Mexico

Everardo González P., Instituto Nacional de Investigaciones Pecurias, Palo Alto, Mexico

Nancie L. González, Program Director for Anthropology, National Science Foundation, Washington, D.C.

Dale D. Harpstead, Department of Crop and Soil Sciences, Michigan State University, East Lansing, Michigan

Robert S. Harris, Professor of Nutrition, Emeritus, Department of Nutrition and Food Science, Massachusetts Institute of Technology, Cambridge, Massachusetts

Richard R. Harwood, Cropping Systems Program, International Rice Institute, Los Baños, Philippines

Fabio Higuita, Instituto Colombiano Agropecuario, Bogotá, Colombia

Joseph H. Hulse, International Development Research Centre, Ottawa, Canada

Derrick B. Jelliffe, Population, Family and International Health Division, School of Public Health, University of California, Los Angeles, California

E. F. Patrice Jelliffe, Population, Family and International Health Division, School of Public Health, University of California, Los Angeles, California

H. H. Kaufmann, Grain Research Laboratory, Cargill, Inc., Minneapolis, Minnesota

Michael C. Latham, Division of Nutritional Sciences, Cornell University, Ithaca, New York

Aaron Lechtig, Human Development Division, Institute of Nutrition of Central America and Panama, Guatemala City, Guatemala

F. James Levinson, International Nutrition Planning Program, Massachusetts Institute of Technology, Cambridge, Massachusetts

J. K. Loosli, University of Florida, Gainesville, Florida

Jerome H. Maner, Centro Internacional de Agricultura Tropical (CIAT), Cali, Colombia

Eugenio Martinez S., Instituto de Ciencia y Tecnologia Agrícolas, Guatemala City, Guatemala

Leonardo J. Mata, Instituto de Investigación en Salud, University of Costa Rica, Costa Rica

Ian A. McGregor, Laboratory for Tropical Community Studies, National Institute for Medical Research, Mill Hill, London, England

Edwin T. Mertz, Department of Biochemistry, Purdue University, Lafayette, Indiana

Fernando Mönckeberg, Departamento de Nutricion y Tecnologia de Alimentos, Universidad de Chile, Santiago, Chile

Arthur D. Odell, Industrial Grain Products, Montreal, Canada

A. E. Olszyna-Marzys, Division of Food Control and Analysis, Institute of Nutrition of Central America and Panama, Guatemala City, Guatemala

H. A. B. Parpia, Food and Agriculture Industries Services, Agricultural Services Division, Food and Agriculture Organization of the United Nations, Rome, Italy

Philip R. Payne, Department of Human Nutrition, London School of Hygiene and Tropical Medicine, London, England

David Pimentel, Department of Entomology and Section of Ecology and Systematics, Cornell University, Ithaca, New York

Antonio M. Pinchinat, Centro Agronómico Tropical de Investigación y Enseñanza, Turrialba, Costa Rica

John A. Pino, Director for Agricultural Sciences, The Rockefeller Foundation, New York, New York

Federico R. Poey, Semillas Poey, S. A., Mexico 6, D. F.

Lewis M. Roberts, Agricultural Sciences, The Rockefeller Foundation, Guatemala City, Guatemala

Manuel E. Ruiz, Centro Agronómico Tropical de Investigación y Enseñanza (CATIE), Turrialba, Costa Rica

Henry J. Schafer, Instituto Tecnológico y de Estudios Superiores de Monterrey, Escuela de Ciencias Maritimas y Tecnologia de Alimentos Guaymas, Bahia de Bacochibampo, Guaymas, Sonora, Mexico

Juan J. Schildknecht, Alimentos, S. A., Guatemala City, Guatemala

Marcelo Selowsky, Development Research Center, World Bank, Washington, D.C.

Malcolm Slesser, Energy Analysis Unit, Strathclyde University, Glasgow, Scotland

Pedro Solana M., Instituto Nacional de Investigaciones Pecuarias, Palo Alto, Mexico

Steven R. Tannenbaum, Department of Nutrition and Food Science, Massachusetts Institute of Technology, Cambridge, Massachusetts

Carl E. Taylor, Department of International Health, School of Hygiene and Public Health, The Johns Hopkins University, Baltimore, Maryland

Carlos Tejada, Director, Institute of Nutrition of Central America and Panama, Guatemala City, Guatemala

Clibas Vieira, Departamento de Fitotecnia, Universidade Federal de Vicosa, Escola Superior de Agricultura, Vicosa, Minas Gerais, Brasil

Javier Perez Villaseñor, Departamento de Biotecnología, Universidad Autonoma Metropolitana-Unidad Iztapalapa, Mexico 13, D. F.

Fernando E. Viteri, Biomedical Division, Institute of Nutrition of Central America and Panama, Guatemala City, Guatemala

George C. Warner, US/AID, Lima, Peru

Robert K. Waugh, Instituto de Ciencia y Tecnologia Agricolas, Guatemala City, Guatemala

Quentin M. West, Economic Research Service, United States Department of Agriculture, Washington, D. C.

Contents

I

Food and Nutrition Problems

1

Man, Food, and Environmental Interrelationships

Lester R. Brown

Worldwatch Institute
Washington, D.C.

Pressure on world food supplies is leading to the emergence of a global politics of food scarcity. The resulting high food prices and shortages are an inconvenience for affluent societies and individuals, but they place poor nations and the poor within them in a dangerous predicament. When global food reserves are low, the ability of the international community to provide relief and respond to emergencies such as droughts or crop failures is greatly diminished. The long-term trend is disturbing; global demand for foodstuffs is outrunning the productive capacity of the world's farmers and fishermen.

Throughout most of the period since World War II the world has had two major reserves of food—carryover stocks of grain in the principal exporting countries and cropland held idle in the United States under government farm programs. Together, these reserves provided a substantial buffer against crop failures (Table I). In 1961 these two reserves combined represented 222 million tons of grain, or 95 days of world consumption. By 1974, these reserves had declined to just 26 days—mere pipeline supplies (Table II).

By late 1974 the world food supply/demand equation was precariously balanced. Under these circumstances, a poor harvest in any major producing country—the United States, the Soviet Union, India, or China—not only will send economic shock waves throughout the food sector of the world economy, but will fuel the fires of inflation in other sectors as well. This delicate balance raises the prospect that climate might replace pollution as a dominant global environmental concern.

Table I. The Changing Pattern of World Grain Trade[a]
(Values in Millions of Metric Tons)

Region	1934–38	1948–52	1960	1966	1973[b]
North America	+ 5	+23	+39	+59	+91
Latin America	+ 9	+ 1	0	+ 5	− 3
Western Europe	−24	−22	−25	−27	−19
Eastern Europe and USSR	+ 5	—	0	− 4	−27
Africa	+ 1	0	− 2	− 7	− 5
Asia	+ 2	− 6	−17	−34	−43
Australia and New Zealand	+ 3	+ 3	+ 6	+ 8	+ 6

[a]Plus sign indicates net exports; minus sign, net imports.
[b]Preliminary.
Source: Based on U.S. Department of Agriculture data.

The extent of global vulnerability is further demonstrated by the degree of the world's dependence on one region, North America, for exportable food supplies. Over the past generation this region, particularly the United States, which accounts for three-fourths of the continent's grain exports, has emerged as the world's breadbasket. The exports of Australia, the only other net exporter of

Table II. Index of World Food Security
(Values in Millions of Metric Tons)

Year	Carryover stocks of grain in principal exporting countries	Grain equivalent of idled U.S. cropland	Total reserves	Reserves as days of grain consumption
1961	154	68	222	95
1962	131	81	212	88
1963	125	70	195	77
1964	128	70	198	77
1965	113	71	184	69
1966	99	79	178	66
1967	100	51	151	55
1968	116	61	177	62
1969	136	73	209	69
1970	146	71	217	69
1971	120	41	161	51
1972	131	78	209	66
1973	106	24	130	40
1974 (proj.)	90	0	90	26

Source: Derived from U.S. Department of Agriculture data.

importance, are only a fraction of North America's. The United States is today the world's major exporter, not only of wheat and feedgrains, but of rice as well. Indeed, North America today controls a larger share of the world's exportable supplies of grain than the Middle East does of current world oil exports.

Between late 1972 and early 1974, food prices escalated rapidly throughout the world in response to the growing excess of world demand over available supplies and the decline in world food reserves. Wheat and rice prices tripled and soybean prices more than doubled. In 1974 soaring food prices contributed to the two-digit inflation that now affects virtually every country in the world. High prices help keep needed food out of the reach of the sizable segment of mankind that spends 80% of its income for food. A doubling in the price of wheat or rice cannot possibly be offset by increased expenditures. It can only drive a subsistence diet below the survival level.

The politics of scarcity leads to such devices as the Soviet use of secrecy to corner the world wheat market in 1972, or restrictions on exports of basic foodstuffs by principal global suppliers. Thailand has limited the export of rice; Brazil has restricted the exports of soybeans and beef; the United States imposed a soybean export embargo in the summer of 1973.

POPULATION AND AFFLUENCE

These events of the early seventies signal a fundamental shift in the structure of the world food economy. Throughout most of the period since World War II, the world food economy has been plagued by chronic excess capacity, surplus stocks, and low food prices. Emerging conditions suggest that this era is being replaced by a period of more or less chronic scarcity and higher prices, with little if any land held out of production. Short-term price fluctuations and temporary commercial surpluses should not obscure the more basic long-term forces at work.

Changing conditions on both the demand and supply sides of the world food equation are contributing to this shift. Throughout most of history, increases in the demand for food derived from growth in population. Since the time of Malthus, the food problem has been viewed as a food/population problem. World population growth continues to be rapid, but rising affluence now has emerged as another major claimant on the world's food-producing resources.

The impact of population growth on the demand for food is easy to understand. A 3% increase in population generates a 3% increase in the demand for food. The impact of rising affluence is not so readily understood. One way to visualize it is in terms of per caput grain requirements. In the less developed countries, only about 400 pounds of grain per year are available to the average person. Almost all of this quantity must be consumed directly merely to meet minimal food-energy needs; very little can be converted into livestock products. By contrast, the average North American uses nearly a ton of grain per year. Of this, only 200 pounds is consumed directly as bread, pastries, and breakfast cereal. The remainder is consumed indirectly in the form of meat, milk, and eggs. Thus, the average North American currently expends five times as many agricultural resources as the average Indian, Nigerian, or Colombian.

The combined effect of population growth and rising affluence is accelerating world food demand at rates without precedent in history. At the turn of the century, the annual growth in global demand for cereals was probably about 4 million tons per year. By 1950 it was about 12 million tons per year. As of 1970, only 20 years later, the world demand for cereals was expanding by 30 million tons per year—the equivalent of the annual wheat crop of Canada, Australia, and Argentina combined. Furthermore, this increase in demand is incessant, occurring in years of good and bad weather alike.

FOUR BASIC RESOURCES

For the first time in modern history, none of the four critical agricultural resources—land, water, energy, and fertilizer—is in abundant supply.

From the beginning of agriculture until about 1950, most of the year-to-year increases in world food output came from expansion of the area under cultivation. Since 1950, however, the major increases—probably four-fifths of the current gains in output—are attributable to intensification of cultivation on existing land area. Most of the good cropland in the world is already under cultivation. Additional opportunities for expanding the world's cultivated area still exist, but they are mainly limited to the interior of Latin America and parts of sub-Saharan Africa. Even in these regions, the cost of food produced on the new land may be much higher than that of food grown in areas cultivated now. Brazil, which occupies much of the interior of Latin America, now has the largest grain trade deficit in the New World.

The principal constraint on efforts to expand world food supplies during the final years of this century may well be water rather than land. In many regions of the world, fertile agricultural land is still available—provided that water can be found to make it productive. Unfortunately, most of the rivers that lend themselves to damming and to irrigation have already been developed. The expansion of irrigated area is slowing as the more desirable sites are exhausted.

Increasing world food production also requires a substantial increment in the amount of energy available for doing so. The recent quadrupling of the world price of energy is certain to affect adversely future food production prospects, but no one can yet foresee exactly how. In the more modern agricultural systems, such as that of the United States, the amount of energy now used to produce food exceeds by several times the amount of food energy the crops themselves yield. As energy-intensive as modern farming is, it consumes less than one-fourth of the energy used in the U.S. food system. The rest is used to transport, process, preserve, and distribute the food. In the developing countries, the future availability of energy will have a profound effect on efforts to provide adequate nutrition, for much greater energy inputs will be necessary if food production in these nations is to increase rapidly.

The fourth major agricultural resource–fertilizer–is also in very short supply. The outlook in this case, too, is for generally higher prices in the future. One reason for the fertilizer shortage is a lag in the construction of new production facilities, but even when supply catches up with demand, the rising cost of energy will undoubtedly keep fertilizer prices well above the historical level. The production of nearly all of the world's nitrogen fertilizer (which accounts for roughly half of all fertilizer used) utilizes natural gas or naphtha as a raw material. In addition, the manufacturing process is energy-intensive, requiring large amounts of electrical power. The combination of soaring energy prices, the enormous capital requirements needed to create new production facilities, and the time required to bring new facilities into production, mean that nitrogen fertilizer will be in critically short supply for many years at least.

ECOLOGICAL UNDERMINING

The ecological undermining of major food-producing systems is also beginning to have an adverse effect on the prospects of increasing world food production. Until recently, the oceans were viewed as an almost limitless source of protein, but the outlook has been sharply altered in the past few years. From 1950 to 1970, the world fish catch climbed steadily, more than tripling over this period from 21 million to 70 million tons. Since then, the catch has declined for three consecutive years, even while the capital and effort expended to bring it in continue to rise. Many marine biologists now feel that the global catch of table-grade fish is at, or near, the maximum sustainable (i.e., self-regenerating) level.

The tragedy unfolding in the African countries south of the Sahara Desert is an example of another type of ecological overstress that is diminishing in the earth's food-producing capacity, although the problem exists elsewhere as well. Over the past 35 years, human and livestock populations along the sub-Saharan fringe have increased rapidly, nearly doubling in some areas. As these populations have multiplied, they have put more pressure on the ecosystem than it could sustain.

Several consecutive years of drought have brought this deteriorating situation to a disastrous climax. If, as some meteorologists believe, the life-giving belt of monsoon rains is shifting southward, then ecological overstress and climatic changes are reinforcing each other with catastrophic human consequences. If the process of more and more land becoming desert is not reversed, then Africa—which has one of the highest population growth rates of all the continents—may lose a large slice of its food-producing capacity.

The Indian subcontinent provides a third dramatic example of ecological overstress. Over the past generation, as human and livestock populations have grown, the subcontinent has been progressively deforested. This trend has increased the incidence and severity of floods. In August of 1973, we read of the worst flood in Pakistan's history. In late summer of 1974, nearly half of Bangladesh was under water, destroying a considerable portion of the rice crop. Unfortunately, the deforestation is accelerating, gradually undermining the subcontinent's food-producing capacity. We know there will be even worse flooding in the Indian subcontinent in the future. The only questions are when and where.

The endangerment of food-producing systems is the most immediately serious ecological consequence of spreading agricultural activities, but by no means the only one. Even where food-producing capacity is not being adversely affected, efforts to increase the food supply, either by expanding the area under cultivation or by intensifying cultivation through the use of agricultural chemicals and irrigation, may cause ecological disasters, such as the inadvertent modification of climate, the eutrophication of freshwater lakes and streams, the rapidly rising incidence of environmentally-induced illnesses, and the threat of extinction of a growing number of wildlife species. New signs of agricultural stress on the earth's ecosystem appear almost daily, as the growing demand for food presses against our ecosystem's limited capacities.

THE LONG-TERM CHALLENGE

The changing nature of the world food problem is forcing us to redefine our understanding of food scarcity. Traditionally, most analysts have viewed the projected demand or need for food against the technological potential for expanding world food production. It is relatively easy to envisage a doubling or tripling of world food output based on known reserves of land and water, achieved through vastly increased inputs of energy and fertilizer. Some even suggest the possibility of a several-fold increase, assuming the uniform application of advanced technology and of the most sophisticated management techniques available. That there is a vast technological opportunity for expanding food supplies is not debatable, but this is not the real problem. The critical issue is at what price the additional resources will be brought into use. We know that most good land in the world is already under cultivation. We know that, with a few exceptions, the most desirable irrigation sites already have been developed. We know that energy, and therefore fertilizer, will be more costly in the future than in the past. We know that in the more advanced countries, where yields are already high, further increases in production will be far more costly than those of the past, in both economic and ecological terms.

In order to bring marginal resources into use, world prices for food must rise above their historic levels. Unfortunately, however, recent food price rises already have far exceeded growth in income among several hundred million of the world's poorest people. As a result, the food intake level of millions of low-income people is being pushed below the survival level—in many regions reversing the long-term trend toward improved nutrition, longer life expectancy, and a decline in infant mortality rates.

Historically, famine has been limited to relatively small geographic areas, as in Ireland in 1847 and West Bengal in 1943. Today, advances in global and national food distribution and transportation systems now ensure that food scarcity is allocated according to income levels, with scarcity concentrated among the world's poor, wherever they are. Even while the threat of traditional famine persists in some areas, a less visible crisis of hunger and malnutrition is emerging among the world's lowest income groups, whether in the Philippines, Bangladesh, sub-Saharan Africa, northeastern Brazil, or among the Andean Indians. The silent crisis of malnutrition may be denying close to a billion human beings the basic right to realize their full genetic potential, their full humanity.

SLOWING GROWTH IN DEMAND

The prospect of a long-term steady climb in food prices, outstripping the purchasing power of a large segment of mankind, presents the international community with a formidable challenge, necessitating a radical shift in the traditional approach to food scarcity. Unless an effort is made to slow the growth in demand for food, the world will be forced farther and farther up the cost curve as ever more marginal resources are brought into use.

The deterioration of the world food situation during the first half of the current decade, together with currently foreseeable trends, makes it quite clear that man cannot remain long on his present demographic path. The choice is between famine and family planning, for future population growth clearly will be reduced by rising death rates, which is already evident in some African and Asian countries, if it is not reduced by declining birth rates. An effort of unprecedented proportions is required to reduce birth rates among the more affluent, who exert such a disproportionately large per caput claim on the earth's scarce resources, as well as among the poor, whose birth rates tend to be high to compensate for the large incidence of infant and child mortality. Programs must be launched immediately to make family planning services available to everyone, to meet the basic social needs of the poor that affect motivation for smaller families, to encourage new social and economic roles for women, and to reorient national economic and social policies in order to promote low fertility.

A simultaneous effort is needed to simplify diets among the more affluent, to reduce, not their nutritional value, but their wasteful per caput claim on the earth's agricultural resources. Important economic, ecological, and health considerations, all involving self-interest, now join the basic moral question of the distribution of scarce resources to argue for the simplification of diets among the rich, particularly for the substitution of high-quality vegetable protein for animal protein.

PRODUCTION POTENTIAL OF POOR COUNTRIES

The changing nature of the food problem also calls for a major shift in geographic emphasis. The opportunity for easily expanding food production in the developed countries has diminished sharply now that idled cropland in the United States has been returned to farming. There is little prospect of quick, easy gains in the United States, Western Europe, the Soviet Union, or Japan, although substantial gains are still possible in all but Japan.

The world's principal unrealized potential for expanding food production is now concentrated in the developing countries. Although soil quality in Bangladesh is as good as in Japan, rice yields are only one-third of those attained in Japan. India's area of cropland is roughly comparable to that of the United States, yet it harvests only 100 million tons of grain per year, while the United States harvests 250 million tons. Corn yields in Brazil and Thailand are still less than one-third those of the United States.

As resources become scarce, the comparative advantage in additional food production shifts toward those areas where it will offer the greatest gains. Today, the increase in food output that can be brought about with an additional ton of fertilizer or gallon of fuel is far higher in the developing countries than in the industrial ones. Because fertilizers are already used very heavily in the agriculturally advanced nations of Europe, in Japan, and in the United States, an additional pound of fertilizer applied in these countries may return no more than five additional pounds of grain. In countries such as India, Indonesia, or Brazil, another pound of fertilizer can yield at least ten additional pounds of grain. It is unfortunate and ironic that, when world fertilizer shortages emerged in 1973, the more advanced nations acted to restrict their fertilizer exports to the poor countries, where the fertilizer could have produced much more food. Neither the rich nor the poor nations gain as world food prices are pushed even higher, intensifying global inflation.

FERTILIZER PRODUCTION AND DISTRIBUTION

Without adequate supplies of fertilizer, there is no prospect of replenishing depleted global food reserves in a meaningful way. In the short run, the inefficient world distribution of available fertilizers needs to be corrected in order to expand total world food production. Policies to that end include an international fertilizer-sharing scheme, as recently proposed by the FAO, in order to meet the more severe shortages in the developing countries, and a reduction in the heavy nonfarm uses of fertilizer in the affluent countries, making more supplies available for the world's farmers. To ensure the adequacy of supplies over the longer term, cooperation is essential between Western firms controlling complex nitrogen fertilizer technology and the countries with surplus energy available, in order to save the natural gas now being wastefully flared, so that it can be used instead for the production of vast quantities of low-cost nitrogen fertilizer.

MANAGING SCARCITY

Over the past two decades, nations have devised numerous means for managing commercial abundance, including special farm subsidy programs and the withholding of cropland from production. It has now become essential to develop the policies and institutions, both national and international, for managing scarcity. Foremost among the new institutions needed is an internationally managed system of food reserves, to be built up in times of relative abundance and drawn upon in times of acute scarcity. This can help support prices for producers during the inevitable periods when supply exceeds immediate world demand, and restrain price increases for consumers during times of scarcity. In effect, the stability that surplus American agricultural capacity has provided for a generation can be restored, at least partially, by a world food reserve system. Clearly, such a system is in the best interests of all nations. It is also obvious that the world community has a basic humanitarian interest in seeing to it that famine does not occur in the densely populated low-income countries following poor crop years. The affluent nations may be less able to provide this assurance in the future if the current system of autonomous, nationally oriented food planning is allowed to continue without modification.

Careful consideration must also be given to the establishment of international standards to govern the conditions under which important food suppliers are permitted to withhold supplies, and to provision of access to needed foods for importing nations. Either revision of present arrangements under the General Agreement on Tariffs and Trade, or creation of new international rules in another forum, should be undertaken to define the circumstances in which principal suppliers would be justified in restricting exports; it could also provide for automatic international consultation and action in the event of international food shortages.

COMPLEXITY, CHANGE, AND LEADERSHIP

An assessment of future food production prospects is an incredibly complex undertaking. One must be at once an agronomist, an economist, an ecologist, a meteorologist, and a political scientist to begin to understand the scope of the problem. This difficulty is reflected in the poor record compiled during the early seventies by those who attempted to forecast changes in the world food economy. Very few anticipated the reversal in the oceanic fish catch. The mass Soviet grain purchase in 1972 took the world almost completely by surprise. No one expected the doubling of world wheat, rice, feed grain, and soybean prices in the 1972–74 period. The U.S. Department of Agriculture, with one of the finest economic analysis units available, projected a 3% annual rate of food price inflation early in 1973; the rate turned out to be closer to 20%. Few foresaw the possibility that the vast acreage of idled U.S. cropland would be called back into use within a two-year period, and it is by no means certain that this step will overcome scarcity and return food prices to a more "normal" level. The leeway that has existed in the world food economy since the end of World War II has now disappeared, at least temporarily.

At a time of rapid change and growing complexity of problems, there is a premium on leadership at all levels. The more rapid the change and the greater the complexity of problems at both the national and the international levels, the greater the need for leadership. The answer to social philosopher Robert Heilbroner's question, "Is there hope for man?" hinges on whether the necessary leadership, both intellectual and political, is forthcoming.

The very pressures that make leadership so necessary make it much more difficult for decision makers to reach intelligent, responsible decisions. Such decisions require time for adequate information and analysis. In the population field, for example, one of the great bottlenecks continues to be the fact that so few leaders understand the dynamics of population growth. Not two national political leaders in a hundred are aware that a 3% annual rate of population growth will result in a 19-fold increase in a century.

We delude ourselves if we think the years ahead will be easy. At best they will be traumatic, and they could be catastrophic. The issues we have outlined will place great stress on the international political fabric. The crucial question is whether we can create a workable order for an increasingly interdependent world. This will require a level of leadership, understanding, and generosity of spirit that few past generations have been called upon to supply.

2

Definition of the Nutrition Problem—Poverty and Malnutrition in Mother and Child

Fernando Mönckeberg

Departamento de Nutrición y Tecnología de Alimentos
Universidad de Chile
Santiago, Chile

Adequate food is essential for every being, but man, up to this time, has not been able to satisfy this need equally well for all of the world's population. Malnutrition and hunger are still his inseparable companions, as they have been since the beginning of history (1). During the last decades, man's knowledge has developed tremendously, and, for the most part, he has applied it for his benefit. No one can deny that he has accumulated sufficient information to provide enough food for humanity. In spite of this, many millions of children and adults continue to suffer from undernourishment and hunger. In fact, the gap seems to be widening between those who are able to produce abundant food and those who cannot.

Repeated failures have shown that fighting malnutrition is not an easy task; the factors conducive to it are numerous and varied. It is a great error to simplify the problem, because this leads to the undertaking of partial or unilateral measures that inevitably end in failure. Malnutrition is never an isolated phenomenon; on the contrary, it enters into every aspect of misery. Undernutrition and poverty are closely interwoven, and it is impossible to eradicate them independently. Malnutrition, disease, lack of education, unsanitary conditions, crowding, and poverty are all interlocked, and solving these problems can only be achieved by approaching these factors together.

The problem is even more complex because chronic malnutrition and poor health damage the individual and make his recovery more difficult. Almost without exception, when malnutrition affects a social group, the ones who suffer most severely are the preschool children who should be undergoing rapid growth. Malnutrition in this age group produces high rates of morbidity and mortality. Severe undernutrition during the first years of life alters the morphology and function of different organs (2) and diminishes the child's capacity for adaptation and defense against an unfavorable environment. The incidence and severity of infectious disease is much greater among malnourished children than in their well-nourished counterparts. Chronic restriction of nutrients also retards the rate of growth and development.

Whether working with experimental animals or humans, researchers agree that severe malnutrition, when it occurs in early life (intra- and extrauterine), affects the development of the central nervous system and impairs performance on tests of mental capacity and behavior (2–7). In recent years, studies of perinatal nutritional status indicate that 8 to 15% of newborns show evidence of intrauterine malnutrition. Several surveys in less developed countries have demonstrated that between 1 and 3% of children experience severe undernutrition during the first months of life. The evidence suggests that both intrauterine and infant malnutrition have permanent sequelae (6). The uncertainties about the effect of chronic undernutrition are of extraordinary importance, because more than 60% of the children in the world suffer from it to some degree. Several investigators have pointed out that in those socioeconomic groups where undernutrition is prevalent, there is also a high incidence of mental retardation. The most obvious manifestation of early chronic undernutrition is physical growth retardation.

Figure 1 shows the growth pattern of three groups of children belonging to different socioeconomic levels. Those showing the greatest growth retardation are those in the lowest socioeconomic group, which also has the highest incidence of retarded psychomotor development (7). Experimental data show clearly that retarded physical growth and maturation are the direct consequence of chronic undernutrition (8). However, we cannot infer a direct causal relationship between undernutrition and retardation of psychomotor development. Although there is a very positive correlation between physical growth retardation and deficits in intelligence quotient (Figure 2), there are many other factors associated with malnutrition that can act negatively on the development of intellectual capacities.

It is a well-known fact that health, intelligence, adequate social behavior, and intellectual efficiency are closely related to the socioeconomic conditions in which the child develops (9). Experiments in animals show that central nervous system development is modified by the presence or lack of stimuli. Rats submitted to isolation and lack of stimulation suffer biochemical alterations of the central nervous system similar to those produced by severe undernutrition

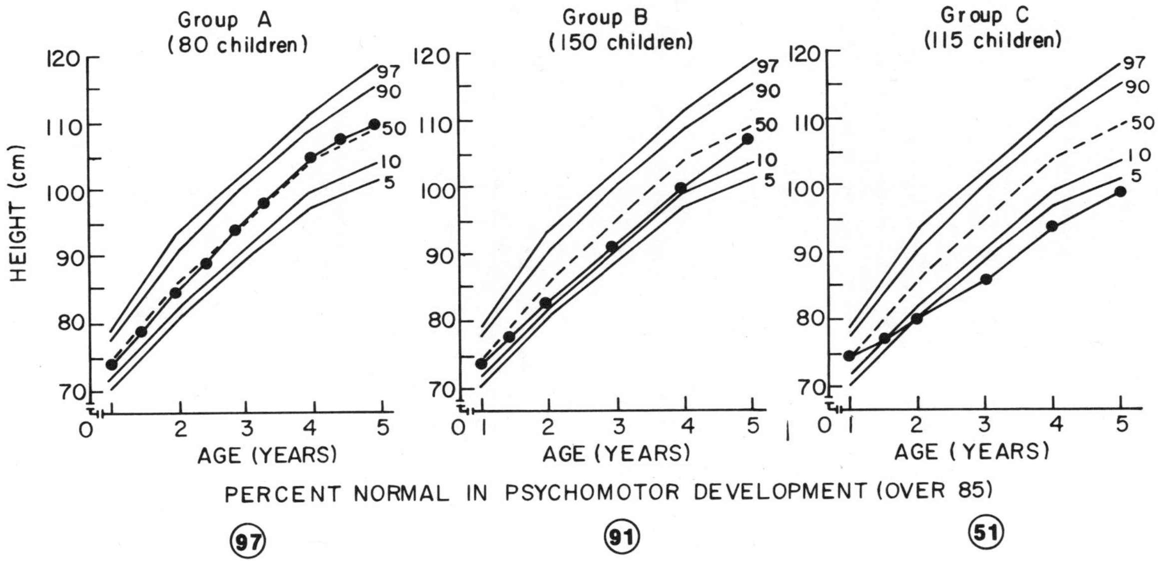

FIG. 1. Growth pattern of three groups of preschool children from different socioeconomic classes in Santiago, relative to percentiles of Iowa growth standard for normal children. Group A is in the highest socioeconomic group and Group C in the lowest. Thus, growth retardation correlated with psychomotor impairment on the Gesell test (normal over 85).

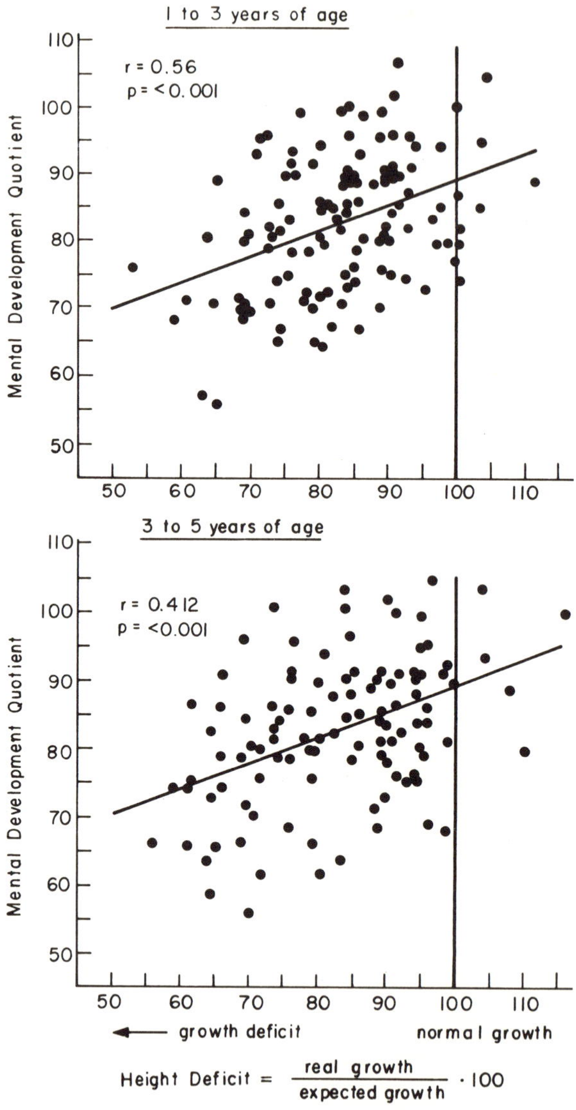

FIG. 2. Height and mental development quotient in preschool children from 1 to 5 years of age. Reproduced by courtesy of *The American Journal of Clinical Nutrition* (reference 7).

(Myron Winick, personal communication). These animals also show abnormal behavior and retarded psychomotor development (10).

Observations in man do not permit such definite conclusions because, from a practical viewpoint, it is impossible to separate the effects of malnutrition and lack of stimulation. It has been possible to observe, however, that even children in an acceptable nutritional state who have lived in an inadequate socioeconomic environment show poorer performance on tests of psychomotor development (Table I). Birren and Hess (11) conclude that poverty affects intellectual development by both social and biological mechanisms. Such children show lower efficiency in intellectual function, poorer performance on specific tests analyzing cognitive conditions, and reduced learning capacity.

It is not logical to think that this intellectual retardation among children in poorer socioeconomic groups is the result of genetic deficiency, because there is evidence that it can be prevented if the children are given adequate food and social stimuli (9, 12).

The environment of poverty is gray and flat; it stimulates neither imagination nor curiosity. There is little color and no toys or games so necessary to initiate the development of the child's abilities. Poor parents have marked limitations in vocabulary, so there is less verbal stimulation for their children. Among the specific cognitive deficiencies observed in these children, verbalization is consistently poor (13, 14). This means an inhibition of symbolic forms and very little abstract or categoric speech (15, 16). Under these conditions, motivation is conditioned by the harsh everyday facts of poverty, with no real incentive for future plans. All this limits the alternative possibilities of behavior for the child.

When poverty is extreme, relations between children and adults are so diminished that there is very little common activity among family members, and even indifference toward the child. Affection and understanding are minimal, which not only is a negative influence upon the development of cognitive functions, but affects personality as well. For example, it has been observed that children belonging to low socioeconomic levels have a very poor self-esteem, which restricts personal motivation and renders them less able to integrate effectively into society (17).

The impoverished family is distorted and disorganized. A frequent finding is

Table I. Intelligence Quotient in Well-Nourished and Malnourished Children of a Closed Population (Slum Area, Santiago, Chile)

Area	Malnourished (IQ)	Well-nourished (IQ)	*P*
Motor	72 ± 12	93 ± 12	< 0.001
Language	68 ± 15	79 ± 14	< 0.001
Adaptability	74 ± 11	86 ± 11	< 0.001
Personal social	70 ± 11	87 ± 11	< 0.001
General	71 ± 9	87 ± 9	< 0.001

a weakening of the father's image (18–20). Generally it is the mother who bears the greater responsibility for the family group (7). Nevertheless, her capacity is limited by her low educational level, by her numerous offspring, and by her hard work, either inside her own house or outside. For example, the intelligence quotient of mothers living in slum areas is consistently low. By Wechsler scale standards, almost 80% of the mothers score less than 79 (Table II).

All of these factors create a very limited environment in which there is lack of stimulation and very few opportunities for the child to learn. Therefore, it seems logical to think that the deficit in psychomotor development is the consequence of the sum total of negative factors: lack of stimulation, little affection, insecurity, undernutrition, and poor health. They potentiate each other in the individual in a way that could properly be called sociogenic biological damage.

The effect of malnutrition is more severe in the younger age groups. The lack of stimulus is also present during this period. For example, different researchers have shown that the intelligence quotient of children belonging to low socioeconomic groups is even lower when early social deprivation has been a factor (21–23). This is particularly important, because probably the damage is the result of cumulative adverse factors beginning during the first months of life, and continuing through the preschool years.

Poverty and malnutrition not only potentiate each other, but they also generate a vicious circle, transmitting the damage from generation to generation. For example, a very significant correlation can be found between the IQ of the mother and the child's growth deficit (Figure 3). In other words, a mother with an important psychic deficit has a very high probability of raising her own child in an undernourished state. Mothers with a normal IQ are more likely to feed their children adequately, even when socioeconomic conditions are not good.

In general, individuals living in a poverty-ridden environment are the products of many generations who have lived in similar circumstances. It is not yet clear whether poverty and its sequelae, repeated through generations, induce more profound changes than in a single generation. Stewart (24) described an experiment in rats in which he provided underfeeding and a restricted environment during nine successive generations. He observed progressive anthro-

Table II. Intelligence Quotient of Mothers Belonging to Middle-Class and Slum Areas, Santiago, Chile

Intelligence quotient	Slum area	Middle class
Normal (over 91)	6%	96%
Subnormal (80 to 89)	17%	4%
Deficient (below 79)	77%	0%

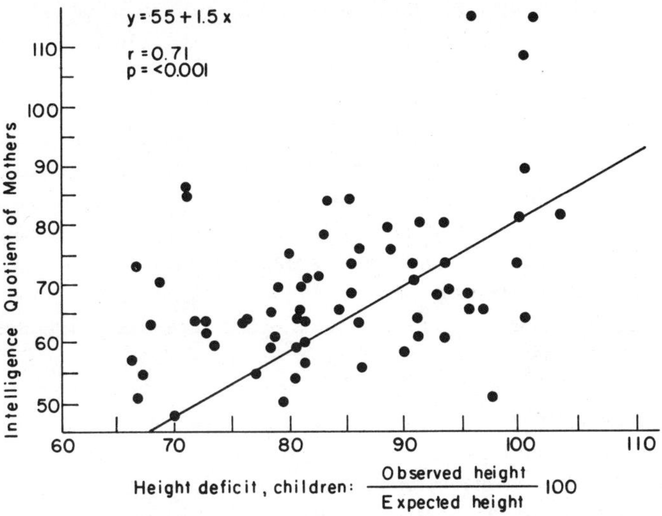

FIG. 3. Intelligence quotient of mothers and height of their children.

pometrical, biochemical, and behavioral changes. He gave the tenth generation of rats a complete diet and observed that many of the alterations took more than two generations to revert to normal. This does not mean that the process is hereditary, because in that case it would be irreversible, but it does mean that it takes more than one generation to restore normality, whatever the cause of the original damage.

It is evident that malnutrition cannot be considered in isolation from the many other factors conducive to poverty and marginal existence. The prevention and treatment of sociobiological damage must be directed at the whole environment. Even assuming a theoretical circumstance in which the infant population could be adequately fed without improving other environmental factors, there might be no improvement in intellectual capacity or in social adaptation. Recent studies done in the slum areas of Cali, Colombia, confirm this assumption (12). Nutritional supplementation and health care improved nutritional status for the children, but produced no significant changes in their intellectual and social capacities. On the other hand, it is important to point out that when the sociocultural situation is so poor, any program designed to prevent malnutrition is inefficient, especially if it is applied to masses of individuals. Unsanitary conditions, poor dietary habits, cultural taboos and beliefs that prohibit consumption of a variety of foods, and limited education of the parents—all come between the theoretical program and the child. This has been shown in Chile, where a program of free milk distribution has existed for more than 20 years. The program, started in 1951, consisted of giving powdered milk to every child under two years of age, in amounts covering more than the total protein requirements and over 80% of the calorie requirements. In 1958 the program was extended to reach children up to 15 years of age, with distribution of 48 million kgs of powdered milk per year. In spite of this enormous effort, which cost over 60 million U.S. dollars every year, there have been no substantial changes in the nutritional status of the population attributable to this program.

It is clear that the only real, short-term possibility for preventing sociobiological damage is the development of integrated programs, consisting of improved nutrition and health conditions, as well as modification of the sociocultural environment by means of direct psychomotor stimulation activities.

It is very important to consider which age groups these programs should reach, because if they are not begun early enough in life, the possibility for recovery is remote. These are the conclusions from an experiment carried out in Chile in the early 1970s, in which the target group was composed of 60 school children ranging in age from seven to nine years. Their socioeconomic level was very low, with a high incidence of malnutrition and poor performance on tests of intellectual function (Table III). Only 9% of the children had an IQ above 90. For one year they received their total caloric and protein requirements at school, with a very well-controlled daily food intake. At the same time, they participated in an educational program especially designed and adapted to their circumstances. At the end of the school year, there was evident progress in growth, height, and weight. Nevertheless, there were no changes evident in the IQs of these children.

Very different results have been obtained with intervention programs begun during early childhood. At present, an integrated program is being carried out with children from birth to two years of age in Santiago. This includes medical care, milk distribution, nutritional education, and psychomotor stimulation in the child's home twice a week. Progress has been very satisfactory thus far, and

Table III. Intelligence Quotient, Weight, and Height in 60 School Children 7 to 9 Years Old, 9-Month Period (Santiago, Chile)

	Study period		
IQ (Gille)	0 month	4 months	9 months
Normal (over 91)	9%	11%	8%
Subnormal (80 to 89)	50%	44%	48%
Deficient (below 79)	41%	45%	44%
Weight increase (average)	0	1.8 kg	2.7 kg
Height increase	0	2.3 cm	4.1 cm

although there are no definite conclusions, after one year of intervention the growth and intellectual levels attained by these children are similar to those of peers in a higher socioeconomic group. Programs of direct intervention must necessarily be continued during all of the preschool years, otherwise the children will experience retardation consequent to the negative influence of the sociocultural environment they continue to live in.

Positive results have also been observed in another similar study of preschool children, carried out in Cali by McKay, McKay, and Sinisterra (12), in which children three to five years of age are given a diet covering every nutrient requirement, health care, and cognitive stimulation. The latter consists of five intervention techniques with the objective of teaching (a) improvement of verbalization and an elementary understanding of quantity and quality; (b) time and space relationships; (c) hand (manipulation) skills; (d) concentration and attention at work and improved memory; and (e) achievement of independent decision-making.

The conclusions of this experiment, which has now been conducted for four years, may be summarized as follows: An adequate feeding and health care program, combined with a psychological and social stimulation program, can produce remarkable changes in social and cognitive development, reversing almost completely the sociobiological damage induced by poverty. When children began participation in the study at age three, their achievement record was very similar to that found among children in higher socioeconomic groups. Even so, recent memory continues to be somewhat impaired in children from poor homes. This also illustrates the need for early introduction of the intervention program in the child's life. Neither nutrition alone nor medical care programs without improved nutrition suffices to improve the results of the different tests measuring the development of intelligence and degree of mental ability in general.

It is probable that the sociobiological damage produced by poverty and its consequences during the infant period, and later during the preschool years, disables the individual for his subsequent integration into society. We now know that learning capacity for such children is very seriously limited during the school years because the child is unable to adapt himself to the demands of his environment. In another recent study a significantly lower school efficiency was observed in children who had been exposed to both nutritional and cultural deprivation. In Latin America, for every 100 children starting primary education, only 20 are able to finish it. It is evident that sociobiological damage is the main cause of this high level of school dropouts (Table IV). Children who are able to finish primary education are those whose environments have been sufficiently generous to allow them to express the greater part of their genetic potential during their growth period. The individual who is not able to complete his primary education is definitely left in the fringes of society. This means that

Table IV. School "Alto Jahuel," Santiago, Chile

	Grades (primary school)			
	1 and 2	3 and 4	5 and 6	7 and 8
Number of students	403	260	160	80
Height deficit for age (average)	10%	7%	7%	3%
Weight deficit for age (average)	15%	8%	9%	3%
Caloric deficit for age (average)	16%	10%	10%	+2%
Animal protein deficit for age (average)	32%	20%	17%	6%
IQ (Wisc.) (average)	81	87	92	101
School performance	50	57	60	66

he must be resigned to obtaining menial employment, at very low wages, or even to unemployment, perpetuating the vicious circle of poverty, disease, and lack of progress from one generation to another, with very little hope of escape.

It is urgent to prevent this damage, because impairment suffered by the individual affects, not only him, but society as a whole. It is especially important to those countries where the great majority of the population lives under these conditions. To fight poverty requires completely new kinds of planning, and great efforts to create integrated programs directed toward populations at risk in the less developed countries. This concept must be clearly understood by economists, sociologists, teachers, and physicians. The complexity of modern society demands more and more every day of the individual if he really wants to contribute to it and enjoy the benefits of human knowledge. Poverty and hunger have accompanied and hampered man during his whole history, but today the increasing gap between those able to enjoy society's benefits and those who are not is all too evident.

REFERENCES

1. Waldorf, C., 1879, *The famine of the world,* Carton Press, London.
2. Mönckeberg, F., 1968, Adaptation to caloric and protein restriction in infants, *in: Calorie deficiencies and protein deficiencies* (Proceedings of a colloquium held in Cambridge, England, April, 1967), R. A. McCance and E. M. Widdowson (eds.), Churchill, London, p. 91.
3. *Nutrition, the nervous system, and behavior,* Proceedings of the Seminar on Malnutrition in Early Life and Subsequent Mental Development, 1972, Mona, Jamaica. Pan American Health Organization Scientific Publication No. 251.
4. Kallen, D. (ed.), 1973, *Nutrition, development, and social behavior: A review of experience,* U.S. Department of Health, Education, and Welfare (NIH) Publication No. 73-242.
5. Richardson, F., 1973, *Brain and intelligence,* National Educational Press, Hyattsville, Maryland.

6. Scrimshaw, N. S., and Gordon, J. E. (eds.), 1968, *Malnutrition, learning, and behavior,* M.I.T. Press, Cambridge, Massachusetts.
7. Mönckeberg, F., Tisler, S., Toro, S., Gattas, V., and Vega, L., 1972, Malnutrition and mental development, *Am. J. Clin. Nutr.* **25:** 766.
8. Salas, E., and Mönckeberg, F., 1974, Nutrición y bioquímica del sistema nervioso durante el desarrollo, *Arch. Latinoam. Nutr.* **24**(3): 321–338.
9. Lesser, G. S., Fifer, G., and Clark, D. H., 1965, Mental abilities of children from different social class and cultural groups, *Monogr. Soc. Res. Child Dev.* **30:** 1–115.
10. Frankova, S., 1974, Interaction between early malnutrition and stimulation in animals, *in: Early malnutrition and mental development.* Symposia of the Swedish Nutrition Foundation, XII., J. Cravioto, L. Hambraeus, and B. Vahlquist (eds.), Almqvist and Wiksell, Stockholm and Uppsala, Sweden, p. 202.
11. Birren, J. E., and Hess, R. D., 1968, Influences of biological, psychological and social deprivation upon learning and performance, *in: Perspectives on human deprivation, biological, psychological and sociological,* U.S. Department of Health, Education, and Welfare, pp. 89–183.
12. McKay, H., McKay, A., and Sinisterra, L., 1973, Behavioral intervention with malnourished children, *in: Nutrition, development, and social behavior: A review of experience,* D. Kallen (ed.), U.S. Department of Health, Education, and Welfare (NIH) Publication No. 73-242, p. 121.
13. Seashore, H. G., 1951, Differences between verbal and performance IQs on the Wechsler intelligence scale for children, *J. Consult. Clin. Psychol.* **15:** 62.
14. Cazden, C. B., 1966, Subcultural differences in child language: An inter-disciplinary review, *Merrill-Palmer Q.* **12:** 185.
15. Bernstein, B., 1961, *Social class and linguistic development: A theory of social learning. Education, economy and society,* Glencoe Free Press, New York.
16. Cazden, C. B., 1968, Three sociolinguistic views of the language and speech of lower-class children—with special attention to the work of Basil Bernstein, *Dev. Med. and Child* **10:** 600.
17. Minuchin, S., Montalva, B., Guerney, B., Rodman, B., and Schumer, F., 1967, *Families of the slums.* Little Brown and Co., Boston, 460 pp.
18. Pollitt, E., 1969, Ecology, malnutrition, and mental development, *Psychosom. Med. XXXI* (3): 193.
19. Graham, G., and Morales, E., 1963, Studies in infantile malnutrition I. Nature of the problem in Peru, *J. Nutr.* **79:** 479.
20. Cravioto, J., Birch, H. G., DeLicardie, E., and Rosales, L., 1967, The ecology of infant weight gain in a pre-industrial society, *Acta Paediatr. Scand.* **56:** 71.
21. Willerman, L., and Broman, S. H., 1970, Infant development, preschool I.Q., and social class, *Child Dev.* **41:** 69.
22. Werner, E., Simonian, K., Bierman, J. M., and French, E., 1967, Cumulative effect of perinatal complications and deprived environment on physical, intellectual, and social development of preschool children, *Pediatrics* **39:** 490.
23. Knobloch, H., 1967, *Prediction from assessment of neuromotor and intellectual status in infancy. Psychopathology of mental development,* Grune & Stratton, New York, pp. 387–400.
24. Stewart, R. J. C., 1973, A marginally malnourished rat colony. The effect of maternal malnutrition on the development of the offspring, *Nutr. Rep. Int.* 7 (5):487–493.

3

Microenvironmental Factors in Severe Protein-Calorie Malnutrition

Joaquin Cravioto and Elsa R. DeLicardie

División de Investigación Scientífica
Institución Mexicana de Asistencia a la Niñez (IMAN)
Mexico, D.F.

Protein-calorie malnutrition (PCM) is a disease complex occurring primarily among the poor in preindustrial societies where the social system, consciously or unconsciously, creates malnourished children, generation after generation, through a series of social misfortunes, among which are limited access to goods and services, limited social mobility, and restricted opportunities for social stimuli at crucial points in life (1).

Given the background of underdevelopment with its resultant economic, cultural, and social disadvantages for a high proportion of the individuals and families of the so-called Third World, it is hardly surprising that more than half of their preschool children have mild to moderate degrees of PCM, and that malnutrition plays a significant role in no less than 50% of the total number of deaths in these children (2).

With so many families at risk of developing malnutrition in such communities, it is surprising that severe, clinically evident PCM almost never reaches a prevalence rate above 10%. This is partly due to the brief duration and high mortality associated with severe malnutrition. However, even when a family is stricken by serious food deprivation, as a rule only one child at a time will show extreme clinical signs of severe malnutrition, the other children seem to be suffering no more than mild to moderate forms of the disease. There is to date no adequate explanation for this phenomenon. One of the main obstacles to finding a reason is the scarcity of pertinent data on the child's environment, and on the child himself, immediately before the development of severe malnutrition. The need for such information stems from the consideration that the presence of a severely malnourished child within the household may be in itself a factor that could change some relevant features of his or her microenvironment. Obviously, such information can only be obtained through longitudinal studies of children and families living in communities at high risk of malnutrition, where a relatively large number of children are followed from birth onward, and where recent collected background data are available for each child.

A unique opportunity for a prospective study of certain host and environmental factors possibly related to the appearance of severe malnutrition in young children presented itself when, in the course of a longitudinal ecology study of 334 children beginning at birth, 14 girls and 8 boys developed clinically severe PCM by five years of age. Fifteen of the 22 patients developed kwashiorkor, the other 7 marasmus. Ten children, 6 with kwashiorkor and 4 with marasmus, were treated at home, while 9 children with kwashiorkor and 3 with marasmus were treated in a pediatric hospital. No deaths occurred in the latter group, but 3 of the 10 children treated at home died.

These cases occurred despite the fact that all children in the cohort studied were medically examined on a biweekly basis. Children who failed to grow normally were identified, their infectious illnesses were treated, and their parents were given advice (which they did not follow) on the appropriate feeding and management of children who failed to thrive. In contrast to its lack of influence on the incidence of clinically severe PCM, this medical attention decreased the infant mortality rate from a figure of 96 per thousand to 46, and reduced the preschool mortality of the cohort by one-half. Incidentally, these data point out, once more, that traditional medical care can strongly influence mortality with minimal or no effect on morbidity.

To assess the influence of environment on the presence of early, severe malnutrition, the analysis focused on a comparison of a series of environmental characteristics recorded for the 22 children who developed PCM, and for a group of children selected from the same birth cohort who were never diagnosed as severely malnourished, and who were matched, at birth, for sex, gestational age, season of birth, body weight, body length, and psychomotor development.

MACROENVIRONMENTAL FACTORS

Three kinds of macroenvironmental factors received consideration. These relate first to the parents as biologic and social organisms; second to the family structure; and third to objective circumstances, such as sources of family income, income per caput, and sanitary facilities present in the household.

Differences in the age, height, or weight of either parent, the mother's number of pregnancies, or the number of live children in the family failed to distinguish between families with and without severely malnourished children.

Moreover, no significant relationship was found between the presence or absence of severe clinical malnutrition and the variables of personal cleanliness, literacy, and educational level.

Contact with mass media was explored through literate parents' newspaper reading and radio listening. The number of mothers or fathers of malnourished children who were regular newspaper readers was not significantly different from the number in the matched control group. Similarly, the number of fathers who listened regularly to the radio was similar in both the malnourished group and the control group.

The situation with the mothers was different. There were almost equal numbers of radio listeners and nonlisteners in the malnourished group, but the number of listeners among the matched control group was more than three times the number of nonlisteners. The difference is significant at the 0.05 level of statistical confidence (chi square = 4.20; $df = 1$; $p < 0.05$).

No significant differences between the malnourished and control groups were found with respect to family size or type of family (nuclear or extended). The socioeconomic status of the families was estimated by using four indicators: main source of family income, sanitary facilities in the household, annual income per caput, and percentage of total income spent on food. No significant associations were found between any of these factors and the presence or absence of severe malnutrition.

Summarizing all features of the macroenvironment, the only differential between severely malnourished children and controls matched at birth for gestational age, body weight, and total body length was the mother's contact with the world outside the village through regular radio listening. None of the other characteristics of the parents (biological, social, or cultural) or family circumstances (including per caput income, main source of income, and family size) was significantly associated with the presence or absence of severe malnourishment.

MICROENVIRONMENTAL FEATURES

Because the features of the macroenvironment did not explain the occurrence of severe malnutrition, our attention was directed toward analysis of the microenvironments of the two sets of children. We selected the potential stimulation of the home as our first general indicator of the quality of child care, and the mother as the principal stimulating agent for young children.

The instrument used for estimating home stimulation was the inventory developed by Bettye Caldwell (3), designed to sample certain aspects of the quantity (and in some ways the quality) of social, emotional, and cognitive stimulation available to a young child within his home. Two inventories were used, one designed for children up to three years of age, and the other for those three to six years old. In both versions the selection of items included has been guided by a set of assumptions about conditions that foster development.

Accordingly, the inventory describes and quantifies the following eight areas of the home environment: (1) frequency and stability of adult contact; (2) vocal stimulation; (3) need gratification; (4) emotional climate; (5) avoidance of restriction; (6) breadth of experience; (7) aspects of the physical environment; and (8) available play materials. In each of these areas almost all items receive binary scores; no attempt is made to rate finer gradations. The total score is the number of items recorded as positive for the child's development. If desired, each area can be scored separately and related to specific features of development.

A trained psychologist recorded the inventory of home stimulation for every child in the cohort at six-month intervals during the first three years of life and at yearly intervals thereafter. At the time of data collection and scoring, the psychologist was unaware of the nutritional histories of the children.

Table I shows the mean scores for total home stimulation in both the malnourished and the matched control groups. At all ages except 18 months the children who had not experienced clinically severe malnutrition also had significantly more favorable environments. Perhaps of even more importance than significant difference in mean scores is the fact that the distribution of scores is markedly different at all ages between the control children and children who

Table I. Mean Values of Total Home Stimulation for Severely Malnourished Children and Controls

Chronological age (months)	Home stimulation score (mean and standard deviation)		
	Severely malnourished children	Control children	t-test
6	32.37 ± 2.57	35.35 ± 4.71	3.46[a]
12	36.41 ± 3.44	39.83 ± 4.71	2.47[b]
18	39.68 ± 4.89	42.43 ± 4.01	1.78[b]
24	39.43 ± 4.81	44.16 ± 6.26	2.48[b]
26	39.46 ± 4.98	44.33 ± 5.69	2.51[b]
31	40.66 ± 7.22	45.86 ± 6.68	2.05[b]
34	44.40 ± 5.31	48.20 ± 5.12	2.00[b]
38	44.40 ± 5.31	48.20 ± 5.12	2.00[b]
46	88.53 ± 16.77	101.40 ± 10.62	2.51[b]
52	90.35 ± 11.83	102.80 ± 11.36	2.88[b]
58	97.71 ± 16.98	109.86 ± 6.38	2.52[b]

[a]Significant at 0.05.
[b]Significant at 0.01.

Table II. Proportion of Future Severely Malnourished Children and Control Children Showing Different Total Home Stimulation Scores at 6 Months of Age

	Proportion of children	
Home score	With future severe PCM	Control
27	0.06	–
28	0.06	–
29	0.12	–
30	0.25	–
31	0.31	–
32	0.56	0.12
33	0.62	0.17
34	0.75	0.41
35	0.87	0.65
36	1.00	0.70
37	–	0.76
38	–	0.94
39	–	0.94
40	–	0.94
41	–	1.00

were to become malnourished, or were malnourished, as well as after their rehabilitation from severe malnutrition.

Table II presents the distribution of scores in home stimulation at 6 months of age, when only one child in the malnourished group was actually severely malnourished. On a range of 27–41 scoring points, one of every four malnourished children had 30 or fewer points, and none scored higher than 36 points. None of the control children had a home with a score of less than 32 points, and at least one of every four homes scored above 36 points. Similarly, at 58 months of age in a range of scores from 55 to 124, almost one-half of those surviving severe malnutrition were in homes with scores below 104 points, and one-fourth of their homes did not exceed 84 points. In contrast, the homes of the control children had a minimum of 100 points, with almost one-half above 110 points (Table III).

The other feature of the microenvironment worth noting is the comparison of the maternal behavior exhibited toward the child before he became severely malnourished and the behavior elicited under similar circumstances in mothers of comparably aged children selected from the same birth cohort who were never diagnosed as severely malnourished.

Starting at birth and at monthly intervals, i.e., each time the infants were

Table III. Proportion of Children with and without Antecedents of Severe Clinical Malnutrition Showing Different Total Home Stimulation Scores at 58 Months of Age

Home score	Antecedents of severe malnutrition	
	Present	Absent
55–59	0.07	–
60–64	0.07	–
65–69	0.07	–
70–74	0.07	–
75–79	0.14	–
80–84	0.21	–
85–89	0.21	–
90–94	0.28	–
95–99	0.36	–
100–104	0.57	0.20
105–109	0.71	0.53
110–114	0.93	0.73
115–119	1.00	0.93
120–124	–	1.00

tested for mental performance, the behavioral responses of the mother during the test situation were independently recorded. Recording and scoring of the maternal behavior was done by adaptation to local conditions of the Maternal Behavior Profile developed by Nancy Bayley at the Laboratory of Psychology, U.S. National Institute of Mental Health. The Maternal Behavior Profile contains 20 variables comprising the majority of transactions occurring during the test situation. Each variable consists of seven scale steps, each designating a relative point of degree or type of manifestation of that variable. Each step is defined as a statement of behavior. The statement that most closely portrayed the reaction of the mother, as her habitual response during the first 12 (monthly) consecutive examinations, was taken as her rating on that particular aspect of behavior.

As may be seen in Tables IVa and IVb, in 15 of the 19 aspects of the test situation the behavioral responses of mothers of infants who later developed severe malnutrition were different from the responses observed in the mothers of the control children. The highest levels of statistical significance were obtained in the behavior displayed by the mother when, in the test situation, her child performed adequately and easily; in the overt signs of sensitivity toward her child; and in the mother's response to the interview.

Significant differences were observed for interest in child performance, response to child's needs, mother's view of her role in the test situation, and

Table IVa. Magnitude of the Behavioral Differences Observed in Mothers of Future Malnourished Children and of Controls

Aspect of test situation	*t*-test (separated)	*P* <
Reaction when child performs easily	4.03	.001
Response to interview	3.61	.001
Sensitivity to child	3.61	.001
Interest in child's test performance	3.19	.01
Responses to child's needs	3.09	.01
Mother's view of her role	2.82	.01
Emotional involvement with child	2.79	.01
Amount of verbal communication with child	2.57	.02
Expressions of affection toward child	2.54	.02
Reaction when child performs extremely well	2.33	.03
Status consciousness	2.18	.04
Cooperation with examiner during testing	2.11	.04

emotional involvement of the mother with her child. The amount of verbal communication and the expressions of affection toward the child were significantly different in mothers of severely malnourished children and controls at the confidence level of 0.02. The mother's reaction when her child performed extremely well, her status consciousness, and her cooperation with the examiner during the test gave differences in behavioral responses at levels greater than 0.02 and less than 0.05.

A mother's behavioral responses when the child had difficulty with a test item, her affective response to the entire situation, and her control of the child during the test, gave differences between the group of mothers of the severely malnourished children and the mothers of control children at the 0.10 level of statistical confidence.

Table IVb. Magnitude of the Behavioral Differences Observed in Mothers of Future Malnourished Children and of Controls

Aspect of test situation	*t*-test (separated)	*P*
Reaction when child had difficult time on item	1.01	.08
Mother's affective response to entire situation	1.74	.09
Control of child during test situation	1.70	.10
Amount of physical contact with child	1.59	.12
Mother's overall general evaluation of child	1.34	.19
Tolerance of child's behavior	1.14	.26
Type of physical contact with child	0.34	.74

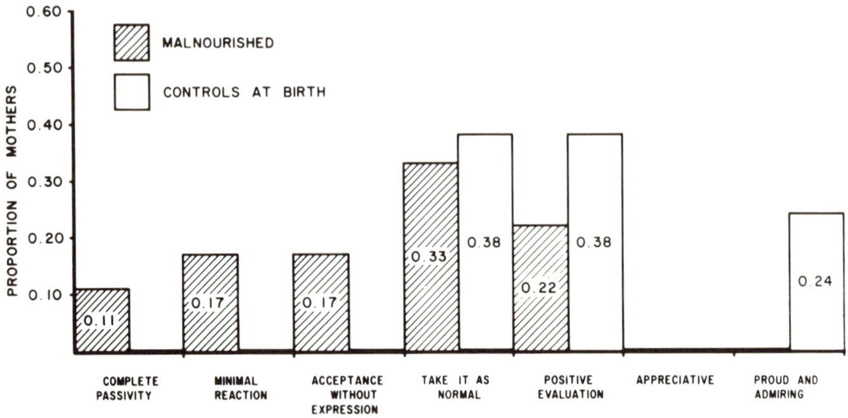

FIG. 1. Behavior exhibited by mothers of children with or without severe malnutrition; mother's reaction when child performs adequately (easily).

Type of physical contact with child, tolerance of child's behavior, the mother's overall general evaluation of the child, and amount of physical contact were the four aspects of the test situation that did not show differences between the two groups of mothers even at the 0.10 level of confidence.

Not only was the average behavior different between the mothers of severely malnourished children and the mothers of the control group, but differences in the proportions of specific behavior within each variable were also found. Figure 1 shows that in regard to the reactions of the mothers when the child performed easily, 4 out of each 10 mothers of severely malnourished children showed complete passivity, little reaction or mild acceptance, and none were appreciative or proud of their children's performance. Conversely, all mothers of the control children at least considered that it was normal for their children to perform adequately and easily, and 25% of these mothers were proud of their children's performance.

On the seven-step ordinal ascending scale of behavioral response to the interview, 5 out of every 10 mothers of severely malnourished children did not go beyond step 3. These mothers were characterized as reserved, defensive, or responding to questions with only slight elaboration. Not a single mother of this group reached step 6. On the other hand, the behavioral responses of the mothers of the control children distributed between steps 3 to 6, with 1 out of every 10 mothers in step 3 (slight elaboration of responses) and 3 in step 6, i.e., mothers who answered enthusiastically and volunteered much information (Figure 2).

As another example of the differences in behavior, Figure 3 illustrates how the amount of verbal communication with the child contrasted between the two

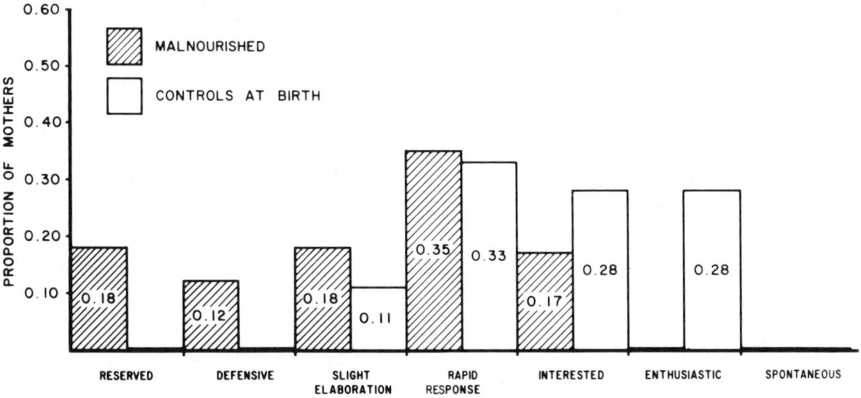

FIG. 2. Behavior exhibited by mothers of children with or without severe malnutrition; reponse to interview.

groups of mothers. Of every 10 mothers of malnourished children, 2 rarely spoke to their children, 4 only occasionally, 3 spoke only when necessary, and one talked with her child, carrying on a two-way conversation. In contrast, the minimal amount of verbal communication of the mothers of the control children corresponded to step 3 of the scale and went all the way up to a real verbal interaction between mother and child.

It is thus apparent that, while data concerning the children's parents, family structure, sources and amounts of family income, sanitary facilities available in

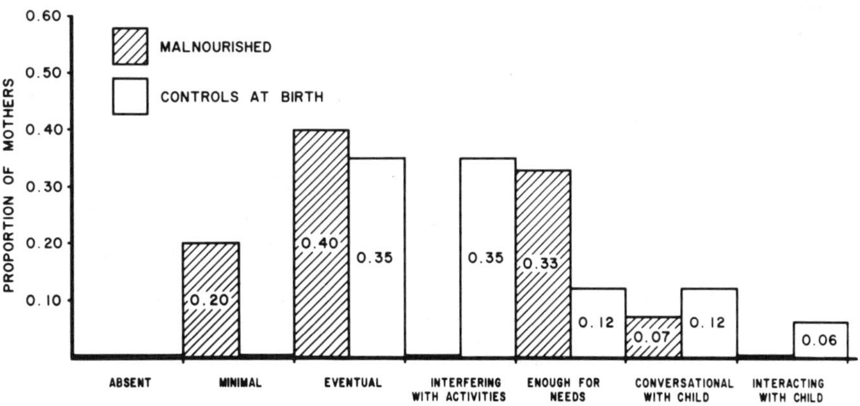

FIG. 3. Behavior exhibited by mothers of children with or without severe malnutrition; mother's amount of verbal communication with child.

the home, and mother's personal cleanliness, literacy, and educational level, failed to show a significant association with the presence or absence of clinically severe malnutrition, radio-listening by the mother, amount and type of stimulation available in the home, and mother's behavior toward her child helped substantially to identify families with and without potentially severely malnourished children long before the appearance of the syndrome.

In a previous study on the ecology of weight gain in infants living in a preindustrial, bilingual village (4), it was observed that besides radio-listening by the mother, the language spoken to the child at home could separate infants with significantly different weight gains in the first six months of their lives. Mothers who addressed their children in the local dialect of the village had infants whose weight gains were significantly lower than infants whose mothers spoke to them in the national language.

It might be considered that listening regularly to the radio, as well as the use of the national language rather than the local dialect, are attributes of a socialization away from traditional behavior. This kind of mother may be more prone to provide her child with a more diversified and stimulating home environment, and to view her mother's role as a continuous series of affective, engaging, and satisfying transactions between mother and child, and not simply as one of a passive, traditional status, to be taken for granted and carried on with a minimum of interaction and novelty.

The data on pattern of the mother's behavioral responses in the test situation allow the identification of different styles of child care within the families having a child at high risk of developing severe malnutrition, and strongly suggest that the occurrence of severe malnutrition among children in the families at high risk is associated with a distinctly inadequate microenvironment.

A low level of home stimulation and a passive, traditional mother, unaware of the needs of her child, and responding to him in a minimal way as if unable to decode the infant's signals, are two characteristic features of this poor microenvironment that lead to severe clinical malnutrition in children of poor families.

If our findings hold for other sociocultural contexts, then the strong association between the presence of severe PCM in children and microenvironmental factors relating mainly to the type of child care and stimulation stresses that changed maternal behavior is an important component of programs aimed at preventing severe protein-calorie malnutrition in high-risk families.

ACKNOWLEDGMENTS

The research was supported in part by grants-in-aid from The Nutrition Foundation Inc., The Foundation for Child Development, The Foundation von Monell, The van Ameringen Foundation, and Carnation de Mexico.

REFERENCES

1. Cravioto, J., and DeLicardie, E. R., 1973, The effect of malnutrition on the individual, *in: Nutrition, national development, and planning,* A. Berg, N. S. Scrimshaw, and D. L. Call (eds.), M.I.T. Press, Cambridge, Massachusetts, pp. 3–21.
2. Béhar, M., Ascoli, W., and Scrimshaw, N. S., 1958, An investigation into the causes of death in children in four rural communities in Guatemala, *Bull. W. H. O.* **19:** 1093.
3. Caldwell, B. M., 1967, Descriptive evaluations of child development and of developmental settings, *Pediatrics* **40:** 46.
4. Cravioto, J., Birch, H. G., DeLicardie, E. R., and Rosales, L., 1967, The ecology of infant weight gain in a preindustrial society, *Acta Paediatr. Scand.* **56:** 71.

4

Perspectives and Priorities in Food and Nutrition Planning

George H. Beaton

Department of Nutrition, School of Hygiene
University of Toronto
Toronto, Canada

Recently there has been major interest in the development and implementation of food and nutrition policy (1–10). The reasons for this interest are readily apparent. The World Food Conference, held in November, 1974, in Rome, gave emphasis to both the crisis now existing in the famine areas and the dire need for a planned husbandry of the world's finite resources if we are to cope with the growing population. Many events in recent years have demonstrated the interlocking effects of events in widely separated parts of the world. The failure of a fishing industry in Peru has exerted a domino effect felt around the world.

Long ago, the epidemiologists pointed out the multifactorial etiology of malnutrition. It has been repeatedly emphasized that nutritional problems must be seen within their social, cultural, economic, and biological setting. The setting in which malnutrition ferments must be altered if lasting improvements are to be obtained. The approach to a multifactorial problem requires multisectoral activity by government.

These notions are not new. The Applied Nutrition Program involving locally coordinated activities of several sectors of government has been with us for many years (11). What is relatively new is the attempt to coordinate these activities at the central level of government rather than the local level—the development of a national food and nutrition policy. Even newer is the attempt to integrate this policy within national development planning. In an agrarian society, in which the economy is based upon agriculture, this implies the placement of food and nutrition policy at the very core of national planning.

Thus, the emphasis in recent years has been on "comprehensive" or "integrated" food and nutrition planning. This emphasis has led to the development of very complex planning models, providing for multiple inputs and including feedback loops from the operational levels. One such model has recently been presented at a Regional Seminar in India (10). It was based upon earlier proposals made at an Inter-Agency Consultation Meeting in Chile (1). Although even more elaborate models have been described, I will discuss this one as an example of trends in planning.

These models play an extremely important role in conceptualizing the problems we face and in illustrating interactions requiring consideration. However, I suggest that at present our ability in model building may well exceed our ability to collect and utilize the multiple data inputs. Conceptually, they are valid; logistically, they are dangerous.

Consider the primary data inputs required by the model cited above. These are shown in Figure 1. Then consider a passage recently written by J. M. Pines (12):

> Establishment of a national nutrition policy and program presents formidable analytical, organizational and political tasks. Recent national nutrition status, expenditure and consumption surveys, available in few developing countries, serve as a statistical base for analysis. Their preparation and review can take years and millions of dollars. Conversion of agricultural data into useful information and its integration with information from other sectors add to analytical burdens.
>
> Current lack of data on consumer habits and attitudes contributes to the difficulties of changing them in nutritionally beneficial ways. Multisectoral nutrition planning, if it is to meet criteria imposed in other sectors, requires years of data collection and analyses that have barely begun in most countries. When nutrition planners are overconcerned with presenting a comprehensive set of proposed activities, *the preparation of required studies can delay actions based on knowledge already available* (Emphasis added).

To these remarks I would add only two additional perspectives (13). First, the implementation of such comprehensive policies would seem to require a superministerial planning and program body—a situation that seems politically improbable. Second, the generation of the policy and recommendations is so complex that once formulated it is more likely to be seen as a fixed directive than as the fluid, evolving program of activities needed to combat ever-changing situations.

Our conceptual developments have outpaced the development of government structures and logistical support systems capable of implementing our concepts. This is a potentially dangerous situation. We must not convince national planners, or ourselves, that a comprehensive approach to food and nutrition planning is the only approach to be considered. Is there not danger that we will persuade the planner to ignore the whole matter if the comprehensive approach is not feasible of implementation?

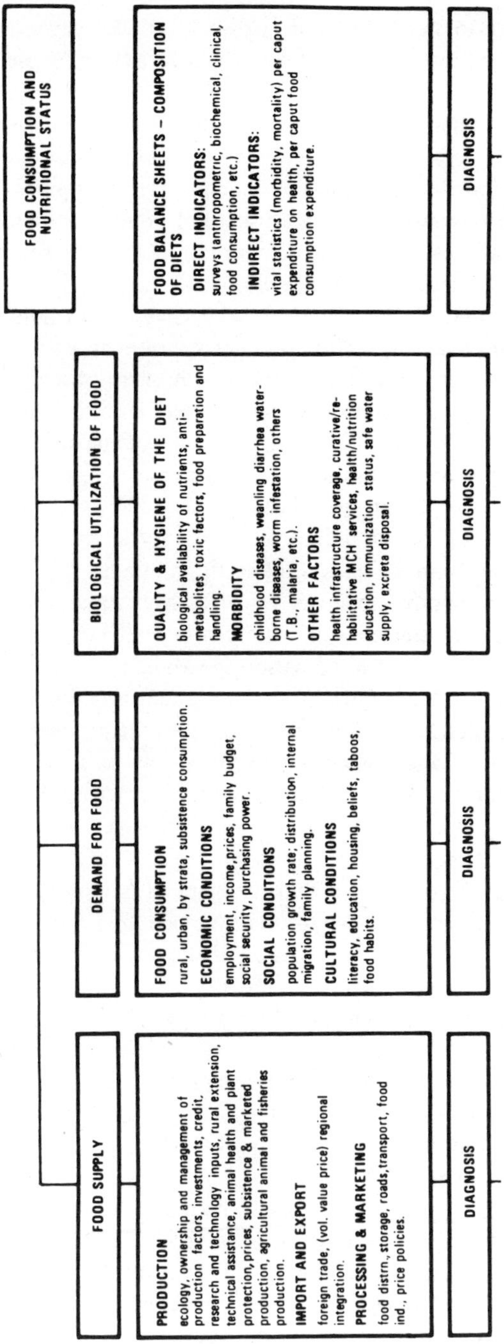

FIG. 1. *Primary data base of the Integrated National Food and Nutrition Policy* (1, 10). Scheme and comprehensive data base are intersectoral in nature.

I do not mean to be a defeatist. However, I do suggest that we must backtrack a little. We must do the best with what is feasible rather than dwell on the "ideal." Nevertheless, we must not lose sight of the comprehensive planning concept. This must remain our long-term goal—present models are beacons to the future.

At present we must continue to consider policy development and program planning within the framework of a multisectoral political structure. We should then work toward the establishment of coordinating bodies functioning at the *inter*ministerial level, rather than the *supra*ministerial level implied by some of the all-inclusive planning models. The role of such a body would not lie in the development of comprehensive national policies; rather it would monitor problems and activities, hoping to influence the development of sectoral policies and programs so that they are complementary, or at least not contradictory. It would serve an advisory role (2). This, then, places the initiation for policy planning and development within the individual sectors.

This discussion has direct relevance to the "definition of the nutrition problem." The precision of the definition must vary in accord with the use to which the definition is to be put. Inherently, there is little or no point in collecting more information than can be effectively used. Furthermore, the nature of the definition—the relevant parameters—will vary with the ministry. Let us consider the definition wanted within the Ministry of Health.

Basically, there are three questions to be asked in defining the nutritional problem: Who is affected? What is wrong? Why does the problem exist? The first two questions, "who" and "what," constitute the definition of the target population(s) and target problem(s) for nutrition programs. They are conveniently considered together because the data bases are generally similar (Figure 2).

However, it must be emphasized that these questions can be answered with varying degrees of precision—and that, in general, the cost of refining the answers may be disproportionate to the increase in precision. Perhaps the simplest to measure is the general condition of the population as assessed by the experienced observer. In areas where malnutrition is severe, this may suffice to define the nature of the problem and its severity. However, successive refinement of the definition may be obtained by considering age-specific mortality rates, hospital and clinic morbidity data, parameters of growth and physical development, detailed examination of the diet (preferably at the level of the individual), and the full-fledged nutrition survey. While we lack generally applicable indicators of functional development, such data as age of menarche may provide a useful index of gross conditions in the population (14).

Observations of the above type may serve to define the nature of the nutritional diseases present in the population. In some cases, additional laboratory or dietary studies may be indicated to confirm the existence of suspected problems (e.g., the type of anemia or the presence of vitamin A depletion).

DEFINITION OF THE PROBLEM

WHO? / WHAT NUTRIENT(S)?

Information Base:	General observation of community Age-specific mortality Morbidity patterns in hospitals/health clinics Height–weight data at convenient ages Birth weight Weight gain in pregnancy Weight change in preschool years Qualitative examination of diet (predicted inadequacies) Detailed nutritional survey - of high risk groups - of general population
Categorized in Terms of:	Age/Sex group Geographic region Population density (urban/periurban/rural) Cultural/ethnic group Income group (family per caput income)

FIG. 2. Some data requirements for the identification of the target group(s) and target problem(s) in nutrition planning. Note that the cost of data collection increases markedly with the precision of data sought.

However, if these are deferred until after the preliminary examination and assessment are complete, it may be possible to apply them to the identified "high-risk groups,' a tactic that should improve the cost/effectiveness of the process.

It is not enough to characterize the nutritional problems. Unless there is reason to believe that they are widely, and uniformly, spread through the population, the particular subgroup of the population affected by nutritional problems must be identified. For program planning purposes, it is appropriate to consider the information in terms of age/sex group, geographic area, city or rural location, cultural/ethnic group, and income level. While the first three of these are relatively straightforward, it is to be recognized that the latter two socio-economic parameters can present a considerable range of refinement of data. Again, the precision to be sought should be seen as a function of the planning capability and probable program approach.

Turning to the third question to be asked in defining the problem, "Why does the problem exist?," the policy planning group encounters the greatest temptation to enter into very complex data collection; here it is of major importance to sort out the roles and interests of the various sectors of government so that the appropriate sector is asking questions that can be of value to its planning activities. Figure 3, using the same groupings as portrayed in the original comprehensive model (Figure 1), portrays some of the features that may

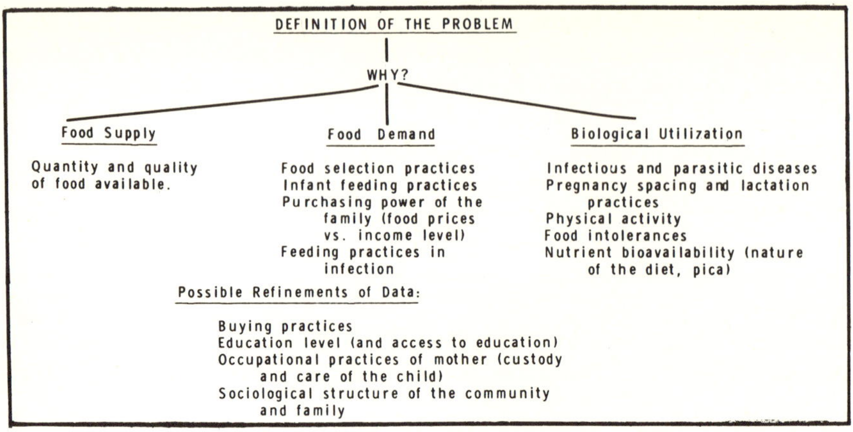

FIG. 3. Parameters of potential interest to the health sector in the examination of causation of nutritional problems in the community. The categorization is based upon that developed in an Interagency Consultative Meeting in Chile (1).

be of particular interest to the health sector in planning programs within its area of responsibility. Obviously these questions can be asked with varying degrees of refinement, ranging from general observation and inquiry to detailed sociological and health surveys. The answers are of fundamental importance to program design; this cannot be challenged. However, it is suggested that in many instances relatively crude observations, coupled with a review of experience in other settings, may serve to define the important components of the problem. Here lies the value of many of the current research studies in the epidemiology of malnutrition–assessment of the role of the microenvironment as well as the macroenvironment (15). As we gain more knowledge and experience, we should be better equipped to "diagnose" a community's underlying problems without resorting to detailed investigations in every setting. Please do not misunderstand. I do not suggest that nutritional problems have the same etiology in all settings. I only propose that, surely, it is more profitable in the long run to invest heavily in studies that may assist us in establishing relatively simple assessment indices–measurements that will serve to categorize the problems–than to dissipate limited resources with detailed studies across a very broad front. We are now approaching the position where we can postulate the root problems in most settings and then put the postulates to the test with limited examinations in the community. Earlier I suggested that precise definition of the problem might be reserved to the "high-risk" population groups. I now suggest that investigation of etiologic factors might be centered on the "high-probability" postulates and that these might be developed through a modest inventory of indices.

In operational programs, data collection does not stop with the definition of the problem. There is a fourth question to be asked: "Is it changing?" Here there is an urgent need to develop meaningful indices of change–not only change in the health situation, but also change in the etiologic factors identified in Figure 3 (14). These indicators should be sufficiently specific to permit meaningful interpretation; they should be simple enough to permit implementation.

It is an inherent argument of this chapter that there is need to refine the methodologic approaches of data collection with the objective of identifying and developing relatively simple assessment tools coupled with meaningful standards of interpretation. Jelliffe (16) and others have described approaches that can be applied at the community level. However, there still remains debate about the proper interpretation of measurements as simple as height and weight (17). Beaton and Swiss (18) have described a simplified approach to the assessment of the nutritional quality of the diet; at present it is applied only to the protein: calorie ratio, but the concepts might be expanded to other nutrients. Resolution of some of the present uncertainties in these matters would greatly facilitate the definition of the problem and the monitoring of change.

SUMMARY

I have taken this opportunity to challenge a trend that I have seen in recent meetings toward the promotion of a holistic, but perhaps impractical, approach to food and nutrition policy planning and implementation. While I support the development of modeling as an approach to the conceptualization of the problems and interactions, it would appear that the data requirements of the integrated nutrition policy approach exceed our present capabilities. I fear that this can result in inactivity at a time when we cannot afford inactivity–inactivity consequent to delay for data collection, or inactivity consequent to a belief that because comprehensive planning is not yet feasible, there is no point in doing any systematic planning.

The precision of the definition of the nutrition problem is a function of the stage of development of the operational planning process. Let us not advocate the collection of data we are not equipped or prepared to interpret and use. In many areas of the world, relatively simple information, often already available, can define the nutrition problem with sufficient precision to permit program development within the individual sectors of government. Surely that must be our immediate goal.

REFERENCES

1. FAO/WHO/PAHO/UNESCO/ECLA Interagency Consultative Meeting on National Food and Nutrition Policies in the Americas, March, 1973, Santiago, Chile.
2. Bengoa, J. M., and Rueda-Williamson, R., in press, 1976, Planning and organization of a

national food and nutrition policy, *in: Nutrition in preventive medicine,* G. H. Beaton and J. M. Bengoa (eds.), WHO Monograph Series, Geneva.

3. Berg, A., and Muscat, R., 1971, Nutrition program planning: An approach, *in: Nutrition, national development, and planning,* A. Berg, N. S. Scrimshaw, and D. L. Call (eds.), M.I.T. Press, Cambridge, Massachusetts.
4. Berg, A., 1973, *The nutrition factor. Its role in national development,* The Brookings Institution, Washington, D.C., 290 pp.
5. Johnston, B. F., and Greaves, J. P., 1969, *Manual on food and nutrition policy,* FAO Nutritional Studies No. 22, Rome.
6. Pan American Health Organization, 1970, *Elements of a food and nutrition policy in Latin America,* PAHO Scientific Publication No. 194, Washington, D.C.
7. Food and Agriculture Organization of the United Nations, Formulation of Food and Nutrition Policies, FAO Nutrition Newsletter 10, No. 2, pp. 1–13.
8. Food and Agriculture Organization of the United Nations, Food Policy and Nutrition Division, 1973, Food and Nutrition: A New View of an Old Problem, FAO Nutrition Newsletter 11, No. 4, pp. 1–16.
9. Protein Advisory Group of the United Nations System, 1973, PAG Statement No. 26, Food and Nutrition Considerations in National Economic Planning, PAG Bulletin 3, No. 4, pp. 7–8.
10. Lunven, P., and Bocobo, D. L., 1974, Food and Nutrition Policy and Planning in Asia and the Far East Region, FAO Nutrition Newsletter 12, No. 2, pp. 12–18.
11. Report of a Joint FAO/WHO Technical Meeting on Methods of Planning and Evaluation in Applied Nutrition Programs, 1966, FAO Nutrition Meetings Report Series No. 39, Rome.
12. Pines, J. M., 1974, Review and advocacy: First steps in nutrition planning, PAG Bulletin 4, No. 3, pp. 35–39.
13. Beaton, G. H., 1974, *Definition of the food and nutrition situation,* Background paper for the FAO/WHO Joint Expert Committee on Nutrition, Ninth Meeting, Rome.
14. Beaton, G. H., and Bengoa, J. M., in press, 1976, Practical population indicators of health and nutrition, *in: Nutrition in preventive medicine,* G. H. Beaton and J. M. Bengoa (eds.), WHO Monograph Series, Geneva.
15. Cravioto, J., 1974, *Interrelación entre nutrición y desarrollo de la personalidad,* Paper presented at the XIV International Congress of Pediatrics, Buenos Aires, Argentina, 3–9 October.
16. Jelliffe, D. B., 1966, *The assessment of the nutritional status of the community,* WHO Monograph Series No. 53, Geneva, 335 pp.
17. Waterlow, J. C., in press, 1976, Classification and definition of protein calorie malnutrition, *in: Nutrition in preventive medicine,* G. H. Beaton and J. M. Bengoa (eds.), WHO Monograph Series, Geneva.
18. Beaton, G. H., and Swiss, L. D., 1974, Evaluation of the nutritional quality of food supplies: Prediction of "desirable" or "safe" protein:calorie ratios, *Am. J. Clin. Nutr.* 27: 485–504.

5

The Environment of the Malnourished Child

Leonardo J. Mata

Instituto de Investigación en Salud
University of Costa Rica
Costa Rica

Patterns of interdependence between man and his environment have differed over time. Man first began to intervene in his environment by organized hunting for food and later he began to domesticate animals and plants. Sedentary societies grew with time, decimating wildlife, destroying or endangering primary forests, and inducing significant soil erosion. Metal craftmanship, the development of complex methods of warfare, and growth of industry and sophisticated technology have led to modern patterns of life in advanced societies. Some of these patterns are now being questioned because, through exploitation of the environment, man is compromising his own survival.

Most of the world's population has lagged behind this process of social evolution, and still subsists on traditional agriculture, using rudimentary technology. Such populations are controlled by governments based in urban areas that enjoy a greater degree of development and hold most of the wealth and political power.

THE ENVIRONMENT OF THE MALNOURISHED MAN

Figure 1 illustrates the present status of the world in relation to famine. Bangladesh, India, and parts of equatorial Africa and of Brazil are experiencing a severe food shortage. Other regions of Africa, Asia, and Latin America face prospective famines. The figure, however, was not intended to illustrate the present food crisis but to point out that the affected areas are in the tropics and subtropics, where environmental forces act more strongly and negatively on man, to decrease and often frustrate the effectiveness of his efforts.

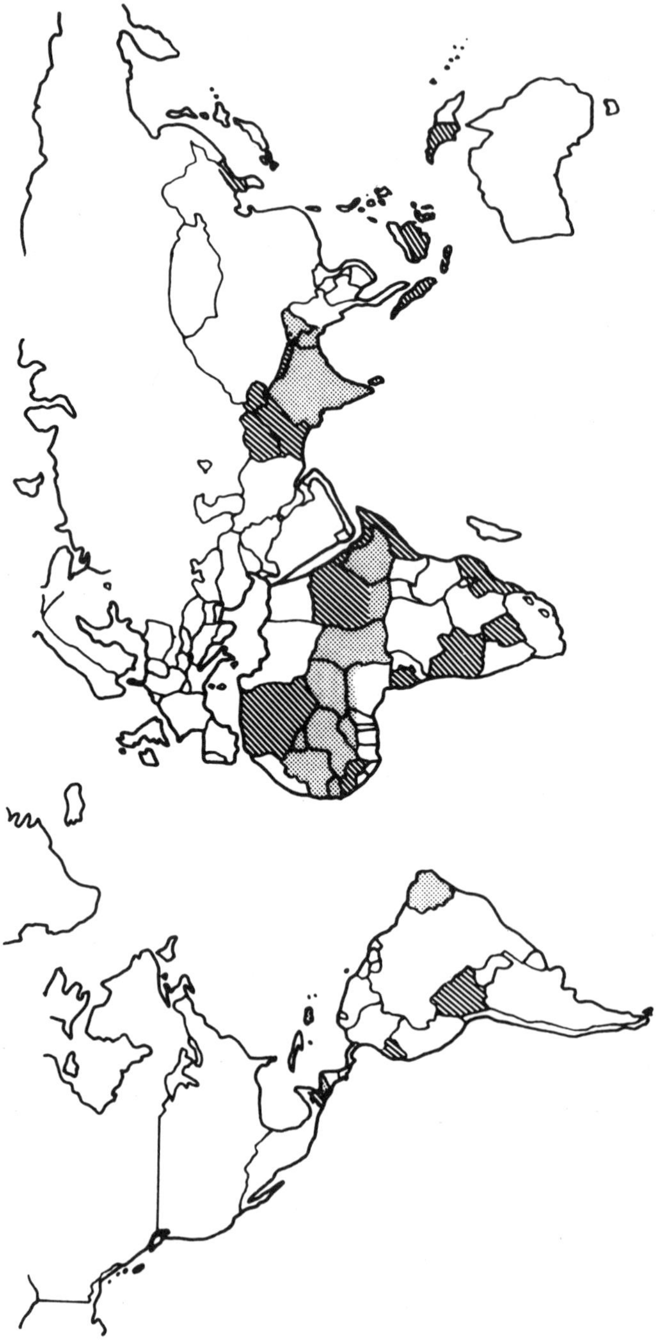

FIG. 1. World map, 1974, showing areas of famine (shaded) and of potential famine (lines).

Environmental factors can be classified as *physical, biological,* and *social,* with a realization that they are closely interdependent and often inseparable from each other. The physical environment includes soil, water, and air. The biological environment includes the viruses, bacteria, and parasites, many of which cause disease and death in man or in the plants and animals on which he depends. The social environment comprises socioeconomic characteristics that result from societal evolution of traditions, beliefs, and forms of social organization.

THE PHYSICAL ENVIRONMENT

In the tropics and subtropics, compared to temperate zones, man is at some disadvantage. In the tropics, steady high temperatures, humidity, rainfall or drought, erosion, and occasional natural disasters are considered deterrents to progress. Such environments diminish the working capacity and creativity of unprotected man (1). They pose greater demands on human body water and electrolytes, and may be a source of nitrogen loss (10). More importantly, tropical environments favor the vectors of blood and tissue parasites and maintenance of the cycles of hookworm, trematodes, and jungle virus infections. In many areas the climate promotes growth of weeds, insects, and fungi detrimental to food crops.

In the tropics Amerindian civilizations remained at a low level of technological development. The arriving Europeans succeeded in improving yields of cash crops and moved some people from subsistence agriculture to large land holdings. The resulting profound changes in social and family life cannot be denied, nor their effects on the economy, health, and welfare of society (14). The important consideration is that populations still living on subsistence agriculture are characteristically poor. Poverty favors deficient sanitation and poor diets, leading to a high incidence of nutritional and infectious disease, and death.

THE BIOLOGICAL ENVIRONMENT

Man living in the tropics is also at greater risk of developing endemic infectious diseases. Some of these infections may affect the human being from gestation onward. The results presented here were derived from long-term prospective observations in a typical village of Guatemala (7,9). A high incidence of infectious disease was recorded among pregnant women in this village: 27 of 100 pregnancies were complicated by bacteriologically confirmed urinary tract infection, an affliction associated with premature birth and low-birth-weight infants (Table I). Furthermore, diarrhea and dysentery appeared in 36 of 100 pregnancies, and lower respiratory disease was present in 30% of the pregnant

Table I. Incidence of Infectious Diseases in 82 Women Observed Prospectively during Pregnancy, Santa María Cauqué, 1972–1973

	Respiratory infection		Diarrhea and dysentery	Urinary tract bacterial infection ($> 10^5$/ml)	Other illnesses[a]
	upper	lower			
Incidence per 100 pregnancies	104 (127%)	25 (30%)	29 (36%)	22 (27%)	20 (25%)

[a]Conjunctivitis, otitis media, stomatitis, skin infection.

females. Deterioration of maternal nutrition during pregnancy because of infection must also affect the developing embryo (15).

Under these circumstances the fetus has greater opportunity to become exposed to infectious agents, or to antigenic components or immunoglobulins synthesized by the mother in the course of her disease. The study of femoral vein blood collected from infants within three to four days after birth revealed 15% of consecutive newborns from four lowland Guatemalan villages with elevated IgM levels (0.19 mg/ml) (Table II), an incidence in excess of occurrence in industrial societies (5). The high rates of elevated IgM values have not yet been explained, but presumably some of these represent congenital infection. In a preliminary study in one Indian village, 1% of the infants were congenitally infected with cytomegalovirus and 1.3% with *Toxoplasma,* while 1.3% were shedding echoviruses at birth (9). The possible consequence of increased risk of fetal antigenic stimulation and congenital infection deserves scrutiny. Intra-

Table II. Incidence of Neonates with High Concentrations of Immunoglobulin M (IgM), Four Guatemalan Ladino Villages, 1972–1973

Village number	Number of infants	Number (and %) with IgM >0.20 mg/ml[a]
1	48	10 (21)
2	52	4 (8)
3	40	6 (15)
4	67	11 (16)
Total	207	31 (15)

[a]Elevated values in cord serum confirmed in blood from infant's femoral vein. IgM was measured by radial immunodiffusion. Data of the Divisions of Environmental Biology and Human Development, INCAP.

uterine infection is known to induce fetal wastage, embryopathy, premature birth, low birth weight, and postnatal sequelae.

The small size of child-bearing women in poor rural areas, their poor nutritional status resulting from deficient diets and frequent episodes of infectious disease, and the presence of fetal antigenic stimulation are factors that help to explain the 7% rate of premature birth and the 32% incidence of fetal growth retardation. By itself, poor fetal growth diminishes survival and retards growth of children (10).

Childbirth in rural areas throughout the world offers many opportunities for contamination of the child with maternal feces, an event made more significant by the high rates of maternal infection. More than 8% of five- and seven-day-old neonates were found to be excreting enteroviruses. Early infection with *Shigella* and protozoa also occurs, but is less frequent (9). These infections, however, generally are asymptomatic and short-lived and disappear in days or a few weeks.

The rural neonate has a remarkable resistance to infection attributable to the adequate nutrition and resistance factors provided by breast milk. The situation changes when weaning begins, at two to five months of age, because supplemental foods are easily contaminated by polluted water or by the mother herself as she prepares them.

Milk output in women who do not supplement their own diets diminishes by the second or third month. Weaning is protracted, extending into the second year of life in most cases, and this coincides with the occurrence of weanling diarrhea, a syndrome caused by a variety of infectious agents and a deteriorated nutritional status. The combined effect of inadequate food intakes and frequent exposure to infectious agents results in a succession of infections, each episode further depleting the child. The magnitude of infection correlates directly with the onset of clinical manifestations.

Particularly high rates of diarrheal diseases and respiratory illnesses are observed (Figure 2). It should be recognized that children are continuously being infected and that clinical manifestations occur virtually in a continuum, as Figure 3 illustrates. Children may be ill for as long as a third of their first year of life. These data correspond to a typical highland region devoid of hookworm and of diseases transmitted by snails and arthropods. In many lowland areas, malaria, flukes, and arboviruses enlarge the morbidity spectrum.

The impact of infection on health is evident in a severe case of whooping cough (Figure 4). The child exhibited pronounced weight loss consequent to anorexia and vomiting and metabolic alterations; the nutritional status deteriorated seriously, favoring clinical manifestations of other infectious agents (9). Recovery of the preillness weight did not occur until 40 weeks later. The arrest in growth of this child at such an early age probably resulted in impairment of biological functions. The nutritional status even in well-nourished individuals deteriorates in the presence of any infectious disease and the effects are of still

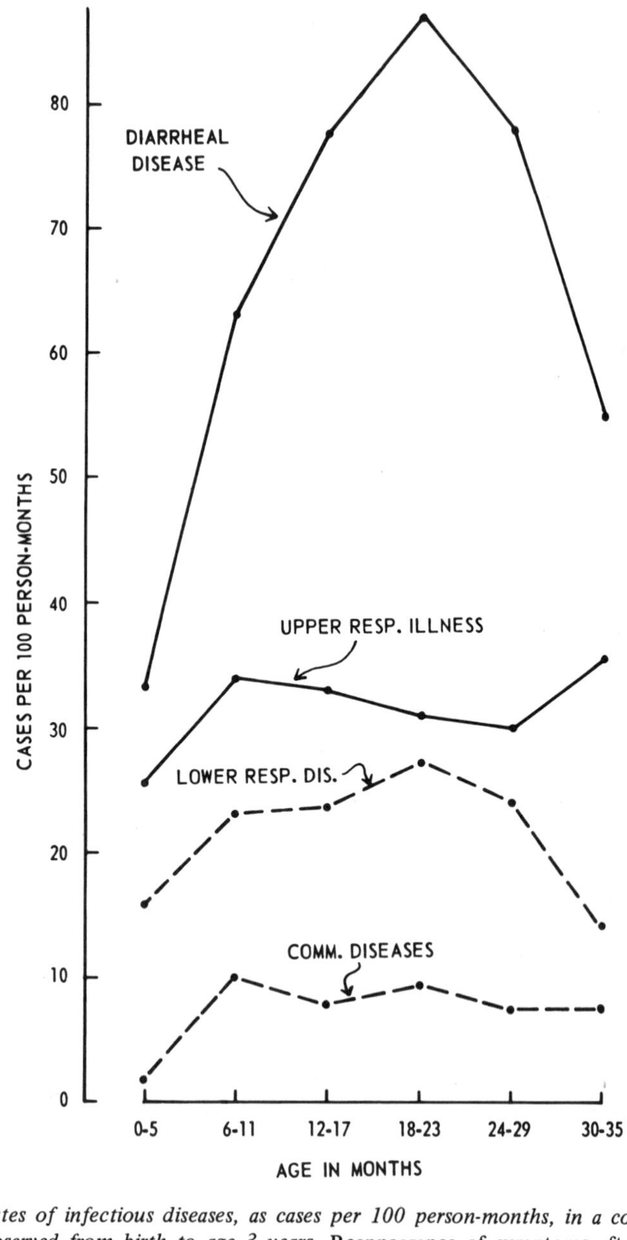

FIG. 2. Rates of infectious diseases, as cases per 100 person-months, in a cohort of 45 children observed from birth to age 3 years. Reappearance of symptoms after 24 hours identified a new case. Santa María Cauqué, 1964–1971.

greater consequence to infants and young children, particularly if they are already malnourished.

In less developed societies, the response to an infectious process in the child is often withdrawal of solid food and sometimes the giving of strong purgatives. Infections commonly are accompanied by anorexia, vomiting, increased peristalsis, and systemic manifestations, often resulting in marked reduction of food intake, impaired digestion and absorption, and nutrient depletion (11). Other alterations are loss of tissue—particularly epithelium, blood, muscle, and liver—depending on the type of infection, its localization and pathogenesis. In both intestinal and systemic diseases there is increased loss of nitrogen, amino acids, electrolytes, and vitamins. Adults experiencing severe infectious disease show impaired performance or inability to work at all (2). However, even subclinical or "silent" infections induce stress responses with increased nitrogen excretion in urine (3).

The metabolic alterations associated with infection have been classed as nutrient overutilization, nutrient sequestration, and nutrient diversion. In overutilization there is increased expenditure of glycogen, mobilization of amino acids from skeletal muscle for gluconeogenesis in the liver, increased synthesis of lipids, and overutilization of vitamins. Sequestration of iron in the liver occurs even in the presence of adequate stores of hemosiderin, a phenomenon apparently mediated by a protein factor released by phagocytes. This perhaps contributes to the anemia in children experiencing recurring infections, even when they live in hookworm-free areas and where dietary iron is only mildly deficient or even adequate. Nutrient diversion includes an uptake of plasma amino acids for abnormal synthesis of haptoglobin, tryptophan-oxygenase, tyroxin-transaminase, and other enzymes. Also, the body diverts its biosynthetic pathways to produce the protein, lipids, and carbohydrates needed for viral replication. Thus, by a variety of mechanisms, the high frequency of infections in developing societies contributes in an indirect way to the food shortage observed in developing regions of the world.

On the other hand, malnutrition, whether primary or secondary to interaction with infection, affects the host's immune capacity, an important issue when one considers that a large proportion of the world's population suffers from varying degrees of malnutrition and is concomitantly exposed to far greater risks of infection than well-nourished populations are (16). Present knowledge indicates that the immunoglobulin system is not affected in persons with mild to moderate forms of malnutrition. However, antibody synthesis is impaired in children with moderate to severe forms of protein-calorie malnutrition (PCM), as evidenced by a failure to elicit a B-cell response with viral and bacterial antigens in untreated kwashiorkor patients.

Alterations in T-cell function and in the amplification of the immune response occur in malnourished persons. In moderate and severe forms of PCM

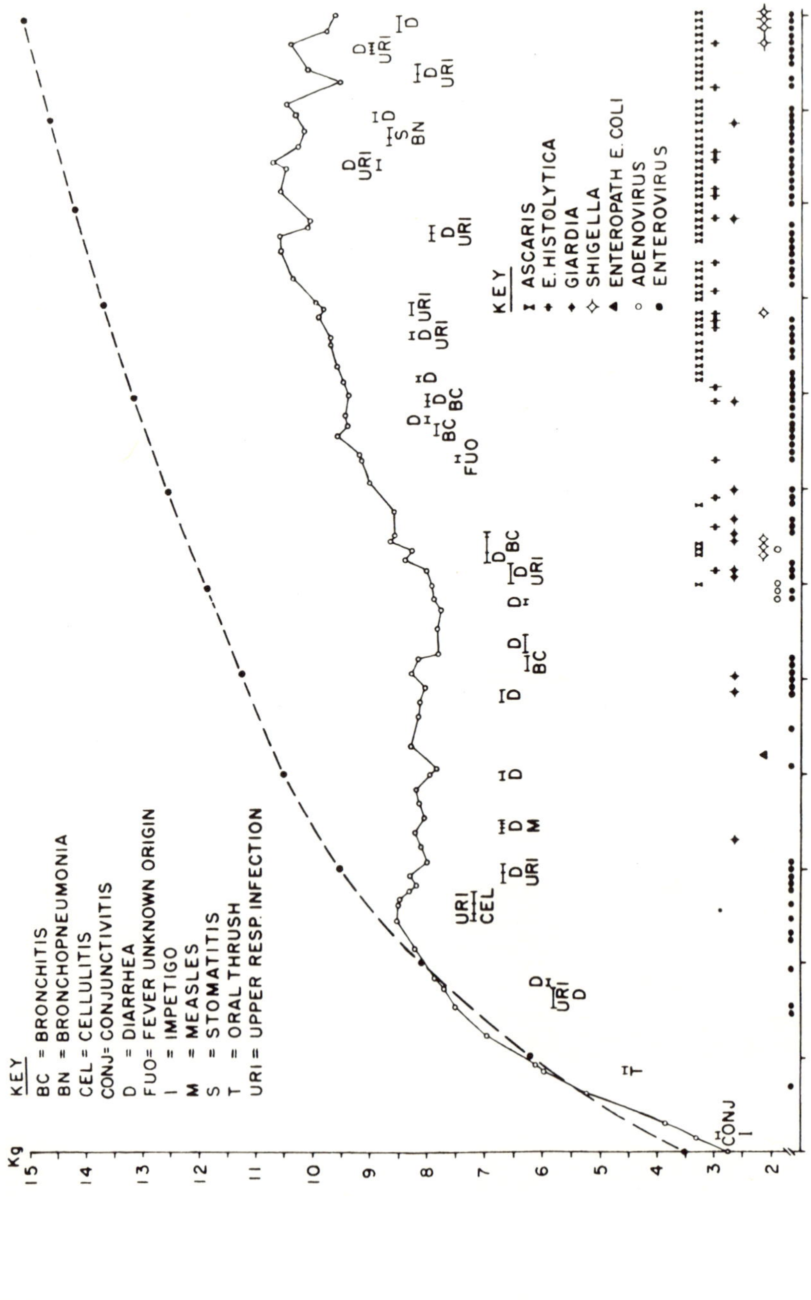
Kg
KEY
BC = BRONCHITIS
BN = BRONCHOPNEUMONIA
CEL = CELLULITIS
CONJ = CONJUNCTIVITIS
D = DIARRHEA
FUO = FEVER UNKNOWN ORIGIN
I = IMPETIGO
M = MEASLES
S = STOMATITIS
T = ORAL THRUSH
URI = UPPER RESP. INFECTION
KEY
I ASCARIS
E. HISTOLYTICA
GIARDIA
SHIGELLA
ENTEROPATH E. COLI
ADENOVIRUS
ENTEROVIRUS

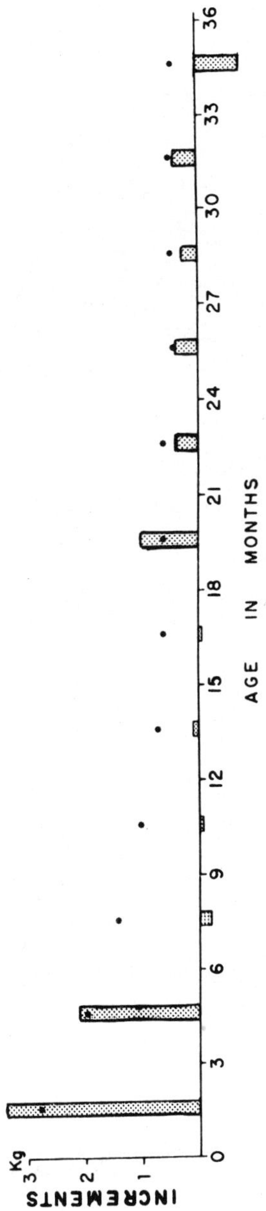

FIG. 3. Weight, infections, and infectious diseases, male child no. 12, Santa María Cauqué. Top: Solid line represents weight of child; broken line is median of the standard. Length of each horizontal line indicates duration of infectious disease. Each mark shows a week positive for the particular infectious agent. Bottom: Observed weight increments (vertical bars) and expected median increments (dots) of the standard (Mata *et al.*, 1971, reference 8).

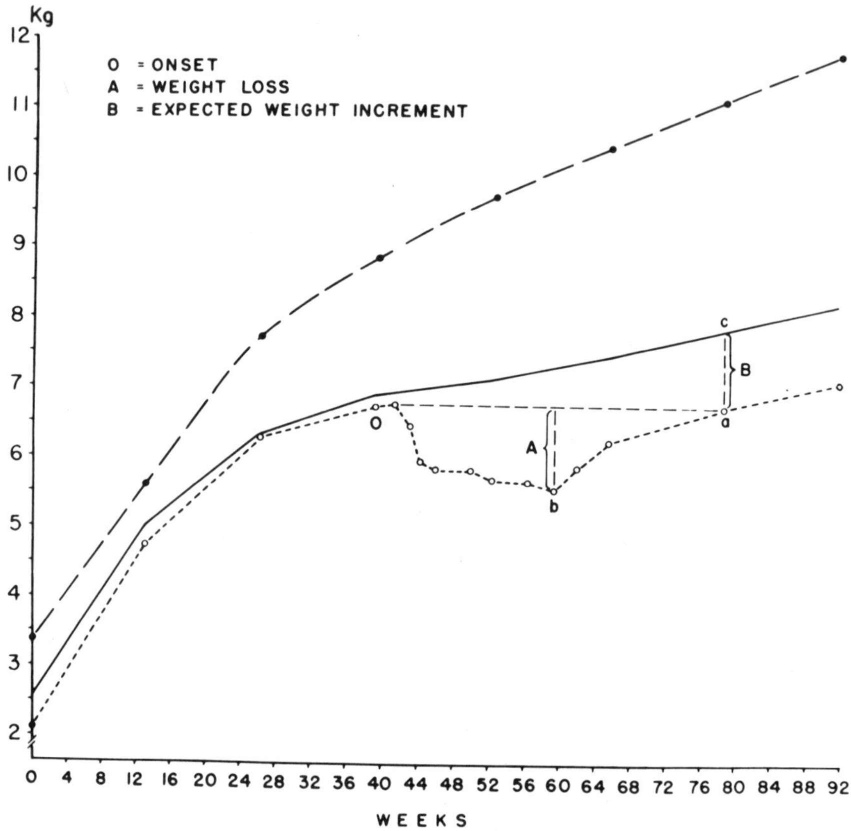

FIG. 4. Whooping cough in a girl of Santa María Cauqué to illustrate deterioration of nutritional status. Adapted from Mata *et al.*, 1972, reference 9).

there is a decrease in the number of immune cells in liver, bone marrow, spleen, Peyer's patches, and lymph nodes; this could explain the failure of malnourished children to mount a leukocyte response to bacterial infection. Alterations in phagocytic cells result in a diminished capacity to ingest and kill bacteria, a phenomenon apparently related more to lack of iron than to protein depletion. It has already been mentioned that iron sequestration occurs during infection.

Furthermore, malnourished individuals have altered or delayed hypersensitivity reactions. Other manifestations of altered cell-mediated immunity in malnutrition are a depressed capacity for blast transformation after challenge with mitogens, a diminished rosette formation, and alterations in factors important for the amplification of the immune response. These are evident, not only in acute PCM, but in underweight children who have experienced fetal growth retardation or early nutritional deprivation (4).

There is no doubt that infection and infectious disease are important factors in determining the occurrence of malnutrition. Conversely, malnutrition diminishes the host's capacity to resist and become immune to infection. The synergistic malnutrition–infection interaction can be considered the most important phenomenon in the genesis of recurring disease, impaired function, and death.

THE SOCIAL ENVIRONMENT

The frequent interactions between infection and malnutrition in the tropics are related to traditions, low educational level, and socioeconomic underdevelopment, as well as to the characteristics of the physical environment. As long as such deficiencies are not corrected, infection and malnutrition will continue to occur at the present rate or even become worse.

To illustrate, Figure 5 shows illiteracy rates in the six Central American countries, showing that in four of them about half or more of the people cannot read or write (12). It is not surprising that in most rural villages of Central America there is little or no knowledge of how disease is transmitted, of the need to boil drinking water, or how to prepare adequate, hygienic food for weaning infants.

Table III summarizes certain characteristics of a typical community in the Guatemalan highlands, pointing out deficiencies in housing, availability of water, and unsanitary disposal of human wastes—all factors related to transmission of infection.

Furthermore, in the same village, a study made 12 years ago showed that land averaged 10 cuerdas (3.3 acres) per family of five members, an amount

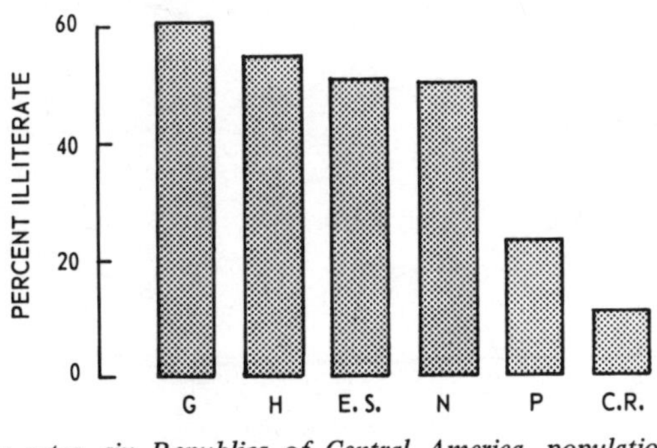

FIG. 5. Illiteracy rates, six Republics of Central America, population census of 1960, SIECA, 1973 (reference 12). (G) Guatemala, (H) Honduras, (E.S.) El Salvador, (N) Nicaragua, (P) Panamá, (C.R.) Costa Rica.

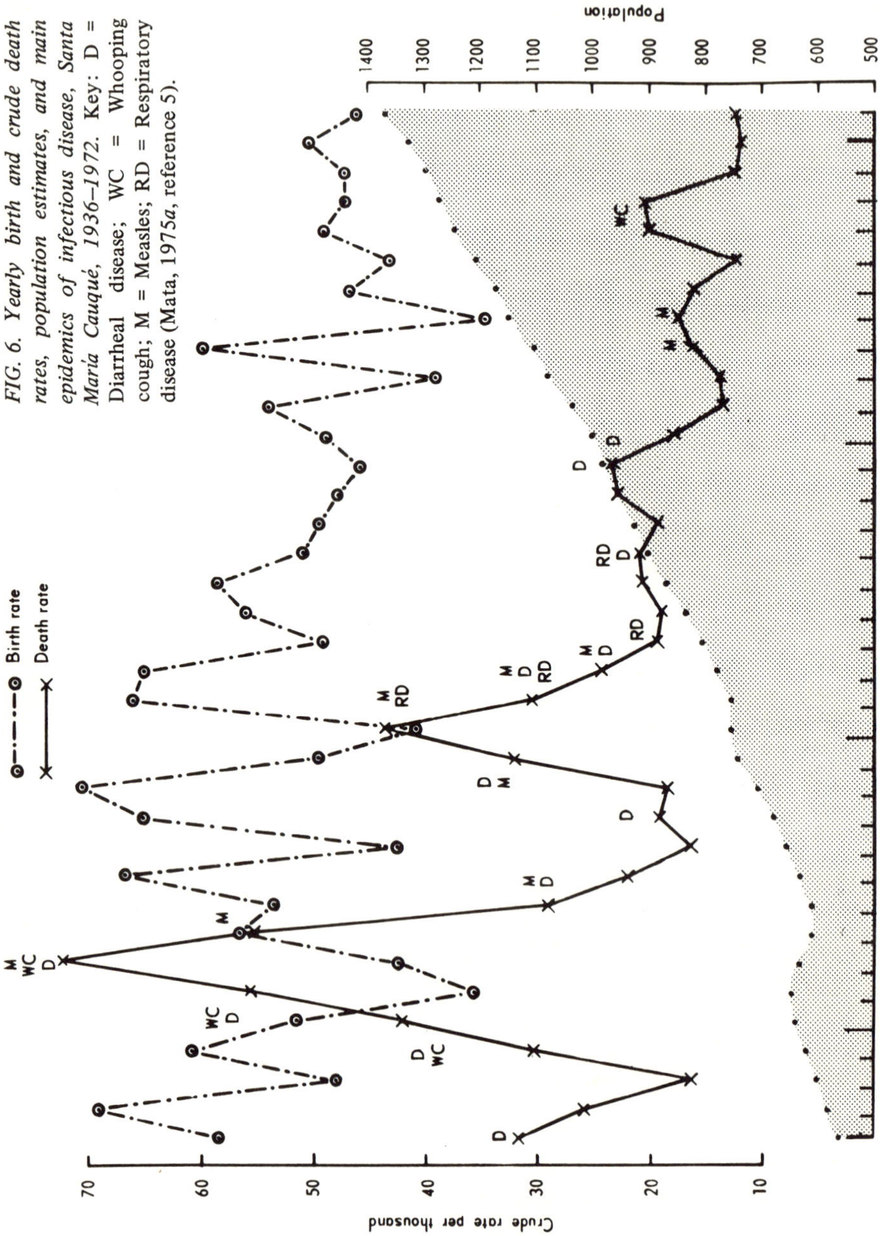

FIG. 6. Yearly birth and crude death rates, population estimates, and main epidemics of infectious disease, Santa María Cauqué, 1936–1972. Key: D = Diarrheal disease; WC = Whooping cough; M = Measles; RD = Respiratory disease (Mata, 1975*a*, reference 5).

Table III. Characteristics of a Typical Highland Village of Guatemala, Santa María Cauaqué, 1967

Features	Percent homes
Earthen floor	86.5
Piped water	7.4
Hearth on floor	88.7
Electricity	30.3
Privy	68.0

permitting cultivation of maize and beans to feed the village for one year. Within a decade the land was subdivided further and many young men in the community are now without land, creating a system of servitude not quite existing a few years ago. In addition, individual men and whole families have migrated to urban centers to live in shantytowns and slums, often under worse conditions than those of the village.

At present, the most pressing problem is the saturation of the carrying capacity of the land. Figure 6 shows that after 1950, deaths primarily due to epidemic diseases declined while birth rates remained high (6). In this village and in Guatemala as a whole the population is growing at a rate greater than 3% per year, without any apparent tendency to decline. Table IV illustrates the present population and population density in Central America and the expectations for the year 2000, figures that speak for themselves.

The economic capacity of villagers is very low, due to population growth, low educational level, primitive methods of agriculture, lack of skill in craftman-

Table IV. Population and Population Density, Central America and Panama[a]

Year	Guatemala	El Salvador	Honduras	Nicaragua	Costa Rica	Panama	Total[b]
			Population in millions				
1974	5.9	3.9	2.9	2.3	1.9	1.5	18.4
2000	15.7	9.6	8.0	5.7	4.4	3.7	47.1
			Inhabitants per km^2				
1974	55	186	26	18	38	20	34
2000	145	457	71	34	88	49	94

[a] SIECA, 1973 (reference 12).
[b] For Central America and Panama.

Table V. Mean Gross Domestic Product, U.S. Dollars per Caput, Selected Regions of Guatemala[a]

Region	1951–1952	1965–1966	% change in 15 years
Dept. Guatemala[b]	847	1071	+ 26
Dept. Sacatepéquez	197	123	– 38
All Guatemala, except three depts.	144	104	– 28
Rural Guatemala	142	105	– 26
All Guatemala	265	329	+ 24

[a]Adapted from Smith, 1973 (reference 13).
[b]Mostly Guatemala City.

ship, and little or no village industry or other types of economic development to employ landless people. The impoverishment of the population is evident in the steady decrease in gross domestic product noted for most of rural Guatemala, even before the recent onset of inflation. The country as a whole shows a gain in the gross domestic product, clearly concentrated in Guatemala City (Table V).

SUMMARY

The study of the relation of man to his environment in developing countries emphasizes the inevitable need for societies to recognize the true causes of infection, malnutrition, and poverty. The need is for improvement in the quality of human life in less developed nations, a recommendation easy to prescribe but difficult to accomplish. Although our pool of knowledge is incomplete, it is adequate to suggest ways to diminish infection, increase food production, utilize food more efficiently, improve education, and provide systems of justice to protect the classes most in need.

The physical environment in tropical and subtropical regions, and the socioeconomic characteristics of the population inhabiting such regions, favor maintenance and transmission of a variety of viruses, bacteria, and parasites that make agricultural progress and social development difficult, and that contribute to poor fetal growth, nutrient wastage, and deficient postnatal physical growth, accounting for most of the childhood morbidity and mortality. In this regard, infections contribute indirectly to the overall food problem in a similar fashion as pests do in terms of food losses and spoilage. The overall effect could be comparable or greater than that resulting from an inadequate capacity to produce or to purchase the food needed.

Thus, my objective has been to stress, within the whole environment, the importance of infection and the need to diminish it. Ways to control and prevent infection are readily known. They have to do with education of the population to improve personal and environmental hygiene. Economic investment is necessary to improve housing and water supply systems, waste disposal, and such preventive measures as immunization programs. Although such measures may appear expensive when first implemented, they have long-lasting effects and many require minimal expenditure once they are established. Large segments of the population stand to benefit, and other development interventions can then be introduced. However, these measures should not be implemented singly. They should be accompanied by community development, family planning, social legislation–in other words, the holistic approach to health and welfare. To do otherwise may aggravate the problem by stimulating demographic growth, perpetuating malnutrition and infection, and maintaining underdevelopment.

REFERENCES

1. Åstrand, P. O., and Rodahl, K., 1970, *Textbook of work physiology,* McGraw-Hill, York, pp. 517, 523–524.
2. Alluisi, E. A., Beisel, W. R., Bartelloni, P. J., and Coates, G. D., 1973, Behavioral effects of tularemia and sandfly fever in man, *J. Infect. Dis.* **128:** 710–717.
3. Beisel, W. R., 1972, Interrelated changes in host metabolism during generalized infectious illness, *Am. J. Clin. Nutr.* **25:** 1254–1260.
4. Chandra, R. K., 1974, Immunocompetence in low-birth-weight infants after intrauterine malnutrition, *Lancet* **2:** 1393–1394.
5. Mata, L. J., 1975*a*, Malnutrition–infection interactions in the tropics, *Am. J. Trop. Med. Hyg.,* **24:** 564–574.
6. Mata, L. J., 1975*b*, *The children of Santa María Cauqué*, Cornell/M.I.T. International Nutrition Policy Series, in press.
7. Mata, L. J., Urrutia, J. J., and García, B., 1967, Effect of infection and diet on child growth: Experience in a Guatemalan village, *in: Nutrition and infection,* G. E. W. Wolstenholme and C. M. O'Connor (eds.), Ciba Foundation Study Group No. 31, Little Brown, Boston, pp. 112–126.
8. Mata, L. J., Urrutia, J. J., and Lechtig, A., 1971, Infection and nutrition of children of a low socioeconomic rural community, *Am. J. Clin Nutr.* **24:** 249–259.
9. Mata, L. J., Urrutia, J. J., Cáceres, A., and Guzmán, M. A., 1972, The biological environment in a Guatemalan rural community, *in: Proceedings of the Western Hemisphere Nutrition Congress III,* Futura Publishing Co., New York, pp. 257–264.
10. Mata, L. J., Urrutia, J. J., Kronmal, R. A., and Joplin, C., 1975, Survival and physical growth in infancy and early childhood, by birth weight and gestational age. Study in a Guatemalan Indian village, *Am. J. Dis. Child.,* **129:** 561–566.
11. Scrimshaw, N. S., Taylor, C. E., and Gordon, J. E., 1968, *Interactions of nutrition and infection,* World Health Organization Monograph Series No. 57, Geneva, 329 pp.
12. SIECA, 1973, *Estadisticas sociales,* SIECA, Guatemala, 88 pp.
13. Smith, G. H., 1972, *Income and nutrition in the Guatemalan highlands,* A dissertation, Department of Economics and the Graduate School of the University of Oregon, University Microfilms, Ann Arbor, Michigan, xiv + 183 pp.
14. Torres, E., 1973, *Interpretación del desarrollo social Centroamericano,* Educa, Costa Rica, 319 pp.

15. Urrutia, J. J., Mata, L. J., Trent, F., Cruz, J. R., Villatoro, E., and Alexander, R. E., 1975, Infection and low birth weight in a developing country. A study in an Indian village of Guatemala, *Am. J. Dis. Child.* **129**: 558–561.
16. World Health Organization, 1972, A survey of nutritional–immunological interactions, *Bull. W. H. O.* **46**: 537–546.

COMMENTS

Carl E. Taylor · *Department of International Health, School of Hygiene and Public Health, The Johns Hopkins University, Baltimore, Maryland.*

Mata, in his excellent review of the environmental factors influencing malnutrition, concentrated on physical and biological factors. To complement his comments, I will focus on that part of the social environment that relates to social organization and the administration of nutrition and health care.

My major theme is that there is not only a synergism between malnutrition and infections, but an even more practical and important synergism between programs for nutrition and programs for infection control. Our research in India has clearly demonstrated this relationship. There is another program synergism about which we still have a great deal to learn: the relationships between family planning and both nutrition and health programs.

These relationships seem reasonable, and they make common sense to those prepared to believe in them. They are not readily accepted by proponents of categorical or single-approach programs. Specialists trained in one discipline tend to look for solutions in their area of competence. To nutrition specialists, it seemed reasonable to accept that part of the causal synergism suggesting that a nutrition program would limit the severity of infections in addition to improving nutritional status. Similarly, specialists in various means of infection control were able to reinforce their claims for programs such as immunization with the further justification that this would help to prevent malnutrition. Family planning specialists can correctly make the claim that one of the most effective measures for improving maternal and child health and nutrition is to ensure each family's right to have the number of children they can properly care for, with planned spacing of births.

While all of the claims are supported by considerable evidence, there are two serious limitations to their practical relevance:

First, our understanding of how these interactions work in normal populations is so incomplete that we know little about the dynamics or the strengths of particular associations. The relationships are bound together in multiple causation. Most of our measurements are in terms of one-way associations between specific causal factors. For practical program planning and development, we need a new approach to measurement that will provide for parallel quantification of the relative strengths of multiple relationships. When we know the comparative balance among the various associations, we will be able to make a beginning with the cost/effectiveness and benefit/cost judgments that lie at the heart of effective planning.

Second, practical program planning for long-term development is moving away from categorical approaches employing single measures. While mass programs using a single, simple procedure may be extremely productive as initial control measures, they will almost inevitably have to be integrated into a general service for the following reasons:

a. Separately organized categorical programs are usually inefficient in that they involve duplication of logistic requirements, such as travel time of field personnel.
b. They are often less effective than integrated services.
c. Finally, categorical services do not make sense to the people being served. They prefer to get a wider range of care from a worker they have learned to trust than single services from a series of workers divided according to disciplinary distinctions they cannot understand. The objective is to use activities for which there is high spontaneous demand in order to get a change in living patterns relating to needs not yet felt. In most countries, too, the integrated programs have much greater political acceptability.

I turn now to some data from our Rural Health Research Center at Narangwal, India, that show program synergism among services for nutrition, maternal and child health, and family planning. This program was developed as a set of service packages that would fit together naturally within the realities of village life. The estimated total cost for the whole package of integrated care, when research costs were deducted, was calculated to be two dollars per person per year.

At the Narangwal Rural Health Research Center in the Indian Punjab, we had parallel projects, studying the "interactions of malnutrition and infection in weaning age children" and the "integration of maternal and child care and family planning." Groups of villages received the different inputs of specified service packages. In each case routines were evolved that were carried out by a family health worker who had weekly supervision by a nurse and by a physician. Easy referral of complicated cases was arranged for those villages where the family health workers were providing primary medical care. All services were based primarily on routine surveillance. For instance, nutritional supplementation depended on early identification of faltering weight curves by systematically weighing all children under three years of age at intervals of one to three months, depending on age. Similarly, antenatal care focused on identifying specified risk categories, which provided a standardized basis for determining whether puerperal care could be provided by the indigenous midwife, or whether the mother should be referred elsewhere for special attention. Home visiting included morbidity surveillance to ensure early treatment. Preventive measures were stressed, including immunizations and health and nutrition education.

The results show the significant benefits achieved by the synergism of combined programs. Mortality rates of children from 11 to 36 months of age were brought down in three years from 24 per 1000 to 10 per 1000 in groups receiving both nutritional care and infection control. The nutrition-only group of villages had a rate of 23 per 1000. Ten years earlier the equivalent rate in the Khanna Study villages 27 miles away had been 48 per 1000, and it is a safe assumption that this general improvement can be attributed to the socioeconomic development in the Punjab, including the fact that practically every home had acquired a hand pump before the Narangwal project started. Infant mortality rates also went down, although perinatal and neonatal rates did not.

The second major area of demonstrated effect was in anthropometric indices. Both weight and height curves showed clear and consistent effects after nine months. The nutrition-only group weighed only slightly less than the combined care group, and both exceeded the controls by a significant margin. Significant benefits were also observed in related parameters, such as improved hemoglobin levels, and cell-mediated immunity. Analysis of morbidity data has not yet been completed.

The data on the relationship between family planning and the medical and nutritional care of mothers and children are incomplete. Preliminary analysis suggests that family planning practice was greatest in villages where maternal care and family planning were combined, with consistent practice by 45% of all couples 15–49 years of age, after four years of field work.

It seems clear that long-term enhancement of nutrition, health, and population stability demands the rapid development of basic services reaching out to the village home. It is hard to generate the political will and commitment to implement such programs because continuity is important. The most effective health officials long ago recognized the wisdom of using a serious epidemic to get acceptance of programs that would otherwise be deferred. We now have the challenge of using the worldwide awareness of massive hunger and increasing death rates to get long-term commitment to the continuing effort necessary to develop basic delivery systems for health, population control, and nutritional improvement. In fact, the most dramatic achievement during the Bihar famine in 1966 was not the mass distribution of food, but the long-range famine prevention that evolved from the pattern of work programs run by voluntary agencies where food was used to pay for developmental work. Villagers themselves organized to build ponds for irrigation, to dig wells, to construct roads, and generally to increase the potential for helping themselves. Developing village level services and local competence is the best way of meeting long-range challenges for improving human welfare and nutrition.

Ian A. McGregor · *Laboratory for Tropical Community Studies, National Institute for Medical Research, Mill Hill, London, England.*

Mata stressed that physical, biological, and social aspects of the environment can have an important influence in determining nutritional status. I would like to augment his observations, drawing upon experience in tropical Africa, especially The Gambia.

With regard to physical aspects, marked changes may occur in the environment within years as well as between years, and these changes may be associated with profound alterations in rates of survival and growth of young children. It has been suggested (1) that death rates in young children might serve as an index of the nutritional state of a country. In Keneba, a rural village of some 900 inhabitants in The Gambia, we have recorded deaths occurring at all ages since late 1949. A recent analysis of 725 recorded deaths showed that 69% occurred before the age of 5 years and that at all other ages, except the oldest (> 50 years), group mortality was very much lower. A further analysis, that took account of seasonal change within years, showed that death in early life occurred more frequently in the wet, rainy season than in the dry months of each year. Seventy-one percent of all deaths before the age of 5 years occurred in the wet months, June–November, inclusive. In contrast, only 41% of deaths at older ages occurred in these months. By the criterion of mortality, therefore, the nutritional state of Keneba children should be particularly poor each wet season.

Data relating to rates of gain in body weight and height have already been reported (2), confirming that growth of young children in Keneba can be remarkably good in the dry months of the year but that in the rains it may cease completely. Weight increments in pounds per quarter year for Keneba children are shown by age and season in Figure 1 (3). Mean rates of gain over the first three months of life at all seasons exceed values for healthy North American children, and are eloquent testimony to the efficiency of breast feeding by the African mother, and to the benefit of the passive immunity conferred by her to her infant against the important endemic infectious diseases, as Mata described. In the second three months of life, growth rates fall below those of American children, but gains are still made in both wet and dry seasons. However, between 6 and 15 months the pattern changes, and although some weight gain in the dry season persists, increments in the wet months are negligible, even negative. At older ages the pattern again changes and, although wet-season gains remain poor, rates in the dry months increase markedly and surpass American values. These season-associated changes in rates of gain in body weight, in which negligible gains alternate with rapid and spectacular increases, are a regular and characteristic feature of growth of young children in Keneba. Because physical changes in the environment similar to those that occur in the Keneba area are common throughout a large part of the tropical world, surveys intended to assess the

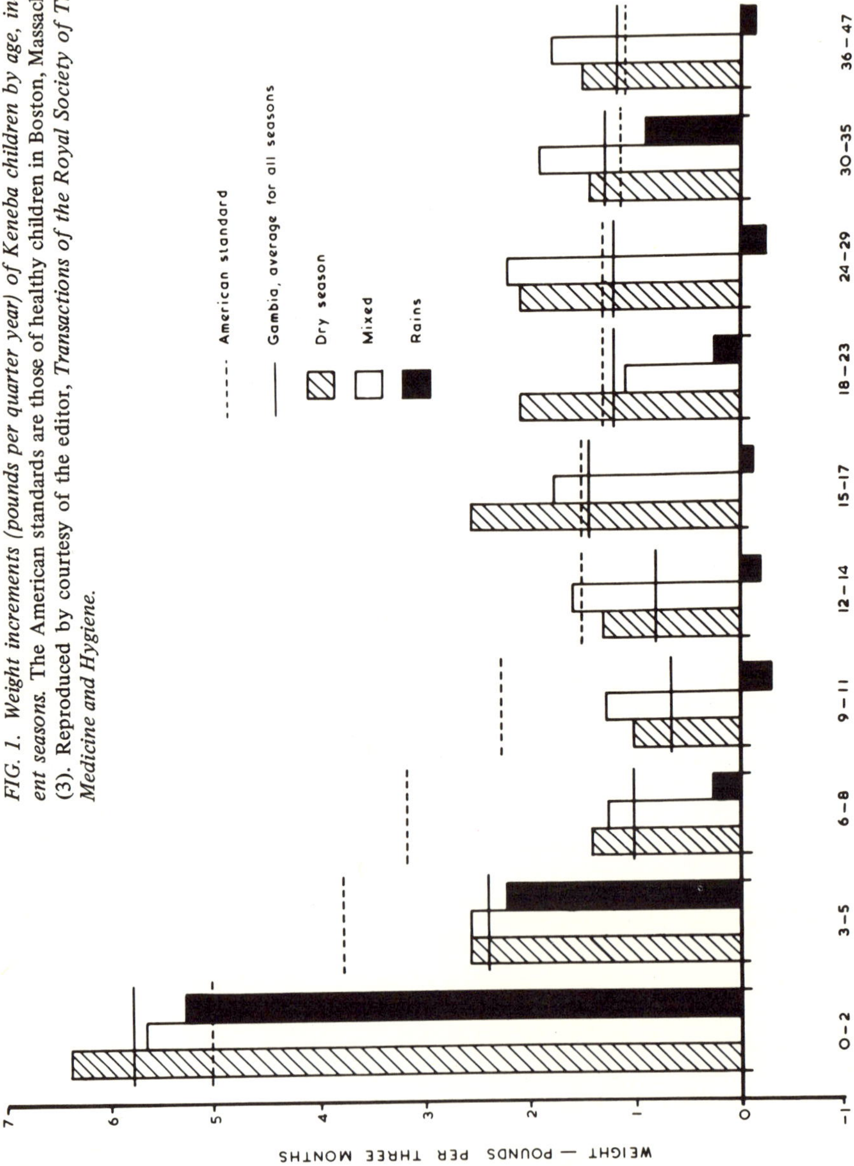

FIG. 1. Weight increments (pounds per quarter year) of Keneba children by age, in different seasons. The American standards are those of healthy children in Boston, Massachusetts (3). Reproduced by courtesy of the editor, *Transactions of the Royal Society of Tropical Medicine and Hygiene.*

nutritional state of children should be planned to take account of their possible effects.

My colleagues and I share Mata's view that physical, biological, and social changes in the environment often interact to influence nutritional state. This is not the place to analyze in detail the factors we believe combine to cause the season-associated changes I have described. Briefly, however, we have no evidence that growth patterns are disrupted during the rains simply because food is not available. However, the transmission of endemic infections such as malaria, filariasis, intestinal helminthiasis, and insect-borne virus diseases increases dramatically at this time, and clinical illness in the young child becomes frequent and severe over the period when passively acquired immunity has been lost and before acquired immunity has become effective. Concomitant anorexia reduces the intake of a bulky, predominantly vegetarian diet below the level necessary to maintain growth, and this effect is further compounded by a marked lowering of standards of care for young children, imposed by an agricultural economy that demands of the parents long hours of unremitting labor during the relatively short crop-growing season.

In dealing with biological aspects of the environment, Mata outlined how malnutrition may depress the functional efficiency of the different components of man's immune response to infection, thus creating a vicious cycle in which malnutrition enhances infection and infection enhances malnutrition. There is also evidence (4–6) that certain pathogens appear to depress, or even suppress, man's immune response to other infectious agents, although as yet there is little information to indicate how important this mechanism is in increasing host susceptibility to secondary infections, or in worsening nutritional state.

Another subject requiring elucidation is the persistence of effective acquired immunity in environments where malnutrition and infectious disease are frequent companions. Our studies in The Gambia (7) show that in adult Africans the daily rates of synthesis and catabolism of the serum protein immunoglobulin G (IgG) are nearly seven times greater than those of adult Caucasian residents of the United Kingdom. IgG functions importantly in antibody activity, and it is possible that its unduly rapid breakdown and resynthesis may curtail the duration of antibody-mediated acquired immunity.

Investigations, as yet unpublished, made in The Gambia in collaboration with Dr. G. Schild of the World Influenza Centre, National Institute for Medical Research, London, have revealed that, between 1968 and 1974, several epidemics of Hong Kong influenza occurred in our study area. Two important observations have been made. First, persistence of specific influenza antibodies in the sera of Gambians following the epidemic is much shorter than that observed following similar epidemics in populations of more developed countries of the Western world. Secondly, reinfection with the same serotype of the virus is common among Gambians, but is rare in Western populations. These observations prompt the question as to whether the standard schedules that have been advocated for immunization campaigns in the developed countries against prevalent infectious diseases will confer an equally effective persistent immunity when used in countries where malnutrition and a high frequency of infection with many different pathogens are common features of childhood.

Finally, Mata described the importance of the social environment. Experience gained in the campaign sponsored by the World Health Organization to eradicate malaria from the world is relevant. Malaria is, in some respects, a simple disease. It can be diagnosed with great precision. Its various vectors can be easily recognized. Drugs that are highly effective against the blood parasite are available, as are residual insecticides that are effective against the mosquito. Yet the global eradication campaign that proved to be so spectacular in developed countries has met with little success in many developing countries, notably those of tropical Africa. Sometimes failure has been attributed to the acquisition of resistance of parasites to drugs or of vectors to insecticides. More usually, however, factors that could be broadly termed *social* have been blamed. These have included widespread poverty, ignorance and superstition, lack of cooperation—even open hostility to remedial measures—nomadism and high population mobility, poor lines of communication, inadequate health and education services, and paucity of reliable executive staff. In this experience the lesson to be learned is simply that when remedial measures are planned in any area, be they nutritional or against infectious disease, a full and detailed knowledge of local beliefs, customs, and social organization is an essential prerequisite of success.

References

1. Wills, V. G., and Waterlow, J. C., 1958, The death-rate in the age group 1–4 years as an index of malnutrition, *J. Trop. Pediatr.* **3:** 167.
2. McGregor, I. A., Rahman, A. K., Thompson, B., Billewicz, W. Z., and Thomson, A. M., 1968, The growth of young children in a Gambian village, *Trans. R. Soc. Trop. Med. Hyg.* **62:** 341.
3. Nelson, W. E., 1969, *Textbook of pediatrics* (9th ed.), W. B. Saunders Company, Philadelphia, pp. 42–43.
4. McGregor, I. A., and Barr, M., 1962, Antibody response to tetanus toxoid inoculation in malarious and non-malarious Gambian children, *Trans. R. Soc. Trop. Med. Hyg.* **56:** 364.
5. Greenwood, B. M., Bradley-Moore, A. M., Palit, A., and Bryceson, A. D. M., 1972, Immunosuppression in children with malaria, *Lancet* **1:** 169.
6. Greenwood, B. M., Whittle, H. C., and Molyneux, D. H., 1973. Immunosuppression in Gambian trypanosomiasis, *Trans. R. Soc. Trop. Med. Hyg.* **67:** 846.
7. Cohen, S., and McGregor, I. A., 1963, Gamma globulin and acquired immunity to malaria, *in: Immunity to protozoa,* P. C. C. Garnham, A. E. Pierce, and I. Roitt (eds.), Blackwell Scientific Publications, Oxford, England, p. 132.

6

The Nutritional Status of Latin American Adults

Antonio Arteaga L.

Nutrition Department
Catholic University
Santiago, Chile

The high prevalence of infant and preschool child undernutrition in Latin America and its important impact on morbidity and mortality have been factors in the neglect of nutritional status in adult populations. This is an oversight that should be corrected, because the efficient working capacity of adults is a principal asset in combating national underdevelopment, which is the basis for most of the undernutrition in less developed countries.

According to the U.N. Demographic Year Book for 1972 (1), an average of only 58.2% of the population in selected countries of Latin America is over 15 years old, and less than 31% of this total can be characterized as economically productive; 80.6% of the men, but only 18.8% of the women, over 15 years old belong in this category (1,2). An estimated 54.4% of the men are engaged in heavy work, 19.6% in work of medium intensity, and 25.8% in sedentary occupations or in work involving only minor physical output. Of the women, 14.1% do heavy work, 20.3% are engaged in work requiring medium activity, and 65.5% have light-activity jobs. It should be noted that housework is not considered in the above categories, which undoubtedly underestimates the degree of activity for many women.

Adolescents between 15 and 19 years of age constitute a large sector of the working population. In this age group, 62.9% of the workers are male and 20.1% are women. This last figure remains the same throughout the years, suggesting that women begin to work at their potential capacity at age 15. There are, of course, important differences in workers in various age groups among individual Latin American countries.

Analysis of the nutritional status of the working population in Latin America has not been easy, because the published investigations and national vital statistics lack uniformity in design and the results are sometimes inconsistent. This discussion is based on the information available for the decade 1960–1970.

Two separate problems emerged as outstanding for Latin America: infant malnutrition with subsequent inadequate growth and development, and nutritional imbalance in the diets of adults. The principal consequences of deficient growth and development are smaller stature, and, possibly, limitation in psychomotor development. Figure 1 illustrates the contrast in the mean statures between adult men and women in various Latin American Countries (3–9) and those in the Iowa State growth and development study (10). The most extreme differences occur in Ecuador, where men are 18.5 cm shorter than American males and women are 16 cm smaller than their North American counterparts. Much has been said about the role of genetics in determining height. We believe that there is sufficient evidence that the height of population groups is closely related to infant and child nutrition.

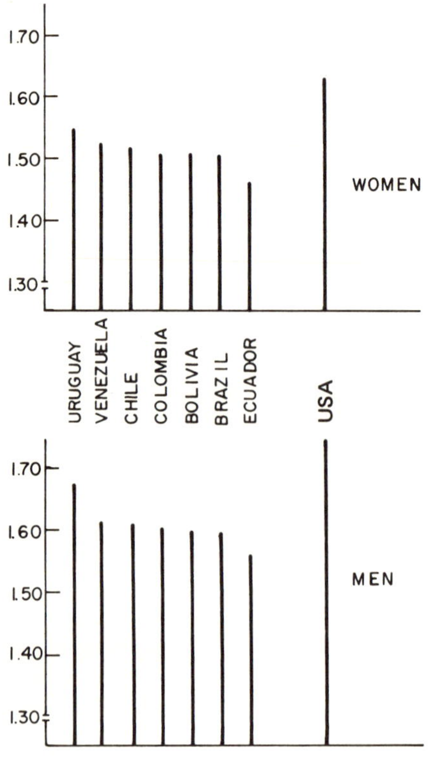

FIG. 1. Average height, Latin American population over 15 years of age, by sex, 1960–70. (Interdepartmental Committee on Nutrition for National Defense, civilian population).

Although there is general agreement that good nutrition in the first year of life plays a part in the structural development of the brain, its role in conditioning levels of intellectual development is still being investigated. Present information (11,12) regarding the low level of intellectual development of preschool and school children is based on poorer than normal performance on a battery of psychometric tests. It is very probable that adults are affected by this limitation as well. Whether this is a result of cultural deprivation, of poor nutrition in the first years of life, or both factors combined is difficult to answer. However, the association suggests an ominous consequence of undernutrition in the child's growing years.

The principal nutrition problem for adults is caloric deficiency and, paradoxically, for some, obesity. The frequencies of undernutrition and obesity in five South American countries are inversely correlated (Table I); undernutrition ranges between 8.7 and 21.2%, while obesity varies from 7.3 to 30%. Figure 2 shows the frequencies of undernutrition and obesity in various adult populations of Santiago, Chile (13). It is apparent that undernutrition is intimately related to socioeconomic level; the highest incidence of malnutrition is observed in the slums and the lowest among executives. On the other hand, obesity does not follow the same pattern: The lowest incidence exists among farm workers. Office workers show the most obesity, but it is also common among slum dwellers.

The frequency of obesity and undernutrition in a population of factory workers in Santiago (13) according to sex and age is given in Figure 3. In this population, women are more apt to suffer from calorie deficiency and are most often undernourished during the reproductive years. Obesity in women tends to occur in those over 35 years of age, reaching its maximum incidence in the sixth

Table I. Undernutrition and Obesity in Latin American Populations (>15 Years of Age), 1960–70

Undernutrition (%)	Country (No. of persons in parentheses)	Obesity (%)
21.2	Ecuador (1010)	8.4
18.9	Colombia (3627)	7.3
17.4	Bolivia (5787)	12.3
16.4	Chile (2911)	17.0
8.7	Uruguay (3627)	30.0

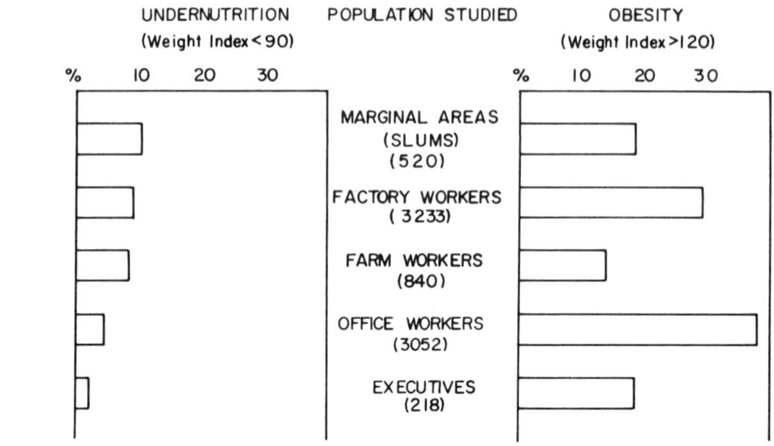

FIG. 2. Undernutrition and obesity in Chilean workers, 1960–70.

decade. Adolescents and young people between 20 and 24 years are least apt to be obese. The majority of those undernourished are less than 10% below desirable weight, 63.1% for men and 65.1% for women. Only 10.8% of the men and 8.5% of the women are severely undernourished. The same general ratio exists for obesity: 63.1% of the men and 54.2% of the women are up to 20% above normal body weight, while 13.6% of the men and 15.2% of the women are severely obese (more than 50% overweight).

In an effort to analyze the causes of calorie deficiency, we show, in Figure 4, the daily per caput availability of calories, the percentage of the population

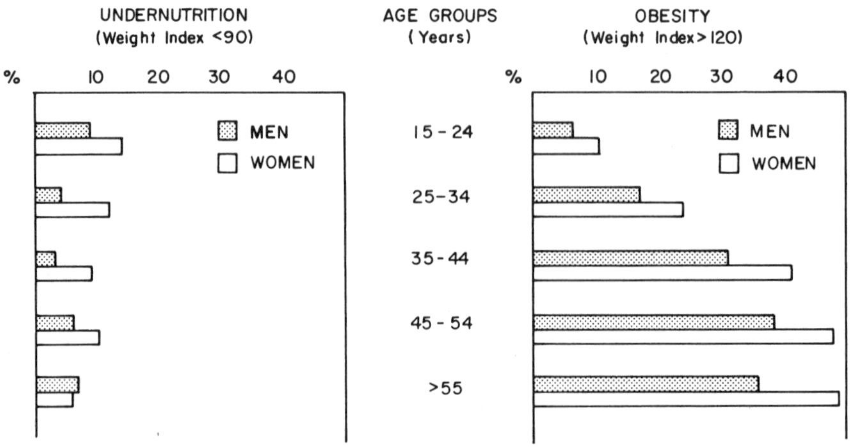

FIG. 3. Undernutrition and obesity by sex and age, Chilean factory workers, 1960–70.

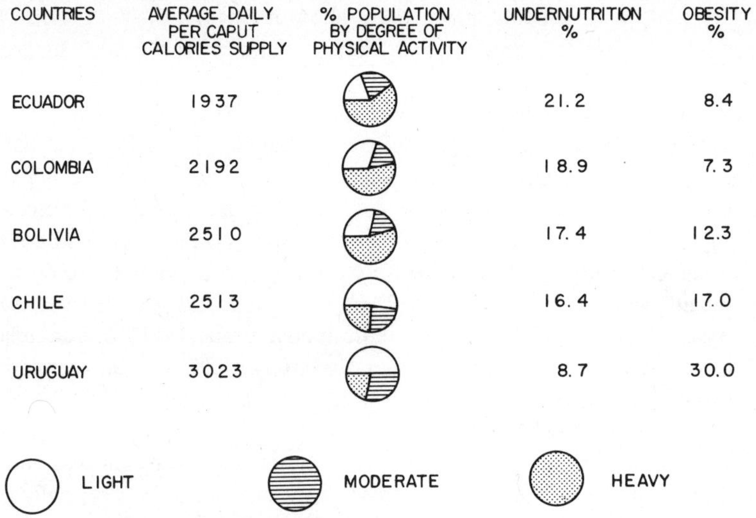

FIG. 4. Average daily per caput calorie supply, degree of physical activity, undernutrition, and obesity in five Latin American countries, 1960–70.

engaged in heavy, moderate, and light activities, and the frequency of undernutrition and obesity in five South American countries. Clearly, the segment of the population performing the hardest work has the fewest available calories, the most malnutrition, and the least amount of obesity. Conversely, the more well-to-do who have sedentary occupations also have more food available and have a higher incidence of obesity.

Table II shows how the level of nutrition knowledge influences the occurrence of adult malnutrition in a middle-income group. The population is stratified according to income per caput and the degree of awareness of sound dietary

Table II. Personal Income, Food Knowledge, and Coverage of Nutrient Allowances in 100 Middle-Class Chilean Women, 1960–70

	Coverage of nutrient allowances (%)			
	Adequate food knowledge (points 30–15)		Inadequate food knowledge (points <15)	
Per caput daily income (Tertiles)	No.	%	No.	%
High	14	108	7	132
Medium	23	104	19	102
Low	15	108	22	87

habits in relation to recommended daily allowances for nutrients. There is an inverse relation between income and dietary intake in those with inadequate knowledge of food (14).

Another of the problems observed in the working population was nutritional anemia, predominantly iron deficiency anemia. Table III gives the percentage of cases of frank iron deficiency anemia as well as those who were considered to be iron-deficient. These data are from a cooperative Latin American study (15) involving Argentina, Brazil, Colombia, Guatemala, Mexico, Peru, and Venezuela, plus those obtained by us (16) in a population of fertile, nonpregnant women. Both iron deficiency anemia and iron deficiency are frequent, especially in women in their reproductive years: 17.3% had anemia and 21.12% were iron-deficient in the cooperative study; 7.2% were anemic and 31% were iron-deficient in Chile. These conditions are less frequent in men; 3.9% had anemia and 3% were iron-deficient.

The common etiology for both problems is inadequate intake and low availability of iron in the foods consumed, intestinal parasites (especially hookworm), and the unmet increased iron requirements for frequent cycles of pregnancy and lactation. This latter factor, together with the poor iron balance in women of reproductive age due to additional iron losses during menstruation, explains the significant magnitude of the problem in these women. In the cooperative study, the possible role of vitamin B_{12} and/or folic acid deficiency in the etiology of nutritional anemias was not considered.

The presence of hypovitaminosis in the adult populations of some Latin American countries is evident in Table IV. The most important fact is the high frequency of very low or deficient levels of serum retinol, ranging from 9.9% in Uruguay to 35.4% in Bolivia. Results from measurement of urinary levels of thiamin, riboflavin, and methylnicotinamide differed among countries. On the whole, ariboflavinosis appears to be the most constant and serious for all countries, while nicotinamide deficiency is infrequent. The Chilean population showed no deficiencies in thiamin or nicotinamide because bread in Chile is enriched with these nutrients.

Table III. Iron Deficiency Anemia in Adults (>15 years) in Some Latin American Countries, 1960–70

Source	Sex	No.	Anemia (%)	Iron-deficiency (%)
Cooperative study[a] (ref. 15)	Men	287	3.9	3.0
	Women	415	17.3	21.2
Chile (ref. 16)	Women	325	7.2	31.0

[a]Includes men and nonlactating nonpregnant women from Argentina, Brazil, Colombia, Guatemala, Mexico, Peru, and Venezuela.

Table IV. Vitamin Deficiencies in Adults (>15 Years) in Some Latin American Countries, 1960–70

Country	Deficient and low levels (%)			
	Serum retinol, μg/100 ml	Urinary thiamin, μg/g creatinine	Urinary riboflavin, μg/g creatinine	Urinary N-methylnicotinamide, μg/g creatinine
Uruguay	9.9	37.5	14.0	2.4
Bolivia	35.4	3.9	20.0	0.7
Chile	22.9	0.0	10.0	0.0
Ecuador	31.0	9.3	13.5	11.4
Colombia	12.0	20.4	22.1	4.2

Uruguay, with the highest levels of calorie and protein ingestion, nevertheless has a high frequency of thiamin and riboflavin deficiency, attributable to consumption of refined products and the absence of enrichment programs. Other nutritional problems with a high incidence in adult Latin American populations—dental caries and endemic goiter—are beyond the scope of this discussion.

In summary, the principal nutritional problems of the Latin American adult population are (1) impaired physical growth and development and (2) probably an associated effect on mental development, learning, and behavior, due to both undernutrition in infancy and early childhood and related environmental and social factors. Caloric undernutrition and obesity vary inversely with the level of socioeconomic development. Iron deficiency, especially in women of reproductive age, is a major problem, as are hypovitaminosis-A, endemic goiter, and dental caries.

To analyze the impact of these principal nutritional problems on the adult Latin American population, only two aspects will be examined: their influence on work capacity and on the general state of health. It is known that work efficiency depends upon many factors, such as training (which implies intellectual level and technical qualification), health status, nutrition, and working conditions. In our Latin American population, in which 46.9% of the working people are engaged in heavy labor and 18.7% in moderate, it is important to examine the effect of malnutrition on capacity to maintain a prolonged effort. In the classical Minnesota study of experimental undernutrition in adults (17), the capacity of subjects to perform the Harvard Fitness Test during semistarvation and rehabilitation (Fig. 5) fell progressively during the 24-week period of food deprivation, and total capacity was not fully restored even by the 20th week of refeeding. An INCAP study (F. E. Viteri, personal communication,

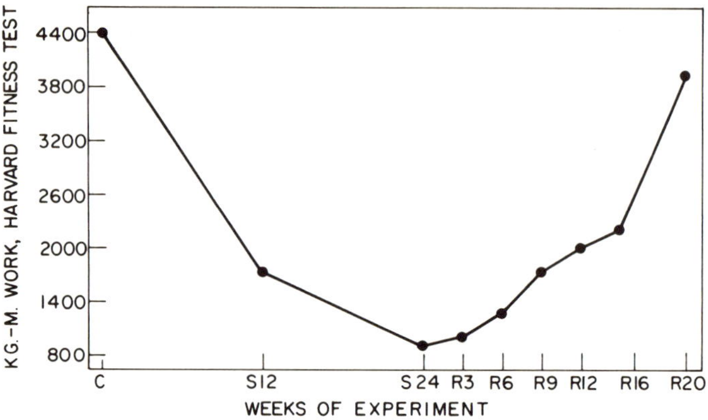

FIG. 5. Total work, as kilogram-meters, performed in the Harvard Fitness Test during semistarvation and rehabilitation. The values represent the averages for 12 subjects. Copyright 1950 by the University of Minnesota, University of Minnesota Press, Minneapolis (reference 17). Used with permission.

1974), showed that adults in a rural population were able to increase their work capacity if they were given nutritional supplements.

Our group has performed studies of physical capacity in Chilean workers using, as an indicator, maximal theoretical aerobic capacity, determined by a submaximum test on a bicycle ergometer, during which pulse rate and oxygen consumption were measured, extrapolating from the experiment of Astrand and Rhyming (18,19). We conclude that the Chilean worker's maximal aerobic capacity is inferior to that of Scandinavian and other workers. There is also a statistically significant correlation, independent of age, between maximal aerobic capacity and the height/weight index, thickness of adipose tissue, and serum hemoglobin level. The correlation is positive for height and hemoglobin, and negative for weight and skinfold thickness (Table V).

The reduced physical capacity of the Chilean worker is fundamentally caused by his short stature and by both lower and higher than normal weight, and variations in acceptable ranges of hemoglobin levels also reduce aerobic capacity during physical effort. Consequently, undernutrition as well as obesity and nutritional anemia appear in individuals of lesser physical development. They compensate for their nutritional inadequacies by reducing work output, a necessary adaptation to a deficient diet.

The interaction between undernutrition and infection has been described in numerous studies (20). Malnutrition augments susceptibility to infectious and parasitic diseases, diminishes the host's defense mechanisms, and reduces the effectiveness of therapeutic agents. Taken together, they contribute to less work capacity, absenteeism, loss of human capital, and even death.

Table V. Correlation of Aerobic Capacity (VO_2 max), Height, Weight Index, Skinfold Thickness, and Hemoglobin in 96 Foundry Workers

Correlated variables	Simple correlation coefficient	Partial correlation coefficient effect of age removed	
		Value	Significance
Height (cm)	0.24	0.46	$P < 0.01$
Weight index	–0.48	–0.24	$P < 0.05$
Skinfold thickness (mm)	–0.60	–0.63	$P < 0.01$
Hemoglobin (g/100 ml blood)	0.55	0.36	$P < 0.01$

To solve these problems, the social, economic, and technological development of countries in Latin America must be promoted by all of the resources we have available. This will mean major increases in food production, strong efforts to increase the economic status of the population, and nutrition education programs. We must also undertake studies of the nutritional status of adults, using standard survey methods. Cooperative multinational studies are necessary to investigate the epidemiology of the problems caused by under- and overnutrition. We must explore programs to supplement adolescents and those involved in heavy labor with calories, especially in countries with low per caput calorie availability. We also suggest the enrichment of foods with iron, vitamin A (or retinol), thiamin, riboflavin, and niacin.

REFERENCES

1. United Nations, 1972, Demographic Yearbook, United Nations, New York.
2. Secretaría General de Organización de Estados Americanos, 1972, América en cifras 1972, Situación económica, Washington, D.C.
3. Nutrition Survey, Chile, March 1960, A report by the Interdepartmental Committee on Nutrition for National Defense, U.S. Government Printing Office, Washington, D.C., August, 1961.
4. Nutrition Survey, Bolivia, May 1962, A report by the Interdepartmental Committee on Nutrition for National Defense, U.S. Government Printing Office, Washington, D.C., June, 1964.
5. Nutrition Survey, Colombia, May 1960, A report by the Interdepartmental Committee on Nutrition for National Defense, U.S. Government Printing Office, Washington, D.C., December, 1961.
6. Nutrition Survey, North East Brazil, May 1963, A report by the Interdepartmental Committee on Nutrition for National Defense, U.S. Government Printing Office, Washington, D.C., May, 1965.
7. Nutrition Survey, Venezuela, May 1963, A report by the Interdepartmental Committee

on Nutrition for National Defense, U.S. Government Printing Office, Washington, D.C., June, 1964.

8. Nutrition Survey, Ecuador, July, 1959, A report by the Interdepartmental Committee on Nutrition for National Defense, U.S. Government Printing Office, Washington, D.C., July, 1960.
9. Nutrition Survey, Uruguay, March–April, 1962, A report by the Interdepartmental Committee on Nutrition for National Defense, U.S. Government Printing Office, Washington, D.C., May, 1963.
10. Stuart, H. C., and Meredith, H., 1964, *Nelson's Textbook of Pediatrics* (8th ed.), W. B. Saunders Co., Philadelphia.
11. Mönckeberg, F., 1973, *Nutrición y conducta,* Nutrición y Desarrollo y Comportamiento Social, Publicación Científica 269, 78, Panamerican Health Organization, Washington, D.C.
12. Padua, A., Valiente, S., Arteaga, A., Castro, E., Michelli, C., and Rosales, E., 1970, *Nutrición y desarrollo psicomotor en escolares Chilenos,* Publicación Departamento de Nutrición, Sede Norte, Universidad de Chile.
13. Arteaga, A., Valiente, S., and Rosales, E., 1966, *Situación nutricional de la población adulta de Santiago de Chile,* Publicación Escuela de Salubridad, Universidad de Chile.
14. Arteaga, A., Malic, M., Monsalvez, A., Troncoso, M., and Santa María, J. V., 1964, *Encuesta por tendencia de consumo de 100 familias de clas media urbana, Nutr. Bromatol. Toxicol.* **3:** 78.
15. Cook, J. D., Alvarado, J., Gutmisky, A., Iamara, M., Sabardini, J., Layrisse, M., Linares, J., Loria, A., Marpes, J., Restrepo, A., Reynafarje, C., Sanchez Medal, L., Velez, H., and Viteri, F., 1971, Nutritional deficiency and anaemia in Latin America—a collaborative study, *Blood* **38:** 591.
16. Winter, A., Taboada, H., Galofré, A., Maiz, A., and Arteaga, A., 1974, Prevalencia de anemia ferropriva y carencia de hierro, en la población materno–infantil del Area Sur Oriente de Santiago, *Rev. Chil. Pediatr.* **45:** 53.
17. Keys, A., Brozek, J., Henschel, A., Mickelsen, O., and Taylor, H. L., 1950, *The biology of human starvation* (Vol. 1), University of Minnesota Press, St. Paul, Minnesota.
18. Arteaga, A., Donoso, H., Apud, E., and Rosales, E., 1971, Relación entre estado nutritivo y capacidad física. Estudio realizado in obreros Chilenos, *Rev. Med. Chile* **99:** 904.
19. Astrand, P. O., and Rhyming, I., 1954, A normogram for calculation of aerobic capacity ("physical fitness") from pulse rate during submaximal work, *J. Appl. Physiol.* **7:** 218.
20. Scrimshaw, N. S., Taylor, C. E., and Gordon, J. E., 1968, *Interactions of nutrition and infection,* World Health Organization Monograph Series No. 57, WHO, Geneva.

7

Nutritional Problems in the Labor Force and Their Relation to Economic Development

Michael C. Latham

Division of Nutritional Sciences
Cornell University
Ithaca, New York

When nutritionists propose a program to improve the health or nutritional status of a population, then economists and planners may ask what the economic benefits of such a program are likely to be. Health is a high human value but one that is difficult to measure in monetary units. One obvious area in which economists and nutritionists have seen a link between nutrition and economic development is that of labor productivity. If poor nutrition is lowering productivity, then an investment in programs to improve nutritional status of workers can be justified on economic grounds alone.

But the hard-nosed economist, using outdated arguments, might also point out that most developing countries have a labor surplus. Therefore the sick and the malnourished are expendable. Either they can be replaced when nonproductive, or, alternatively, payment can be made to them on the basis of the amount of work done. More persons who are less productive can be employed for the same task at no additional cost. Therefore, where there are labor surpluses, individual productivity is relatively unimportant.

In recent years there has been an increased dialogue between economists and nutritionists (1), and this has coincided with a certain disillusionment about the means and the pace of development in the third world, especially when viewed in the narrow context of GNP, GDP, or per caput income. There has, at the same time, been a realization that it is desirable to shift emphasis away from capital-intensive toward labor-intensive development projects.

Dr. Arteaga's chapter, which has concentrated on the problems of Latin America, is surely based on the assumption that the key elements in development are human beings of both sexes. People in most societies place a high priority on their own health and that of their families. The economist has tended to view improved health as a welfare question. Therefore maximization of a country's income (or per caput income) may still be the economist's goal in pushing for national development, and the equity question may remain relatively ignored. Fortunately, perhaps, more so than for most health factors, improved nutrition can be shown to have a favorable effect on both per caput income and improved quality of life for people. Certain nutrition programs can therefore be viewed in these terms.

In development plans, effective nutrition programs deserve support even if they do not contribute to raised national incomes, provided they do contribute to improved lives for the majority of people. Development projects that contribute only to growth in capital but have no effect, or a negative one, on the human well-being of the majority, should not, in my view, be supported. Similarly, expenditure of public funds on nutrition programs that will benefit mainly the elite, or even the middle classes, do not deserve a high priority.

What is the purpose of economic development? Whom is it for? If improved health and nutritional status of people are not considered in development plans, then one might seriously question whether this really is development. Nutrition projects are therefore justified as part of human development programs. A reduced infant and toddler mortality rate, a lowered morbidity, and a healthier population provide better indicators of development than do telephones or number of automobiles per family, or dollars or pesos per head. Who would claim that development is more advanced in Mexico or Brazil than in China or Cuba, simply because per caput incomes are higher in the former countries, while childhood malnutrition has apparently been almost eliminated in the latter?

There will be those who argue that in a given country economic growth and more money per head are the prerequisites of improved nutrition. It is quite clear that those with higher incomes in North and South America do usually have better nutritional status and health. But improved nutrition can take place without raising incomes. All-important, however, is the *distribution* of any benefits that result from economic growth. Too often the major benefits go to a small elite group of the population. Sometimes a moderate benefit seeps through to the middle class or to the families in the employed labor force, but very few of the benefits accrue to those families who are poor and for whom malnutrition is a real problem.

An example of an effort not reaching the poor is the so-called low-cost nutritious food product whose development has often received public financial backing. Commercially processed and packaged food must cost more than commonly eaten local foods processed in the home on the basis of cost per 100 calories or per gram of protein (2). Therefore, for the very poor, or for the laborer eking out an existence on the minimum wage, the purchase of these commercial foods, even if nutritious, may lower, not raise, the family's intake. If anyone other than the manufacturer is benefiting, it is the middle and upper classes.

Decisions by planners concerning nutrition intervention programs should take into consideration the relationship of nutrition to classical economic growth in terms of productivity, and also the equity questions discussed above. Decisions must be influenced by political and social considerations. Staatz (3) has suggested that if the target group is composed primarily of low-income people whose lack of income is the main reason for their malnutrition, then a nutrition intervention program that generates considerable employment and income for them, in addition to increasing their intake of nutrients, probably is preferable to another program (e.g., one based on the free distribution of imported weaning foods) that does not generate much local employment or income. The former program most likely would have a significant indirect effect on nutrition as well as a direct effect, because, as their incomes increased as a result of the new employment, the poor presumably would buy more and better quality food than previously.

NUTRITION IN THE LABOR FORCE

Arteaga has undertaken the difficult task of delineating the nutrition problems of Latin America as they impinge on the working population. He has discussed the obvious links between poor nutrition and productivity—such as lack of calories, poor physical and mental development, and anemia—and also some others including obesity, vitamin A deficiency, and goiter.

At the outset, consideration should be given to what constitutes the labor force of a country. Arteaga neatly used the term *active population* for labor force. Too often economists and others tend to consider first those who are wage earners and second those who produce goods and provide services for the market as constituting the labor force. The role of women in household work and child-rearing tends to be forgotten. But even the work of those who produce food for the family, rather than for the market or for export, are relatively ignored. In many countries women play a major role in agricultural production, especially of traditional crops. President Nyerere of Tanzania put it this way (4):

> The truth is that in the villages the women work very hard. At times they work 12 to 14 hours a day. They even work on Sundays and public holidays. Women who live in the villages work harder than anybody else in Tanzania. But the men who live in the

> villages (and some of the women in the towns) are on leave (holiday) for half of their life.

I am certain that this is true also for many parts of Latin America.

Therefore, when reviewing the relation of nutrition to productivity and development, consideration should be given as much to housewives as to hacienda workers, to the backyard cultivators as to banana and sugarcane cutters.

NUTRITIONAL STATUS AND PRODUCTIVITY

A great deal has been written about the straightforward relationship between calorie and nutrient intakes, and work output. It is, of course, clear that humans have to burn calories in order to perform work. But a careful perusal of the literature shows that relatively few experiments have demonstrated that increased calorie intakes result in increased work output or productivity. The important studies in Germany during and after World War II (5) are often quoted, but are by no means definitive. The so-called Minnesota starvation study of Keys and co-workers (6) increased our knowledge but did not address this question. The recent work in Guatemala by Viteri and his colleagues (7), in which the effects of calorie and iron deficiencies were studied, has broken new ground. Viteri, in one study of the energy expenditure of two groups of Guatemalan peasants, one supplemented and the other unsupplemented, showed a marked increase in energy expenditure in the supplemented group. Both groups, however, had a negative energy balance, the time period was short, and the type of work performed was not identical in both groups.

The World Bank study (8) in Indonesia has shown that even moderate anemia does affect productivity. Treatment of anemia for a period of 60 days led to an increase in productivity of 15% for rubber tappers and 25% for weeders. An earlier report by the same group showed no difference in Harvard Step Test results from those whose hemoglobin was above and below 13 g, but significantly lower Harvard Step Test scores in the group with hemoglobin levels below 11 g/100 ml.

Care must be taken, however, to distinguish between results based on measures of work capacity and physical fitness and those in which work output or productivity was determined. The results are much less clear in studies relating nutrition to work output because other factors, such as motivation, determine how hard people actually work compared to how hard they can work. The extent to which a low-calorie intake by workers reduces the output of goods and services in a poor country is dependent on at least three factors, namely: (a) the extent to which the actual work performed is reduced or limited by calorie deficits; (b) the importance of the work relative to other factors in the whole production process; and (c) the levels of employment or the availability of "surplus labor" in the economy.

MALNUTRITION AND PRODUCTIVITY OF JAMAICAN SUGARCANE CUTTERS

A study of the relationship of certain nutritional and other factors to the productivity of Jamaican sugarcane cutters has recently been completed (9). This was a cooperative investigation involving the Caribbean Food and Nutrition Institute and our group at Cornell, and carried out with the approval of the Jamaican government, the trade unions, and the sugar growers.

The productivity of sugarcane cutters in Jamaica was known to be low. In 1971 the average amount of cane cut per man per day on nine sugar estates in Jamaica was 3.1 tons, whereas it was 8.6 tons on a Florida sugar estate using West Indian cane cutters. This low productivity in Jamaica has resulted in increasing pressure on the government to permit mechanization of harvesting. Mechanization would necessarily result in fewer jobs in a country which, in 1972, had an unemployment rate estimated at 22%.

The field investigation was conducted for the whole of the seven-month 1972–73 crop period on the Parnassus and Innswood sugar estates. The work of the sugarcane cutter lends itself to this kind of study because payment is made on the basis of the amount of sugar cane cut, the amount cut being weighed and recorded each day.

In the study, weight for height (W/H) was chosen as the measure of nutritional status of primary interest, and was used as an independent variable. Weight for height is an index of fatness or thinness, and therefore of energy stores, and can serve as an indicator of work capacity. As the cutting season extends over a period of several months, energy stores may be a major determinant of ability to sustain a high level of productivity for the full crop-harvesting period. The selection of weight for height also implies that energy intake and its interaction with energy stores is the primary nutritional restriction on productivity.

An increase in energy intake (supplementation in the field) was used to test this hypothesis, but supplementation was only possible on one estate (Parnassus). Several nutritional variables including hemoglobin, hematocrit, height, weight, skinfold thickness, and arm circumference, and many social variables, such as off-season income, number of dependents, distance from work, and other factors were also recorded. The relation of these variables to productivity and to each other was determined.

On Parnassus estate, where supplementation was provided in the second half of the season, there was a significant effect of weight for height on productivity, both before and after supplementation. The cutters whose W/H was below 85% cut significantly less cane than those whose W/H was above 95%. This significant relationship remained when factors such as age, weight, height, and skinfold thickness were controlled.

The persons in the lowest W/H group have, on the whole, lower weights and lesser arm circumference and skinfold thickness than the other two groups have. This could affect their productivity because (a) the lower energy stores may prevent a constant level of production in the face of possible fluctuation and occasional deficiencies in energy intake, and (b) the lower weight of the lowest W/H group indicates a lower $\dot{V}O_2$ max. This may be an important determinant of work output, because of the restricted amount of work available and the competitive way in which extra tasks are allocated. In this study, loss of weight over the season was, in general, insignificant, and anemia was not a common problem.

On Parnassus estate there was a significant increase in productivity during the second portion of the crop season in which supplementation was given. In many studies it would have been concluded that supplementation produced this rise in productivity by increasing food intake. However, the measurements of food intake made suggest that the supplement given in the field did not increase total 24-hour nutrient intake. Therefore, the large increase in production in the second period was due to a "time" effect, especially, perhaps, to increased work availability in the second period, to the timing of when food is eaten, or to some other unexplained factors. The calorie-rich supplement taken during work breaks could have had some positive effect even if it resulted in reduced consumption of food during nonworking hours. The supplement could have had a motivational or placebo effect; i.e., the results might indicate a kind of Hawthorne effect rather than a nutritional one. A third factor significantly related to productivity was the "gang effect." There were significant differences in productivity among gangs, and yet gangs did not differ in any of the other variables that we tested relating to income, health, nutritional status, age, and others. We can only conclude that gang leadership, social interaction among workers, morale, and other human factors contributed to these differences.

We would conclude that nutritional status is an important factor influencing work productivity of Jamaican cane cutters. This relationship would very likely be even more strongly positive, and supplementation would be likely to have a definite effect, in a situation where unlimited work is available at all times to the workers being studied.

HEALTH AND NUTRITIONAL FACTORS AS DETERRENTS TO EMPLOYMENT

In five counties in upstate New York we have investigated the health and nutritional status of low-income working and nonworking women (10). These 400 women all had children, and all either had been or were eligible for welfare payments.

Among the unemployed, poor health was a major stated reason for not working. A detailed medical, nutritional, and sociological investigation was undertaken for each woman. The nonworking women were found to have much higher rates of disease and of physical disabilities. Several of these were nutrition-related and contributed to failure to obtain or hold a paid job.

Other scientists are beginning to ask the question: Is big better? In our study size was a definite handicap in obtaining or holding employment—size of girth that is! Obesity was a major problem, and overweight women were much less likely to be working. The fat woman was at a disadvantage when applying for a job, she may have been less efficient on the job, and she had more difficulty holding the job. Our investigation of major employers in the area revealed that many discriminated against obese subjects in their employment practices.

Another major health problem related to nutrition was dental caries. These women had appalling teeth, and over half had lost all of their teeth by 50 years of age. The average woman who still had some teeth required over $250 worth of dental treatment, at Medicare rates, to restore her teeth to some semblance of satisfactory appearance and function. The expense and lack of availability of dental services for the poor was found to be a major deterrent to receiving dental care. Dental problems resulted in loss of work for those who were employed, and in some cases was a deterrent to obtaining a job in those who were unemployed. An edentulous middle-aged woman without dentures does not feel encouraged to seek employment and is likely, because of her appearance, to be discriminated against when interviewed for a job. A young woman with some front teeth missing is not likely to be successful in obtaining a job, such as that of waitress, in competition with someone with a complete set of teeth.

Other conditions that commonly affected employment were hypertension, psychological problems, and diseases of the musculoskeletal system, some of which may be related to obesity and to nutritional deficiencies.

Undoubtedly, in low-income women in an industrialized country, ill health and poor nutrition are related to both employment and earning capacity, especially in the case of the untrained and unskilled, and those with poor educations.

CONCLUSION

Both work capacity and work output are influenced by the nutrient intake and the nutritional status of those who perform work, be they housewives, persons engaged in subsistence agriculture, or wage earners in the labor force. There is no doubt that the sequelae of childhood malnutrition may also affect the future capacity of individuals for work. Obvious examples have been cited by Dr. Arteaga, and include blindness or poor vision following xerophthalmia; stunting of physical, and perhaps mental, development resulting from protein-calorie malnutrition; skeletal deformities caused by rickets or fluorosis; and several others.

But good nutrition for the work force, and for those who one day will enter it, is important not only in terms of productivity. Programs to improve nutrition and health form the cornerstone for human development. It may be that family-planning efforts and population-control programs will fail in most societies that have not attained some fairly good level of health and nutrition for their people. In countries where there is much unemployment and underemployment, labor-intensive rather than capital-intensive development schemes deserve priority. In many of these, agricultural development activities can provide work, can make available more food, and can improve the economy. Economic development must be for the benefit of the majority of people and must be designed to improve their quality of life. It should not be for the benefit of the elite alone, and should not be measured simply in monetary terms. The widening gap between rich and poor individuals, families, and nations has not only economic and political consequences, but also very important nutritional and health implications.

ACKNOWLEDGMENTS

I thank Dr. Peter Heywood, Dr. Barry Popkin, and Mr. John Staatz for ideas that they shared with me while graduate students at Cornell, and that have been liberally used here. The results of the productivity study in Jamaica discussed in this chapter are based largely on the Ph.D. thesis of Dr. Heywood. Drs. Daphne Roe, David Call, and Robert Cook also deserve acknowledgment as partners in some of the research reported here.

REFERENCES

1. Berg, A., Scrimshaw, N. S., and Call, D. L. (eds.), 1973, *Nutrition, national development, and planning,* M.I.T. Press, Cambridge, Massachusetts.
2. Popkin, B. M., and Latham, M. C., 1973, The limitations and dangers of commerciogenic nutritious foods, *Am. J. Clin. Nutr.* **26**: 1015.
3. Staatz, J., Unpublished thesis draft.
4. Nyerere, J. K., 1967, *The Arusha Declaration and TANU's Policy on Socialism and Self Reliance,* Address by President Julius K. Nyerere, Feb. 5.
5. Keller, W. D., and Kraut, H. A., 1959, Work and nutrition, *in: World review of nutrition and dietetics,* G. Bourne (ed.), Hafner Publishing Co., New York, pp. 69–81.
6. Keys, A., Brozek, J., Henschel, A., Mickelsen, O., and Taylor, H. L., 1950, *The biology of human starvation,* University of Minnesota Press, Minneapolis, Minnesota.
7. Viteri, F. E., 1971, Considerations on the effect of nutrition on the body composition and physical working capacity of young Guatemalan adults, *in: Amino acid fortification of protein foods,* N. S. Scrimshaw and A. M. Altschul (eds.), M.I.T. Press, Cambridge, Massachusetts, pp. 350–375.
8. International Bank for Reconstruction and Development, Staff Working Paper No. 152, 1973, and No. 175, 1974; S. S. Basta and Soekirman, 1974, personal communication.

9. Heywood, P. F., 1974, *Malnutrition and productivity in Jamaican sugar cane cutters,* Ph.D. thesis, Cornell University, Ithaca, New York.
10. Roe, D., Eickwort, K., and Latham, M., 1973, *Report on study of health and nutrition status of working and non-working mothers in poverty groups,* Unpublished report for the U.S. Department of Labor.

8

Definition of the Nutrition Problem in the Labor Force

Fernando E. Viteri

Biomedical Division
Institute of Nutrition of Central America and Panama
Guatemala City, Guatemala

Arteaga made reference to the fact that many of the adult laborers in Latin America are suboptimally nourished, and proposed a series of measures aimed at correcting this situation. I will present a very brief summary of our findings on the nutrition, body composition, work performance, and energy balance of rural agricultural workers in Guatemala to illustrate some of the negative interactions between nutritional deficiencies and work performance, productivity, and socio-economic development. The characteristics that stand out most clearly among male agricultural laborers in a tropical, developing area are their small size, leanness, slow working pace, and, in the lowlands, often their pallor. Over 30% of them have hookworm infection (1). Dietary surveys indicate that their calorie intakes are frequently less than 2700 per day (2), with protein intakes ranging between 70 and 90 g per day (2,3). Often riboflavin, folate, and vitamin A are inadequate (2). Further observations and inquiries bring about other so-called characteristics: They are often referred to as "lazy, inefficient workers," and as people who find it difficult to engage in after-work activities aimed at individual or communal betterment. In other words, they are apathetic human beings.

We investigated some of the relations between these characteristics and nutrition, starting with the two nutrients that seemed most limiting: calories and iron.

Table I. Body Composition of Supplemented and Unsupplemented Agricultural Laborers in the Highlands of Guatemala

Subjects	Body weight (kg)	Height (cm)	Lean body mass (g/cm)	Muscle mass (g/cm)	Adiposity (g/cm)
Supplemented	60.1[a]	161	322	153	50
($N = 18$)	1.3[b]	1	7	6	3
Unsupplemented	50.8	158	294	119	26
($N = 18$)	1.0	1	6	6	1

[a]Mean.
[b]SE.

CALORIES

From previous work (3–5), as well as from work in progress (6), the following specific points appear pertinent.

1. Agricultural workers subsisting on an average intake of 2700 calories per day have lower body weight, less adipose tissue, and reduced lean body mass (LBM) and muscle mass compared to similar agricultural workers receiving a nutritional supplement that increased their calorie intake to 3550 per day (Table I). It is worth noting that none of the latter workers were obese.

2. Supplemented laborers also have more total circulating hemoglobin, and display superior performance on tests of physiological functions indicative of physical work capacity, including maximal oxygen consumption ($\dot{V}O_2$ max.) and cardiac output at $\dot{V}O_2$ max. In Table II, both populations have been

Table II. Pertinent Variables Involved in Work Performance of Agricultural Workers in Guatemala (Grouped by Lean Body Mass)

	Lean body mass (kg)		Hemoglobin concentration (g/100 ml)		Total circulating hemoglobin (g)		Maximal O_2 consumption (ml/min)		Maximal cardiac output[a] (liters/min)
	Mean	SD	Mean	SD	Mean	SD	Mean	SD	Mean
< 45 ($N = 15$)	42.7	1.5	15.0	1.7	622	87	2145	308	16.1
45–49.9 ($N = 19$)	47.3	1.4	15.8	1.4	721	75	2302	253	17.0
50–54.9 ($N = 16$)	52.6	1.4	15.6	1.2	752	73	2498	335	18.0
55 and + ($N = 14$)	58.2	2.8	16.2	0.8	917	117	2934	269	20.5

[a]Calculated on the basis of Hermansen, *Acta Physiol. Scand., Suppl.* 339, 1973.

grouped into LBM categories to indicate the relationship between body composition and physiological performance in these populations.

The linear regression and scattergram between LBM and $\dot{V}O_2$ max. is shown in Figure 1. Table III presents the interrelation between total circulating hemoglobin and $\dot{V}O_2$ max. in absolute terms. This relationship disappears when the last variable is expressed as per kilogram of lean body mass (Table IV). This, plus the fact that the correlation coefficient between LBM and $\dot{V}O_2$ max. is higher than between total circulating hemoglobin and $\dot{V}O_2$ max. (r = 0.692 and r = 0.534, respectively), suggests that the primary effect of caloric supplementation in these populations has been an increase in LBM, which possibly induced elevations in both $\dot{V}O_2$ max. and total circulating hemoglobin. This type of response has also been documented in children recovering from malnutrition, whose rate of increase in total circulating hemoglobin is governed by the rate of increment in LBM (7,8).

The increment in LBM and muscularity that accompanied the nutritional supplement made the laborers better able to handle work situations that demanded strength and repeated large muscle action. Being not only short in stature but also having a relatively reduced muscle mass and LBM, suboptimally nourished workers do not respond to high-energy-demanding work situations with full efficiency. Furthermore, in active individuals, LBM correlates highly significantly with $\dot{V}O_2$ max. and tissue oxygen delivery (cardiac output and total circulating hemoglobin) (Figure 2).

The mechanisms by which calorie supplementation brought about such changes in LBM are not yet clear. One possible mechanism could be increased activity, leading to an effect similar to that of physical training. Caloric supplementation may also have played an important role in the complex phenomenon of physical endurance, which is markedly dependent on availability of energy for muscle action derived either from body energy reserves (for the most part, adipose tissue) or from available food energy. The following data indicate that food energy may have an important role in defining the activity level of agricultural populations.

3. Supplemented laborers reach a new energy equilibrium by increasing their energy expenditure. This is achieved almost exclusively by becoming more active physically.

Results of time/motion studies in both supplemented and unsupplemented laborers indicate that the latter group lost weight during the period of observation when they increased their energy expenditure above their level of intake. In spite of greater effort, they were unable to continue to be active after work; they usually took long naps in the afternoon. In contrast, the supplemented men were more active, worked at a higher energy expenditure level (3–5), and did not interrupt their work in midafternoon. Furthermore, in spite of spending more calories than the unsupplemented group, they did not lose significant

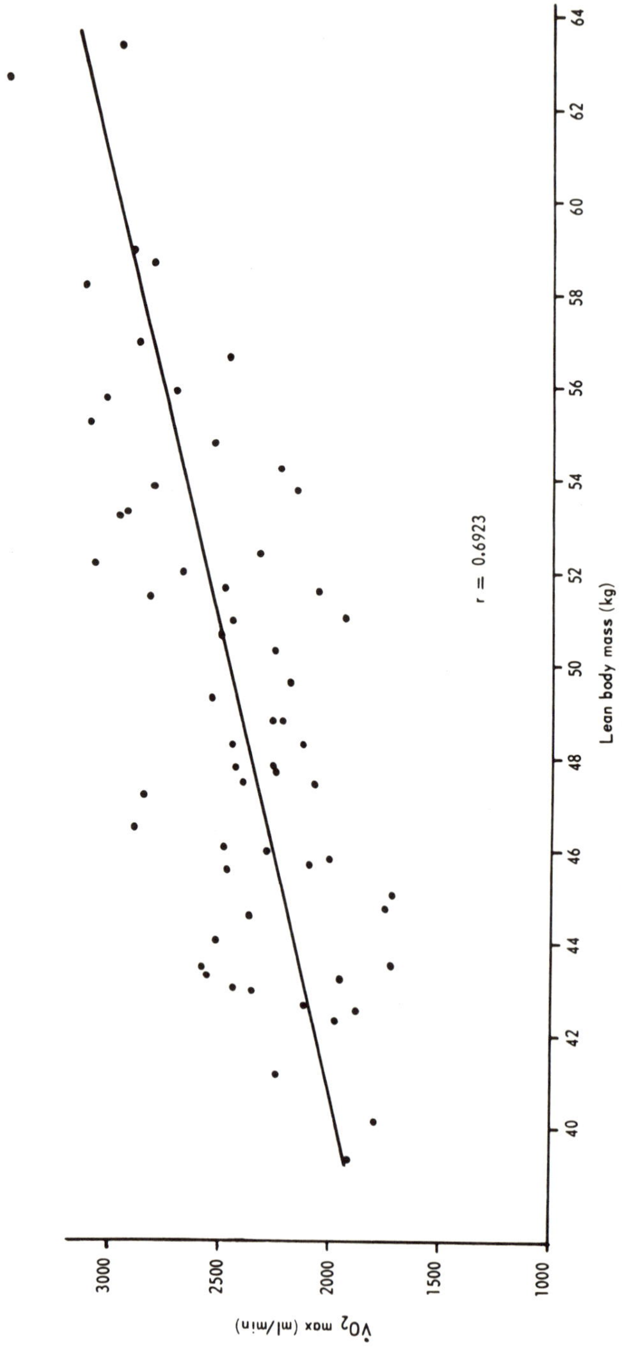

FIG. 1. Lean body mass and maximal oxygen consumption of agricultural laborers in Guatemala.

Table III. Maximal Oxygen Consumption ($\dot{V}O_2$ max.) for Different Values of Total Circulating Hemoglobin of Agricultural Workers in Guatemala

Total circulating hgb. (g)	*N*	$\dot{V}O_2$ max. (ml/min)	
< 600	7	2009[a]	184[b]
600–699	20	2302	333
700–799	20	2446	341
800–899	11	2538	275
900+	6	2931	336

[a]Mean.
[b]SD.

amounts of weight (Table V). Additional data derived from these studies are that one standard, representative task requires approximately 990 calories spent in physical activity during a period of four to six hours.

Based on this and other available information, the following generalizations can be made (Figure 2):

a. The average agricultural laborer in Guatemala requires 1612 calories per day in order to compensate his basal energy expenditure. Such energy expenditure can be further divided into that spent during a night's sleep (8 hours), which amounts to 540 calories, and 1072 calories that are expended during the rest of the 24 hours.

b. He requires 990 extra calories for the activity increment involved in performing one standard, representative task for 4 to 6 hours. Adding these energy expenditures to that in sleep, plus performance of one task in the

Table IV. Maximal Oxygen Consumption per kilogram Lean Body Mass for Different Values of Total Circulating Hemoglobin of Agricultural Workers in Guatemala

Total circulating hgb. (g)	*N*	VO_2 max. (ml/min) / LBM (kg)	
< 600	6	46.2[a]	5.3[b]
600–699	18	49.6	6.9
700–799	19	48.7	6.0
800–899	10	49.4	4.6
900+	6	49.8	4.1

[a]Mean.
[b]SD.

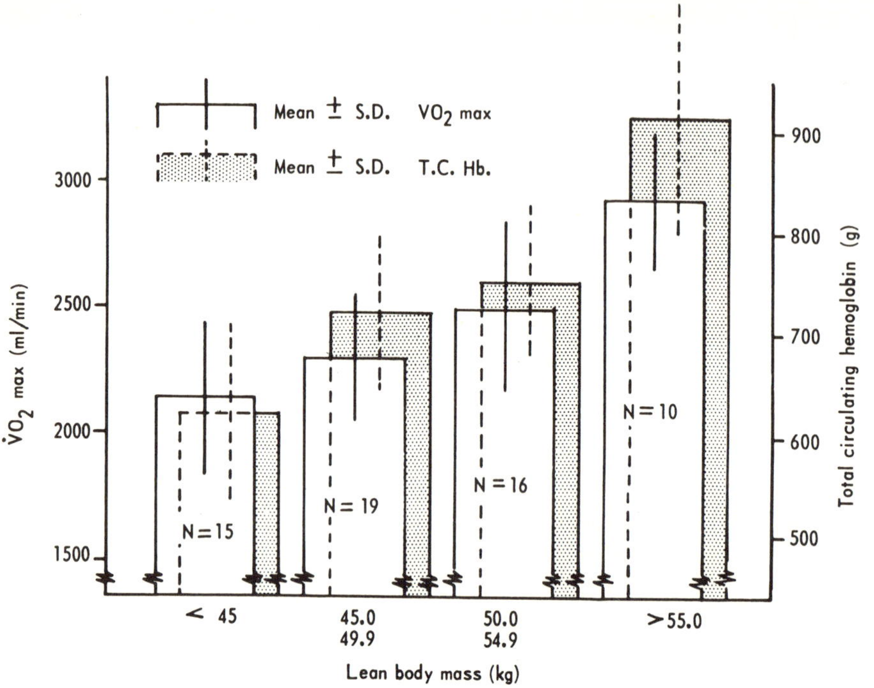

FIG. 2. Maximal oxygen consumption and total circulating hemoglobin for different amounts of lean body mass of agricultural laborers in Guatemala.

Table V. Caloric Intake, Expenditure, and Balance, and Body Weight Changes of Agricultural Workers in Guatemala (Period of Observation = 3 Days per Subject during Time/Motion Studies)

	Groups			
	Supplemented (N = 18)		Unsupplemented (N = 18)	
	Mean	SE	Mean	SE
Energy intake (cal/day)	3555	168	2695	118
Energy expenditure (cal/day)	3694	109	3396	128
Energy balance (cal/day)	–138	180	–707	110
Change in weight (g/3 days)	–29	64	–346	174
Expected weight change (g/3 days)[a]	–22	29	–316	46

[a] 1 g of weight loss is assumed to yield 6.2 calories.

morning, it becomes evident that a laborer who eats 2600 calories per day has spent all available food energy for performing that task. Consequently, he must remain very inactive after work in order to maintain energy balance. The only way he can achieve this is by spending this time napping or just sitting, doing nothing. Another alternative is, of course, to do less than one task a day, or do an inadequate job at it.

From our studies it is also evident that an active worker engaged in

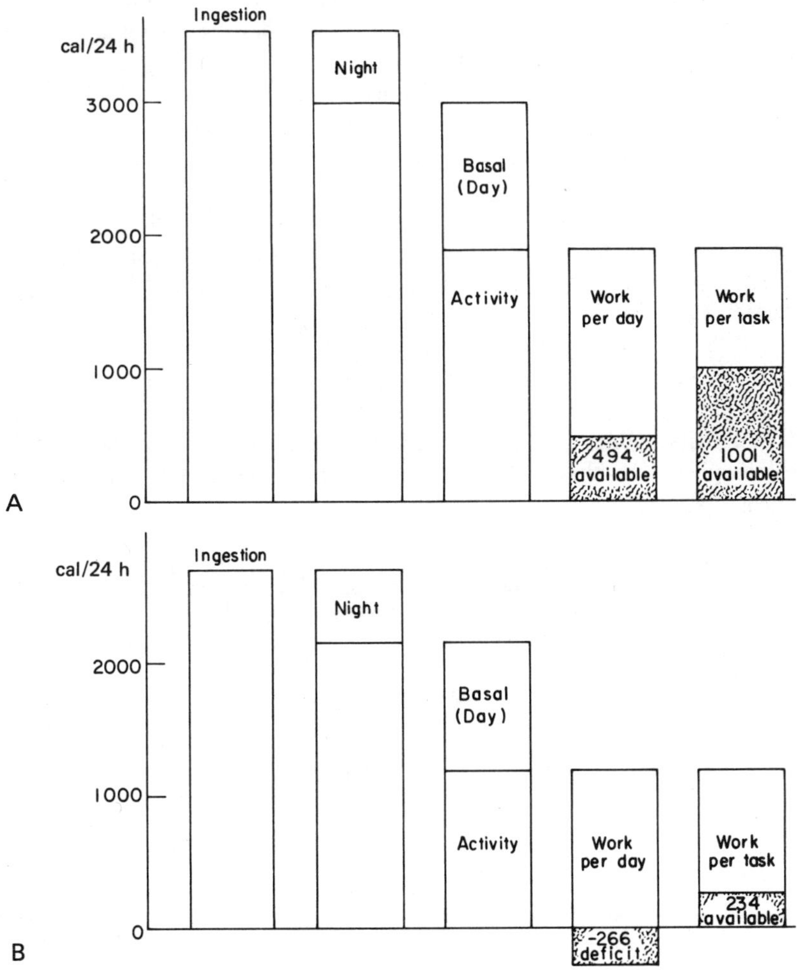

FIG. 3. Energy balance of supplemented (A) and unsupplemented (B) agricultural workers in Guatemala. Values represent an average day and are broken down into different energy expenditure categories.

agricultural activities on an 8-hour-per-day basis spends close to 1500 calories on top of his basal caloric expenditure in farming chores. The total energy expenditure comes up to 3110 calories in 16 hours, there being 8 additional after-work hours left. If a laborer is to remain active during this time, he requires at least 1 calorie per minute beyond his basal energy expenditure, or nearly 480 additional calories. The total energy expenditure would then amount to 3590 calories per day. The calorically supplemented group working an 8-hour day spent very close to this amount (Table V). It is obvious that, thermodynamically, the unsupplemented group (eating 2700 calories) could not be efficient workers on an 8-hour-per-day work schedule, and that on a task-per-day basis, their after-work activity is reduced to essentially nil (Figure 3).

This also explains why hired laborers are not contracted on an 8-hour-per-day schedule and why the agricultural labor force is often characterized as "lazy and apathetic," without the drive to participate in after-work activities.

The actual work pattern of agricultural laborers demands effective use of strength, near maximal work capacity, and endurance. For example, the use of a hoe, an ax, or a machete demands strength and endurance; walking up a hill with a load also demands near-maximum effort. Such efforts, however, take up only a short period throughout the day because most manual laborers work at close to one-half of their maximum aerobic capacity (½ $\dot{V}O_2$ max.).

In brief, insufficient caloric intake imposes a ceiling on the total energy expenditure in agricultural laboring populations that, in the long run, results in low productivity, which in turn contributes significantly to socioeconomic underdevelopment. Furthermore, by making the individual less muscular, caloric insufficiency also renders him less able to perform high-energy-demanding tasks,

Table VI. Maximal Predicted Work Load (cal/min) That Can Be Sustained by Individuals with Various Levels of Hemoglobin Concentration and Three Different Maximal Cardiac Outputs

Hgb. concentration (g/100 ml blood)	Maximal work load (cal/min) for maximal cardiac output		
	15	20	25
4	3.2	4.2	5.3
6	4.8	6.4	8.0
8	6.4	8.5	10.6
10	8.0	10.6	13.2
12	9.6	12.7	15.9
14	11.1	14.8	18.5
16	12.7	17.0	21.2

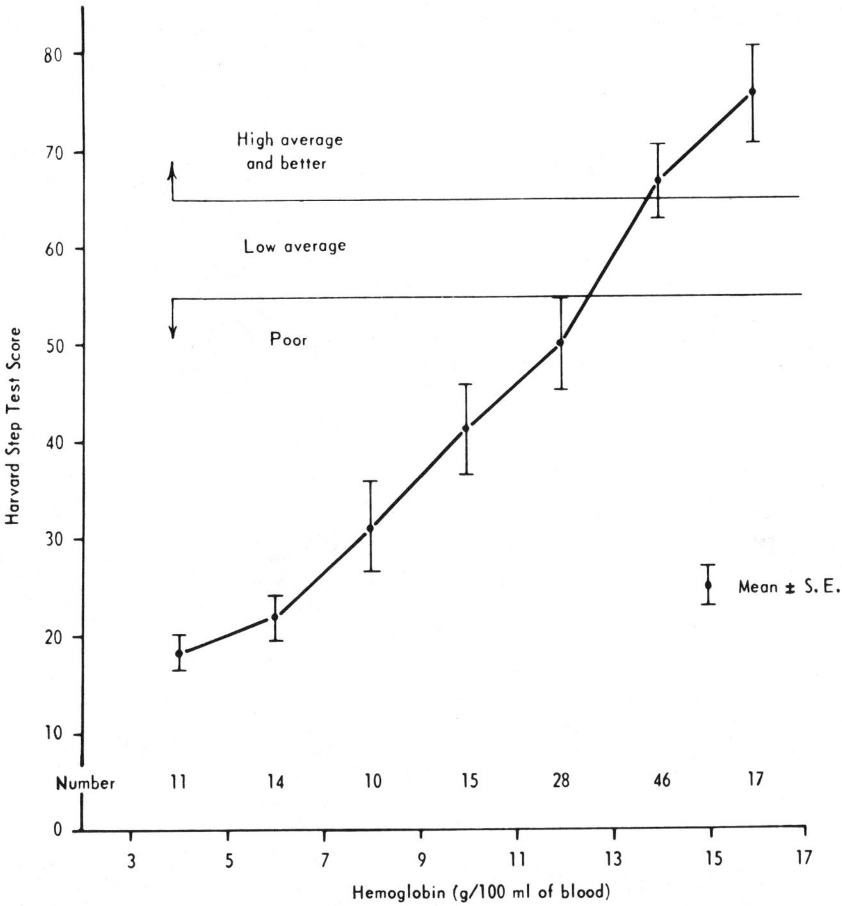

FIG. 4. Physical fitness in relation to hemoglobin concentration in Guatemalan agricultural workers.

and his smaller LBM also limits his maximal oxygen delivery to tissues and, therefore, acts synergistically with anemia.

IRON

Chronic iron deficiency anemia diminishes tissue oxygen delivery for a given cardiac output. A known compensating mechanism for anemia is an increased cardiac output at rest and during submaximal work situations. This results in meeting tissue oxygen demands by means of a more rapid circulation of blood, with reduced levels of hemoglobin. However, maximal cardiac output is not

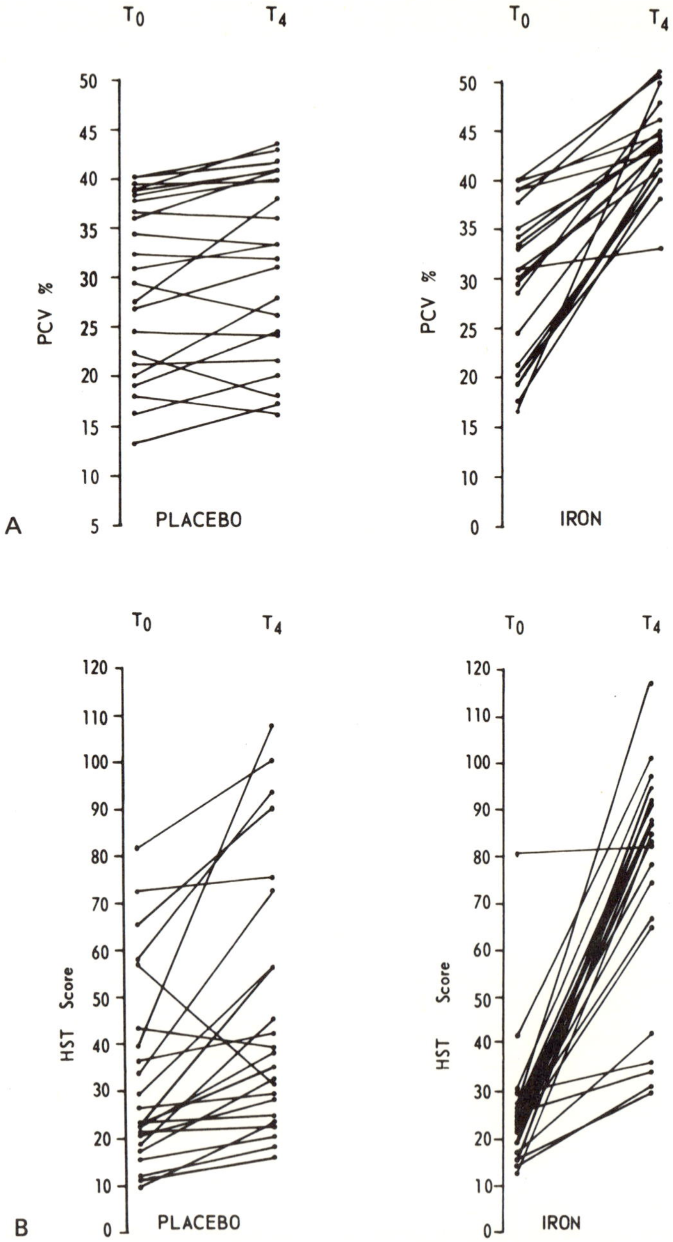

FIG. 5. Changes in packed cell volume (PCV) and in Harvard Step Test score (HST score) in two groups of Guatemalan agricultural workers, before (A) and after (B) 4 months of treatment with placebo or with oral iron.

increased in anemia, so that maximal, or near-maximal, oxygen delivery to tissues is reduced. The end result of anemia on work performance will necessarily depend on two factors: (a) tissue oxygen demands, and (b) maximal oxygen delivery capacity. The first of these factors is directly proportional to the intensity of physical effort; the second is inversely proportional to the degree of anemia, or directly proportional to the hemoglobin concentration in the blood. It is also directly proportional to the maximal cardiac output. This last variable, as described earlier, is proportional to LBM in active populations.

These basic concepts allow us to predict the maximal energy output a laborer can sustain for a given period of time, on the basis of body size and hemoglobin concentration (9) (Table VI). Furthermore, the lack of proper understanding of these physiological considerations has resulted in contradictory reports on the effect of anemia on physical working capacity and productivity.

Our own experience in evaluating physical fitness in active populations with anemia before and after treatment with oral iron (10–12) indicates that the capacity to perform a short, near-maximal effort correlates inversely, and very significantly, with the degree of anemia (Figure 4). Treating the anemia without any other intervention results in a marked improvement of this physiologic test (Figure 5).

In summary, anemia decreases the capacity to perform energy-demanding tasks. Mild to moderate degrees of anemia (hemoglobin concentrations between 9 and 13 gm per 100 ml of blood in adult males) only decrease the capacity to perform hard to extreme physical efforts. More severe anemia impairs performance during even mild efforts.

Anemia and insufficient calorie intake thus decrease work capacity by different mechanisms, both leading, finally, to decreased productivity and to hampered agricultural and general socioeconomic development.

REFERENCES

1. Viteri, F. E., Guzmán, M. A., and Mata, L. J., 1973, Anemias nutricionales en Centro América; influencia de infección por uncinaria, *Arch. Latinoam. Nutr.* **23:** 33–53.
2. *Nutritional evaluation of the population of Central America and Panama. Regional summary,* Institute of Nutrition of Central America and Panama (INCAP) and Nutrition Program, Center for Disease Control (formerly Interdepartmental Committee on Nutrition for National Development). Washington, D.C., U.S. Department of Health, Education and Welfare, 1972, 165 pp. (DHEW Publication No. (HSM) 72-8120).
3. Viteri, F. E., 1971, Considerations on the effect of nutrition on the body composition and physical working capacity of young Guatemalan adults, *in: Amino acid fortification of protein foods,* N. S. Scrimshaw and A. M. Altschul (eds.), M.I.T. Press, Cambridge, Massachusetts, pp. 350–375.
4. Viteri, F. E., Torún, B., Galicia, J. C., and Herrera, E., 1971, Determining energy costs of agricultural activities by respirometer and energy balance techniques, *Am. J. Clin. Nutr.* **24:** 1418–1430.

5. Viteri, F. E., and Torún, B., 1975, Ingestión calórica y trabajo físico de obreros agrícolas en Guatemala. Efecto de la suplementación alimentaria y su lugar en los programas de salud, *Bol. Of. Sanit. Panam.* 78: 58–74.
6. Viteri, F. E., Torún, B., and Immink, M. D. C., 1975, Nutrition and productivity. Effect of energy intake and supplementation on the productivity of agricultural workers in Central America. Preliminary report. Presented at the 14th Meeting of the Pan American Health Organization (PAHO), Washington, D.C., Advisory Committee on Medical Research.
7. Viteri, F. E., and Alvarado, J., 1970, Aspectos fisiológicos y respuestas adaptivas en la desnutrición calórica y en la desnutrición proteínica, *Rev. Col. Med. Guatemala* **21**: 175–230.
8. Viteri, F. E., and Pineda, O., 1971, Effects on body composition and body function, *in: Famine. A symposium dealing with nutrition and relief operations in times of disaster,* G. Blix, Y. Hofvander, and B. Vahlquist (eds.), Symposia of the Swedish Nutrition Foundation IX, Almqvist and Wiksell, Uppsala, pp. 25–40.
9. Viteri, F. E., and Torún, B., 1974, Anaemia and physical work capacity, *Clin. Haemat.* **3**: 609–626.
10. Viteri, F. E., 1973, Physical fitness and anemia, *in:* Malnutrition and functions of blood cells, N. Shimazono and T. Arakawa (eds.), Proceedings of the Symposium sponsored by the Malnutrition Panels of the United States–Japan Cooperative Medical Science Program, The National Institute of Nutrition, Tokyo, Japan, pp. 559–583.
11. Viteri, F. E., 1973, Hematological status of the Central American population: Iron and folate deficiencies, *12th Meeting of the Pan American Health Organization (PAHO),* Washington, D.C., Advisory Committee on Medical Research.
12. Cifuentes, E., and Viteri, F. E., 1972, Physical fitness, iron deficiency and anemia in agricultural laborers of Central America, *Fed. Proc.* **31**: 719 (Abstract 2843).

9

Nutrition and Development: The Dynamics of Commitment *

John Osgood Field and F. James Levinson

International Nutrition Planning Program
Massachusetts Institute of Technology
Cambridge, Massachusetts

International concern with problems of malnutrition manifests itself in a variety of ways. More persons are discussing it; more conferences are held; more studies and surveys are undertaken. Yet program development and resource allocation remain inadequate. Fewer than half a dozen low-income countries are pursuing serious national nutrition programs, and the future of some of these is in question.

The problem, in some ways, probably differs little from that which confronted nutrition advocates 25 years ago when INCAP was established. Most planning commissions still equate growth, with the development of capital stock and expenditures on human resources, with consumption rather than investment. Seen in this light, malnutrition is an indicator of underdevelopment, the solution to which lies in the very process of development for which capital accumulation is necessary. With development, the problem solves itself; to address malnutrition explicitly or "prematurely" is a wasteful diversion of scarce resources, and hence counterproductive in the long run. Historical confirmation for this perspective is provided by the development patterns characteristic of Western Europe, North America, Japan, and, most recently, Taiwan.

Accordingly, nutrition advocates attempted, through the decade of the 1960s, to cast the rationale for nutrition in this mold—to justify nutrition in

* A variation on this paper has been published in *Food Policy* **1**(1): 53–61, 1975.

terms of its contributory effects on the process of economic growth. In some ways, the stimulus for this came from Theodore Schultz (1) and others who postulated that capital stock has a human as well as a physical component. According to this view, expenditures on education and health are as legitimate an investment as plant equipment for purposes of increasing productivity and, in turn, a nation's wealth.

With respect to nutrition, this human capital argument was related to the nutritional status of both adults and children. In adults, improved nutrition increases physical capacity and perhaps time spent on the job, and may boost productivity as a result. In children, early malnutrition not only leads to physical limitations, but also affects learning and behavior. Inadequate nutrition during the period of most rapid brain growth may be manifest in neurological damage. Perhaps more important, malnutrition and its accompanying apathy and listlessness may limit the child's social and emotional interaction with his family and environment. The child's mental development largely determines his learning capacity and, in turn, the extent to which he will be able to take advantage of educational opportunities. Finally, learning ability is postulated to have an important effect on future productivity (2).

The nutrition–human capital argument, while plausible and in many ways attractive, has not, in fact, succeeded in eliciting major public resource commitment. In the context of labor-surplus economies, planners often conceptualize increased productivity, not as an asset, but as an additional problem in terms of its exacerbating effect on unemployment. In addition, planners tend to equate their most serious productivity problems, not with labor capacity, but rather with the availability and cost of petroleum imports, nitrogenous fertilizer, and industrial spare parts.

This paper represents an initial attempt to identify some of the ways in which nutrition may come to enjoy a higher priority in the developmental concerns of low-income countries. Our discussion focuses on three dynamics that, singly or in combination, appear to have the potential to reintegrate nutrition with development planning on a new and higher footing. These dynamics are: (1) a growing awareness of the extent to which malnutrition impedes fulfillment of various social programs already undertaken by most governments; (2) the new momentum in international development thinking and assistance emphasizing equity over growth; and (3) certain patterns and trends within many low-income countries that hold out the possibility of a distinctly political motivation to improved nutrition as a goal of public policy.

Against these "enabling" factors must be cited a major operational constraint: the limited institutional capability of many governments, particularly in Asia and Africa, to effect the kind of outreach that permits a sustained and multisectoral assault on malnutrition. We shall say a few words about this as well. First, let us elaborate on the three dynamics.

DYNAMIC NO. 1: MALNUTRITION AND SOCIAL SECTOR INVESTMENTS

Although the direct nutrition–economic growth argument has not been entirely convincing to government decision makers, some planners have begun to view nutrition as a means of conditioning effectiveness in other areas of existing governmental expenditure and have justified nutrition investment on these grounds. If, for example, the relationship between malnutrition and learning capacity is valid, and if a government is committed to the provision of education to an ever-expanding proportion of society, there would seem to be a clear rationale for similar government financing of nutrition to utilize more fully a country's educational capacity.

Similarly, there is considerable evidence demonstrating the synergistic relationship between malnutrition and infectious disease, with strong reason to believe that both health and health care can be affected positively by nutrition intervention (3). In most countries today, the bulk of the health budget is directed toward curing infectious disease. Yet, the demand for expensive treatment of infectious disease would be decreased if, as a preventive measure, malnutrition were reduced.

There has also been much discussion of nutrition–family planning relationships. Nutrition advocates have argued that high infant and child mortality rates have an adverse effect on the willingness of reproductive-age parents to practice family planning and, in turn, that most of this high mortality is a function of malnutrition. The linkage probably is quite complex, with reductions in infant and child mortality representing one of several prerequisite thresholds (including, perhaps, particular levels of education, income, and urbanization, along with heightened status of women) inducing family planning acceptance (4). It also is likely that the process is not automatic but requires the existence of an effective system for the delivery of family planning services. Nonetheless, the role of nutrition as a determinant of family planning effectiveness may be an important stimulant to nutrition investment, particularly as the longer-term consequences of high population growth rates are increasingly appreciated.

The essence of this dynamic, in short, is that nutrition comes to be perceived as important in the context of policy concerns that most governments have in the often frustrating pursuit of development (5). At issue is not what nutrition means for productivity and other statistical indicators of development as such, but what it means for components of the process that already enjoy reasonably high priority, such as education, disease control, family planning, and–increasingly–attempts to influence rural-to-urban migration (6). Nutrition comes to the fore not as a new, isolated preoccupation but because of growing appreciation for the suppressant side effects of malnutrition, best addressed by efforts to prevent malnutrition.

There is a lesson here for the nutrition community. Having held the "nutrition factor" up as a new concern deserving explicit governmental attention, we should also encourage its return to the policy contexts in which responsible government officials will find it most compelling.

DYNAMIC NO. 2: INTERNATIONAL MOMENTUM

The second dynamic is epitomized by this book: an accumulation of scientific evidence revealing the ravaging effects of malnutrition on infant and childhood mortality, its relation to physical and possibly even mental stunting, and the impact it has on social stimulation and learning ability, on the one hand, and the possibilities for effective counteraction based on judicious applications of technical and scientific knowledge, on the other.

To be sure, the notion that scientific evidence produces concern and then commitment may have an abstract cogency, but the response is hardly the same everywhere. In fact, there is a certain litany to the claim, the kind that often introduces an appeal for funds. Yet, the work done at institutions like INCAP, international meetings of scholars and officials, and the increasing relevance of bilateral and multilateral assistance as stimuli for new programmatic departures have all generated a momentum giving malnutrition a visibility and salience it has never known before. Moreover, these activities have at least begun to specify viable options for governments to act upon in combating malnutrition.

There is reason to believe that this momentum will stimulate action, granted a very big "if" to which we shall return later. In the first instance, nutrition advocacy is not a "position issue" in the sense that people divide on the basic idea as they do on the question of birth control. Nobody is *for* malnutrition. Then, too, most political leaders like to think of themselves as benign, devoted trustees of their people. Some even have notions of national honor against which the reality of widespread malnutrition, morbidity, and infant mortality may be defined as sources of shame. If many governments have done little to combat malnutrition to date, this probably stems as much from bewilderment concerning what to do as from the vague hope that economic development will solve the problem in some automatic fashion.

One effect of what is going on, therefore, is to give a heightened urgency to the problem while at the same time offering practical, empirically tested ways of dealing with it. For example, experimental interventions conducted by the Rural Health Research Centre in Narangwal, Punjab, have become the basis for the new integrated nutrition/public health/family planning delivery system recently announced by the government of India. The Candelaria project has generated similar interest in Colombia. As a result, things are starting to happen, even in growth-oriented countries like Brazil, that would have been unthinkable as recently as five years ago. If this momentum can be sustained, we might witness something on the order of a steamroller effect, with even the most conservative countries doing something about malnutrition to save face and avoid international embarrassment.

The big "if," in our judgment, is the current world food crisis. This crisis is, quite literally, a two-edged sword. It could be the principal catalytic event to galvanize national and international energies behind programs to end starvation and the malnutrition that lies behind it. On the other hand, it could very easily become a major diversion if countries define the problem as merely one concerning the international distribution of food and neglect the more fundamental issues of domestic distribution and development priorities generally. At the moment, the world food crisis forms a large unknown, conditioning the future vitality of the international push against malnutrition.

NUTRITION AS A POLITICAL ISSUE

Politics is the key to fulfilling the promise of the two dynamics discussed above. When nutrition is taken out of the laboratory or home economics curriculum and is made an explicit focus of government planning, it becomes, by definition, intensely political; and the more prominent nutritional concerns are in the planning efforts of a country, the more political they become. This is because planning, like politics generally, is concerned with who gets what from whom, and how (7,8). Yet before planners can decide what to do, they must first have a mandate to do something. The reverse is possible as well: Planners can decide what should be done if certain goals are to be achieved and then wait for political leadership to give the green light. This, presumably, is one of the functions of INAN in Brazil and certain other national institutes of nutrition. In effect, the planners become advocates.

The relevance of politics to nutritionists follows from the fact that any allocation of resources by government (particularly any large-scale allocation) is a product of political decisions. Moreover, such decisions are usually made for political reasons. At each step in the process, from authorization to planning and resource allocation and on to implementation, politics in one guise or another is a constant companion.

In our judgment, the question of political commitment is basic. With it, much can be done; without it, nutrition activities are likely to be constrained by policy tokenism—a symbolic gesture, another pilot project or general survey, a new crumb to the social sector, and so on. Most of us know this only too well. Without commitment, nutritionists labor on the fringes of development. With commitment, they can be in the forefront. When all is said and done, the orientation of a country's political leadership is the most important determinant of the nature, magnitude, and possibly even success of programs addressed to malnutrition, public health, and problems of the poor.

Aside from conceptual barriers concerning the nature of economic development and structural barriers arising because nutrition is not a "sector," and hence cuts across and is interpreted differently by the substantive ministries involved (usually agriculture, health, and education), there are political limitations that have impeded nutrition's claim to be taken seriously. As a science it seems remote and somewhat esoteric; as a practical matter, it is normally associated with dieticians, home economics teachers, and others far removed from the centers of power. More importantly, the political priorities of most national leaderships lie elsewhere. Perhaps the most basic reason for this is that the malnourished, along with others making up the "peripheral poor," tend to be politically inarticulate and passive. They are not part of the leadership's functional constituency; they are not members of its coalition of interest. In the competition for scarce resources, they lose out (9).

It might be thought that the major differential explaining why some governments are committed to the relief of malnutrition while others are not has to do with ideology. Perhaps the most common hypothesis is that explicit policy attention to public health, nutrition, mass education, and the like (and significant resource allocations for these purposes) is a product of socialism. Most governments in low income countries profess to be "socialist"; and while this is a slippery label indeed, it does seem to connote a shared concern for the well-being of people and their protection against the multiple inequities of the marketplace. When the socialist ethos is strongly held, social inequalities and human deprivations like malnutrition are simply not acceptable conditions; abject poverty in its many manifestations is associated with fundamental injustice and its eradication becomes a cardinal objective of public policy. The very conception of citizenship is often broadened to include the notion of social rights (livelihood) along with civil (legal) and political rights (the franchise, or some equivalent) (10).

Corroborating evidence is not hard to find. There are socialist regimes in low-income countries that have sustained a commitment to popular well-being at the expense of elite privilege and conventionally conceived economic growth, and this emphasis has manifested itself, among other ways, in the extension of health care to all citizens regardless of location or status. A number of countries come readily to mind: China (11–13), Cuba (14–16), Chile (particularly under Allende) (17), and—in aspiration, at least—India, Tanzania (18,19), and Peru (20). Thus, Article 47 of the Constitution of India, under the Directive Principles of State Policy declares: "The State shall regard the raising of the level of nutrition and the standard of living of its people and the improvement of public health as among its primary duties. . . ." The present (fifth) five-year plan contains an entire chapter on nutrition.

There are several problems with such a comprehensive explanation, however. It is strong on intent but, in many instances, weak on capability. Also, one does not have to be a socialist to desire an end to injustice and human misery. Then, too, many political leaders who claim to be socialists—usually with some diluting ethnic or regional prefix—have little that is tangible to show for their rhetoric. The actualities are more complex than the imagery.

In most countries commitment is not an either/or proposition. It exists in degrees and with variation over time. Even so, it is perhaps useful to think of commitment to the alleviation of malnutrition in terms of a threshold, above which nutrition becomes a major thrust of policy, not merely a sideshow. Where that threshold is, what level of commitment is necessary, cannot be identified in the abstract. Yet the record to date suggests that few countries have crossed it. Hence the growing art and science of nutrition planning implicitly accepts a workaday world of uncertain commitment, competition for attention and sustenance, and the often burdensome need to show quick results in order to carry on.

Will this always be so? Perhaps yes, but if it is the fate of the nutrition planner to be a "patient revolutionary," biding his time with pilot projects and marginal influence on what others do until a change in priorities propels him onto center stage (21), his moment of opportunity may not be far off.

DYNAMIC NO. 3: POLITICAL MOTIVATION

The third dynamic is less explicitly concerned with nutrition than the prior two are, but it could become quite significant to nutrition, especially in concert with the international momentum and policy synergism noted above. The essence of this dynamic may be summarized as follows:

Basic change →	**Political challenge** →	**Political response**
Popular politicization	(a) New demands on government (b) Legitimacy crisis	(a) Repression, forced depoliticization
	Implications for nutrition Nutrition planning and other initiatives to improve conditions of the poor	{ (b) Increased priority to equity (c) Attempt to mobilize rural support

There are several problems with this scenario. The final link in the chain is the weakest. Indeed, the entire dynamic may be snuffed out at any point along the way. Even where it does occur more or less as shown, it may not lead to nutritional benefits. On the other hand, both the frequency of political challenge and the possibility of the kinds of political response indicated are sufficiently realistic to warrant serious consideration.

In most developing countries people are being politicized. For all sorts of reasons having to do with particular crises, the impetus of modernization, and the deliberate efforts of political elites to reach and mobilize their populations, a larger world of politics is becoming relevant to remote villages and tribes, and increasing numbers of people are being brought into contact with new leaders, institutions, symbols, and ideas. The political awakening and activation taking place has been called a "participation explosion" (22), although participation per se is only one element. What is occurring is something greater and more pervasive. "Politicization explosion" is perhaps a more appropriate designation, in that it implies new perspectives, orientations, and wants, as well as new behaviors.

The significance of politicization is twofold. It stimulates a host of new demands upon government, and in many instances it either produces or accentuates a legitimacy crisis for political elites and the institutions through which they rule (23). As numerous scholars have observed, changes in regime have occurred with greater frequency in low-income countries than changes in leadership within an ongoing regime. Politicized people are prone to associate the solution to their many needs and wants with the workings of the political system. To a degree previously unknown, government is called upon to cope with a wide range of problems arising out of traditional deprivation–no longer to be accepted passively–and from the very process of change itself. This is the context in which debates over growth versus distribution acquire a measure of political urgency (24). The responsiveness of political elites to these demands is often the key to their survival in office. Confirmation of the vulnerability of many holding political office has been provided by the results of elections held recently in Kenya and Brazil.

Politicization without expanding legitimacy is destabilizing. Most leaders in low-income countries derive their support from a limited social base, while the political system as a whole functions in almost total isolation from the broad masses of people now beginning to claim relevance. If these claims are pressed and demands for governmental attention are vocalized, the opportunity exists to broaden support for the regime. Of course, the reverse side of opportunity is the threat to legitimacy that typically follows upon neglect or failure of effort. The political need to do something meaningful in the countryside represents an opportunity for well-timed advocacy and possibly for meaningful nutrition programming as well.

THE QUESTION OF CAPABILITY

Some nutrition interventions require relatively little in the way of coordination, sustained effort, or popular responsiveness, e.g., food fortification. Most, however, assume effective outreach, a long-term presence, and a capacity to enlist popular support and energies behind prescribed activities (mothercraft centers, sanitation, crop experimentation, public works in general). In these instances political commitment alone is not enough. Also needed is the ability by governmental bodies to penetrate society and to implement planned programs and projects. Capability converts commitment into impact.

Let us illustrate this point by reference to two case studies in the nutrition–public health literature. During his recent visit to China, Wray found no evidence of malnutrition in that large and poor society. He did observe children 18 months of age in nursery school and some form of health care available at close range everywhere he went (11). Wray's account is more than one of commitment (expressed in the Chinese Communist ethos that the country's most valuable resource is its people). It is an account of successful penetration of a vast hinterland by political institutions and their ability to organize the population behind a whole range of self-help programs. The picture goes beyond mere information dissemination and the building of health facilities in the formal sense. It suggests constant reinforcement; not benign neglect, but an endless barrage of social and sociopolitical inputs capable of reorienting thought, guiding behavior, and providing services of high quality throughout the society.

Vincente Navarro's analysis of the health system in Cuba has a similar message (14). Following the Castro take-over the Cuban government pursued twin goals of equalizing access to medical services across the country (they had been largely concentrated in Havana) and providing comprehensive coverage, both based on the simple belief that health is a human right to be guaranteed by the state. Navarro's paper provides a rich overview of the system in action, along with evidence that it has had a profound effect on the incidence of malnutrition and other public health problems. Making the system work are its mechanisms of control and, equally important, its capacity for eliciting public cooperation and support. The latter is not merely or even principally a function of coercion. One senses in the Cuban case, as in the Chinese, that a fundamental change has taken place in the popular image of government, from being distant, aloof, and essentially extractive (the tax collector), to being proximate, involved, and essentially distributive. As a result there has been a redistribution of effort and emphasis within the health system along with dominance over and resocialization of the medical profession.

The combination of commitment and capability is so rare in low income countries that, quite possibly, it forms a distinctive achievement of Communist governments in the present period. In each respect and in almost every detail the nature, scope, coverage, and results of the public health systems of countries like Cuba and China far exceed what one typically finds elsewhere (25). Moreover, these systems function as they do despite resource scarcities (14).

The key to these nutrition success stories is organization, and it is precisely organization and its attendant capabilities–penetration, coordination, and impact–that are lacking in most low-income countries. Political scientists have long been impressed with the prevalence in the Third World of authoritarian regimes with little real authority, either in the sense of legitimacy for the leadership and system of rule or in the sense of capacity to see that decisions made at the center will give rise to actions having the intended effect on the periphery (26). Power may be concentrated, but there is precious little of it. The capital city is functionally far removed from the rest of society, and the mechanisms do not exist politically, administratively, or otherwise to bridge the gap. Center–periphery cleavages plague democratic countries like India as well as more authoritarian countries (27).

For nutrition, the question is the extent to which governments can really accomplish what they might plan to accomplish, given the resources, expertise, and institutional infrastructure at their command. The new thrust of international assistance—targeting on the poorest people of the poorest countries—merely underlines the question. Almost by definition, the poorest countries are the most difficult to work in, and the poorest people in those countries are the most difficult to reach and have an impact upon. Our impression is that in the countries where nutrition and health needs are greatest and where a technical "turning of the spigot" is not the answer, governmental capacity to penetrate (in the functional sense) is so limited that even with political commitment, erudite planning, operational consensus, and a pliant public, implementation of nutrition programs is likely to be an Achilles heel of awesome proportions.

This circumstance may help to explain why in so many low-income countries nutrition and other socially oriented programs are often evaluated in terms of activities, not impact. The latter is a frightening standard when capabilities are so low. It is safer to count the number of school children receiving officially sponsored lunches than to question whether such an elaborate distribution system has any nutritional merit or answers the real nutritional needs of the society at large. The same is true for construction of nutrition rehabilitation centers, health clinics, and the like. Their very existence is held up as evidence of progress, even though their impact on the problem is often miniscule.

On the other hand, the capability gap would seem to ensure the constructive role nutrition planners are likely to play in most low-income countries should there be a major upgrading in official circles of the attention given to malnutrition. As the case of China indicates, nutrition goals can be achieved without benefit of nutrition planning per se. When nutrition is so embedded in a matrix of public health services, and when the extension of these services is complemented by well-chosen inputs in agriculture, education, local public works, and community development generally, nutritional problems tend to be addressed almost as a matter of course. Such instances are uncommon, however. So long as there remain serious constraints on what can be done, the nutrition planner will be necessary both to diagnose the dynamics of the problem and to chart the most cost-effective solutions to it. If the new equity-oriented push of international assistance is matched by a corresponding effort in the same direction by national governments, the nutrition planner should be a viable, indeed vital, commodity in most low-income countries for some time to come. It is also possible that good nutrition planning may become an important means of strengthening the capabilities as well as the popular image of the governments adopting it.

CONCLUSION

There are grounds for qualified optimism concerning the future role of nutrition in national development programs. While generalization beyond national boundaries is difficult and often misleading, one can state with some confidence that the dynamics outlined in this chapter will represent important elements in policy formation, and that they may well be persuasive in the inclusion of nutrition in national planning.

Whatever form these and other dynamics take in individual countries, it is clear that major nutrition allocation decisions will be political decisions. Different governments will react to them in different ways and for a different combination of reasons. The possibility exists that nothing of consequence will happen. Taken alone, each of these dynamics is vulnerable to a token response, especially given the multiplicity of pressures with which governments must cope. In combination, however, and in certain political environments they could bring about significant change.

Even with an upgrading of commitment to nutrition, local capabilities will condition what it is possible to accomplish. Ironically perhaps, the nutrition planner's contribution, as he moves beyond advocacy, is likely to lie in the promotion of institutional development and what we have termed *effective outreach* as well as in the formulation of nutrition programs for their own sake. This would represent a return to a basic proposition in development thinking—often lost sight of in practice—that true development is interactive and reinforcing. Indeed, the capability–impact linkage could be politically attractive in its own right.

REFERENCES

1. Schultz, T. S., 1961, Investment in human capital, *Am. Econ. Rev.* **51**: 1–17.
2. Scrimshaw, N. S., and Gordon, J. E. (eds.), 1968, *Malnutrition learning, and behavior,* M.I.T. Press, Cambridge, Massachusetts, 566 pp.
3. Scrimshaw, N. S., Taylor, C. E., and Gordon, J. E., 1968, *Interactions of nutrition and infection,* World Health Organization Monogr. Ser. No. 57, WHO, Geneva, 329 pp.
4. Austin, J. E., and Levinson, F. J., 1974, Population and nutrition: A case for integration, *Milbank Mem. Fund Q.* **52**(2): 169–184.

5. Berg, A., 1973, *The nutrition factor: its role in national development,* The Brookings Institution, Washington, D.C., 290 pp.
6. Weiner, M., 1974, *Internal migration policies: Purposes, interests, instruments, effects,* Working Paper, Center for International Studies, Massachusetts Institute of Technology, Cambridge, Massachusetts.
7. Lasswell, H. D., 1958, *Politics: Who gets what, when, how,* Meridian Books, New York, 222 pp.
8. Mott, J. F., 1974, Politics and international planning, *Soc. Sci. Med.* **8**: 271–274.
9. Weiner, M., 1962, *The politics of scarcity: Public pressure and political response in India,* University of Chicago Press, Chicago, Illinois, 251 pp.
10. Marshall, T. H., 1965, *Class, citizenship, and social development,* Chapter 4, Citizenship and social class, pp. 365, Anchor Press, Garden City, New York.
11. Wray, J. D., 1974, *Health and nutritional factors in early childhood development in the People's Republic of China,* Paper prepared for the Report of the Early Childhood Development Delegation Visit to the People's Republic of China, November–December, 1973. unpublished.
12. Heller, P. S., 1972, *The strategy of health-sector planning in the People's Republic of China,* Discussion Paper 24, July, 1972, Center for Research and Economic Development, University of Michigan, Ann Arbor.
13. Arena, J. M., 1974, Nutritional status of China's children: An overview, *Nutr. Rev.* **32** (10): 289–295.
14. Navarro, V., 1972, *Health, health services, and health planning in Cuba,* Unpublished manuscript, Department of Medical Care and Hospitals and International Health, Johns Hopkins University, Baltimore, Maryland.
15. Navarro, V., 1972, Health services in Cuba–an initial appraisal, *N. Engl. J. Med.* **287**: 954–959.
16. Fagen, R. R., 1969, *The transformation of political culture in Cuba,* Stanford University Press, Stanford, California, 271 pp.
17. Solimano, G., 1973, *Nutrición en el sector salud: Diagnostico, programas y realizaciones en Chile, años 1971–1973,* Paper presented at I Conferencia Sub-Regional Sobre Politicas de Alimentación y Nutrición, Lima, Peru, 9–14 de Julio, 1973, unpublished.
18. Gish, O., 1973, Doctor auxiliaries in Tanzania, *Lancet* **ii**: 1251–1254 (Dec. 1).
19. Gish, O., 1973, Resource allocation, equality of access, and health, *Int. J. Hlth. Services* **3** (3): 399–412.
20. Peru: Diagnostico Nutricional (Lima: Instituto Nacional de Planificación), 1973.
21. Pines, J. M., 1974, *Review and advocacy: First steps in nutrition planning,* Paper presented to the Protein Advisory Group of the United Nations System, 22nd Meeting, Rome, 24–27 June, 1974, Document 1.17/13, PAG, United Nations Headquarters, New York, New York 10017.
22. Almond, G. A., and Verba, S., 1963, *The civic culture: Political attitudes and democracy in five nations,* Princeton University Press, Princeton, New Jersey, p. 2.
23. Field, J. O., 1974, *Politicization and system support in India: The role of partisanship,* Paper presented at the Annual Meeting of the American Political Science Association, Palmer House, Chicago, August 29–September 2, 1974, and reissued as Monograph C/74-12 by the Center for International Studies, Massachusetts Institute of Technology, Cambridge, Massachusetts.
24. DeSchweinitz, K., Jr., 1964, *Industrialization and democracy: Economic necessities and political possibilities,* The Free Press, Glencoe, New York, 309 pp.
25. Scrimshaw, N. S., French, D., and Levinson, J. M., 1973, *Relief and rehabilitation of*

war victims in Indochina, Part III: North Vietnam and Laos, Hearing before the Subcommittee to Investigate Problems Connected with Refugees and Escapees of the Committee on the Judiciary, United States Senate, Ninety-Third Congress, First Session, July 31, 1973. U.S. Government Printing Office, Washington, D.C., 1973, pp. 33–49, and Scrimshaw, N.S., Appendix I, pp. 63–67.

26. Zolberg, Z., 1966, *Creating political order: The party-states of West Africa,* Rand McNally, Chicago, 168 pp.
27. Field, J. O., 1973, *Partisanship in India: A survey analysis,* Doctoral dissertation, Stanford University, Palo Alto, California.

COMMENTS

Robert F. Chandler, Jr. • *The Asian Vegetable Research and Development Center, Shanhua, Taiwan.*

During the first three days of the FAO/UNDP-sponsored conference on *The Use of Improved Technology for Food Production in Rainfed Areas of Tropical Asia* in Hyderabad, India in November, 1974, several prominent Indian agricultural officials presented their programs for increasing crop yields under rainfed conditions in India. Not one of them ever mentioned that there is any food crisis in India, nor did they discuss the plight of the small farmer and ways by which their programs could be tailored to his needs. They gave no indication of how they were attempting to bridge the gap between agricultural research and the farmer. The conclusion one reached was that their principal objective was to present well the results of their work to their peers in agricultural science and to their superior officers in the Indian Council for Agricultural Research so that their positions and programs would continue to be funded by the government. They did not seem to be concerned about the fact that progress in the adoption of modern technology by Indian farmers is exceedingly slow.

In my opinion, one of the real needs in promoting agricultural development in the poorer countries is to identify the factors at the farm level that limit progress, and this can only be done by increasing the communication among the research scientist, the extension worker, and the farmer. Too often the various segments of the chain of communication spend much time talking to each other and not enough time getting into the field where the problems are. Without the latter there cannot be understanding of the basic factors responsible for either progress, or the lack of it, in increasing yields on land now being cultivated.

Pedro Belli • *Instituto Centroamericano de Administración de Empresas, Managua, Nicaragua.*

Field and Levinson have addressed themselves to an important question: Why have resources for improving nutrition remained inadequate? There is international concern for the problem, more persons are discussing it, more conferences are being held, more studies and surveys are being undertaken, yet program development and resource allocation remain inadequate. Why? The authors would have us believe that it is mainly the planners' and politicians' fault, and that those of us concerned with nutrition and socioeconomic development do not share in the blame.

Most economic planning commissions, the authors claim, view problems concerned with malnutrition in one of two lights: (a) They see the solution of malnutrition as a byproduct of economic development, something that will disappear as countries grow richer; or (b) they view malnutrition as an impediment to economic growth and hence consider expenditures on food and nutrition programs as investment in human capital. Under this latter view, dollars spent on nutrition and food programs must compete on equal terms with dollars spent on roads, hospitals, schools, electrification programs, for example.

The first approach, of course, does not elicit much sympathy from nutrition planners. Alleviation of malnutrition will come of itself as the roads, schools, and electric plants provide employment and living wages for the poor, who will then be able to buy more and better food. The second approach, the authors claim, "has not, in fact, succeeded in eliciting major public resource commitment," because (a) economic planners view increases in productivity as potential sources of additional unemployment, and (b) economic planners are not convinced that investment in food and nutrition programs is all that productive in economic terms anyway. But, the authors argue, let us not despair, for things may change. Three "dynamics" indicate that there may be better times ahead.

First, planners are beginning to realize that a dollar spent on food and nutrition programs may save two or more in other programs that rank higher among the planners' priorities. Health and family planning programs are cited as examples.

Second, there is an international effervescence that is culminating in the flowering of scientific evidence revealing the negative effects of malnutrition on infant and childhood mortality, physical and possibly mental growth, and social stimulation and learning ability. This new knowledge, together with the possibilities for effective counteractions, has given malnutrition a visibility it has never enjoyed before.

Third, in most developing countries people are becoming politicized and making new demands upon governments. As politicization expands, the political leadership finds it necessary to win allegiance in the countryside. "Nutrition interventions and related improvements in the living conditions of the rural poor", the authors claim, "are means to this end."

These three "dynamics", the authors think, presage better times for food and nutrition programs. To be sure, even though the "dynamics" have been unleashed, their effects will not be automatic. First, there has to be a political commitment: "With it, much can be done; without it, nutrition activities are likely to be considered political tokenism." Second, the political commitment, although necessary, may not be sufficient to improve nutritional status: Governments must have the capability to implement plans.

It is quite difficult to assess the authors' arguments without the evidence that they used to reach their conclusions; however, we can accept their basic premise without much difficulty: Resources for improving nutrition have been inadequate. Their most important conclusion—governments of low-income countries will not incorporate nutrition planning in their development programs unless there is a political commitment—is certainly plausible. Nevertheless, their analysis of nutrition planners' failure to obtain government funding leaves much to be desired. Moreover, much more than what the authors have stated has to be done in order to obtain a political commitment.

Regarding past efforts, I think that we are more at fault than the planners are. Take, for example, the relationship between malnutrition and low productivity. Has that relationship been established conclusively? Although there has been much research in the area and the causal connection seems eminently reasonable, has it been established beyond a shadow of doubt? Moreover, even if we accept that there is a causal connection, do we have at our disposal the weapons to convince the planners that a dollar spent on improving nutrition will be better spent than one expended on preventing malaria, or polio, or on constructing a hospital? If we do not have the answers to these questions, can we reasonably expect a planner allocating scarce resources among competing goals to give nutrition a high priority? Perhaps, but the grounds for doing so would clearly not be economic grounds. Planners, however, have a clear bias toward economic criteria.

Concerning the future, I think that the authors are right in stating that a political commitment is necessary in order to raise nutrition and food programs on the planners' list of priorities, although I am somewhat skeptical about the inevitability of the process that the authors sense is beginning to emerge.

I can think of three reasons why the political commitment could be forthcoming: (a) for humanitarian purposes; (b) for economic reasons; or (c) for political survival. The authors have discussed the third reason. I will make a few remarks about the first two.

On a humanitarian basis, planners may opt for increased expenditure on food and nutrition programs simply because any thinking person aware of the possible consequences of malnutrition will find it repugnant to know that it exists. This has probably been the basis for most extant food and nutrition programs. Given the results obtained, I would hazard the guess that either humanitarian grounds are not convincing enough or planners are not sufficiently aware of the possible consequences of malnutrition. There is not much that those of us concerned with the problem can do about the first factor, but there is much that we could do, but have not done, about the second.

In Central America, for example, in spite of INCAP's presence and influence, it is my experience that the political and economic decision makers are not sufficiently aware of either the extent or the possible consequences of malnutrition. The knowledge accumulated by nutrition experts around the world has remained mostly on the shelves of scientific libraries. Perhaps some has seeped through to the ministries of health. Neither the planners, however, nor the influential decision makers seem to have a thorough grasp of the importance of the problem. My experience in Central America suggests that we have been somewhat derelict in our duties.

On economic grounds again, the case for allocating more resources to alleviate malnutrition is possibly a strong one, but little research has been done to prove it. Once more, the political commitment could be accelerated if we could show the planners, in their own framework of thinking, that a dollar spent on food and nutrition programs is a dollar well spent.

In summary, whereas winds of change may be blowing, in order to augment resources devoted to food and nutrition programs, we need to do a bit more homework concerning the relationship between nutrition and economic productivity, and also a share of proselytizing to stress the consequences of malnutrition.

The authors of the article could have done us an important service in identifying, at least in preliminary form, the direction our research should take and which unanswered questions planners most often ask. Unfortunately, the authors did not take advantage of this opportunity, and no such guidelines appear in their discussion.

Marcelo Selowsky* · *Development Research Center, World Bank, Washington, D.C.*

The Field–Levinson chapter represents an effort at spelling out several approaches that eventually could lead to a larger commitment of government resources to the nutrition sector.

The first approach–which I would define as the most pragmatic one–explores how the commitment to nutrition could be increased in the context of present objectives of governments in relation to nutrition-related sectors, i.e., health and education. In this context an increased commitment to nutrition can be justified on the grounds that existing programs in these sectors could be made more effective.

*These comments represent the view of the author, not necessarily those of the World Bank.

These comments discuss the dynamics of commitment in the realm of this first approach. It represents, at least in the short run, the most realistic scenario in which nutrition planners will have to operate. The task is how to make the best of a situation where the commitment to nutrition is rather weak, either because it involves redistributive policies that are politically resisted, or because the government does not wish to invest in what it considers a non-growth-oriented sector.

From the point of view of a development economist interested in nutrition, I would like to address briefly three issues that could bear on the success of the nutritionist in obtaining a higher national commitment under the scenario described above. Some of them are of a substantive character; others are of a more tactical nature.

Presenting the Nutrition Problem to the Policy Maker: The Problem of Trade-Offs with Other Planning Objectives

The introduction of nutrition programs into an economy can have strong effects on the reallocation of productive resources among different sectors of the economy. Very probably such reallocations will involve a trade-off with other planning objectives of governments and therefore will be resisted.

The following question should be raised: Is there something in the way nutritionists present policy proposals that unduly exaggerates the perception of those trade-offs on the part of the overall planner or policy maker? My experience is that this is often the case. An illustrative, though extreme case, is when the nutrition problem is presented as a global objective with overtones that imply "planning the economy in terms of nutrition." This is perhaps the least promising tactical approach for any interaction between nutritionists and the overall planner. In this case the issue of the trade-off is likely to be perceived as insurmountable.

It is obvious that in such presentation the need to define objectives and priorities in terms of target groups becomes crucial. However, even with better defined targets, an exaggerated perception of the trade-offs can occur. This happens when the policies suggested by nutritionists so as to reach the target groups involve the use of indirect policy instruments with wide-range economic effects such as those on balance of payments and reallocation of resources in agriculture.

The irony of the above discussion is that the more indirect the policy instrument selected to reach the target group (*indirect policies* like subsidies to particular inputs used in agriculture or differential exchange rates for food imports vis à vis *direct programs* like food stamp programs)—and therefore less in the realm of professional expertise of the nutritionist—the larger becomes the trade-off with other planning objectives.

The Need for Defining Target Group-Oriented Policies: The Problem of the Fiscal Cost

Formulating nutrition policies in terms of target group-oriented programs, i.e., programs that reach the target group without heavily subsidizing other (nontarget) groups has two advantages: First, not only does it make the trade-off with other planning objectives less serious, but second, it will also reduce the fiscal cost (or cost to the budget) of such programs, another important consideration in the receptivity of nutrition objectives by the overall planner. The identification of such programs by nutritionists has, in my view, the highest payoff in terms of inducing short-run changes in a country's commitment to nutrition objectives.

In order to illustrate the importance of identifying such programs, some estimates of the cost-effectiveness of general and target group-oriented food programs are presented (1). Table I shows the cost of achieving an extra unit of food consumption by the target group (initially consuming 20% of urban food supplies) under different types of programs. The *general* price subsidy program consists of a general food price subsidy benefiting all urban consumers. As can be seen, the cost of target group-oriented programs is substantially lower, particularly when additional total consumption can only be obtained at an increased cost (under a supply elasticity of one instead of infinity). Table II evaluates the *general* price subsidy program specifically for cereals, and expresses the cost of the program as a fraction of the GNP of the country. For a country like India, with a per caput income of approximately $100, such a figure is at least 5.6%, which makes the program prohibitively expensive.

The above results clearly illustrate that target group-oriented programs are potentially much more cost-effective and probably the only feasible solution to the elimination of malnutrition in subgroups of the population.

Table I. Cost Effectiveness of a Target Group-Oriented Food Program and a General Food Subsidy (in Terms of the Initial Price of the Food Commodity)[a]

	Supply elasticity	
	(Constant cost)	(Increasing cost)[b]
Target group		
Food stamp	1.0	1.2
Price subsidy	1.6	1.8
Income transfer	2.0	2.3
General price subsidy	7.5	11.0

[a]See reference 1.
[b]Assumes a supply elasticity equal to one.

Table II. Fiscal Cost of a General Price Subsidy Required to Induce a 20% Increase in Cereal Consumption in the Urban Area (as a Fraction of GNP of the Country)[a]

Per caput income of the country (in dollars)	World price of cereals (per ton)	
	$200	$300
100	5.4%	7.1%
300	1.8%	2.5%

[a]See reference 1.

The Availability of Programs under Increases in the Fiscal Budget

Several developing countries are undertaking changes in their tax structures that would yield substantially higher government revenues. In other countries these increases are sometimes a short-run phenomenon due to changes in the prices of their main exports. Has the nutrition sector always been ready to take advantage of some of these increases in government funds? Do nutritionists always have available a package of realistic programs—in terms of the financing required—that can be quickly submitted to the overall planner under such circumstances? Agility in project identification is crucial if the nutrition sector wants to be successful in competing for government financing under increases in the size of the fiscal budget.

Reference

1. Reutlinger, S., and Selowsky, M., 1975, *Undernutrition and Poverty: Magnitude and Target Group Oriented Policies,* Working Paper No. 202, World Bank. Revised version, January, 1976.

Aaron Lechtig · *Human Development Division, Institute of Nutrition of Central America and Panama, Guatemala City, Guatemala.*

Field and Levinson stressed that political commitment from government is necessary in order to implement nutrition programs. I have two comments that relate to proposed actions to bring about such commitments.

The first has to do with the alternative of "political survival," one of the proposed strategies to induce government action in the nutrition area. This approach may be purely opportunistic and may lead to actions exclusively oriented to mask the real problem and to dilute the pressure for progressive social and economic change in the developing countries. Would it not be better to work actively to change the social structures that are the main factors in the causal complex of poverty and malnutrition?

The three alternatives, or options, proposed by the authors to produce such a political commitment from governments are based on the assumption that social and political structures will remain unchanged in the less developed countries. Given the changes that have already occurred in them during the last 20 years, this basic assumption does not necessarily hold. My inclination would be to take advantage of the lessons from recent history in Asia, Africa, and Latin America in order to develop a set of alternative approaches that would not only consider that present social structures must change, but would also be specifically oriented to produce these changes.

H. A. B. Parpia · *Food and Agriculture Industries Services, Agricultural Services Division, Food and Agriculture Organization, Rome.*

The concern of Levinson and Field for children of developing countries is appreciated. It is, however, difficult to agree with their proposals for subsidized feeding programs as a short- and long-term measure, and for inclusion of such provisions in bilateral and international assistance. Developing countries face hard reality with regard to policy choices, and such proposals cannot be considered in isolation. It is well known that the developing countries' share of world income is only about 16%, while they have 71% of the world population. It would, therefore, be very difficult to give priority to any subsidized or charity feeding program over other important development activities that would have impact on the overall well-being of the people. Only those nutrition programs can receive priority that can be geared to economic development activities that would result in improved food supplies, provision of more employment, and greater self-sufficiency. Such programs must be clearly identified so that they receive priority in allocation of resources. The countries generally know best how to allocate their own resources as well as those received under bilateral and international assistance. It is not proper for aid-giving agencies to decide for a country how it should allocate priorities and resources except, perhaps, under emergency conditions.

II

Technological and Ecological Problems Limiting the Production of Food

10

Technological and Ecological Limitations to Production of Food Crops

Robert K. Waugh and Eugenio Martinez S.

Instituto de Ciencia y Tecnología Agrícolas
Guatemala City, Guatemala

The gap that exists between actual food production and production potential is analogous to having useful and valuable manufacturing patents but no factories making use of them. Technology is already making great contributions to production, but we can produce far more food with our present knowledge. The problem is that available and new technologies are not used to best advantage. Why is this so? Are farmers so resistant to change that they will not use better technology? Has the farmer been approached in an effective manner? What are the technological limitations to food production?

The restraints can be classified into two highly interrelated general groups: the technological, ecological, and/or biological, and the nontechnical–conditions and situations that exist within our social, economic, and governmental structures that limit food production.

ARABLE LAND

There is increasing awareness that the planet on which we live is not a never-ending, inexhaustible source of materials. The two most important means of increasing production are increasing land area cultivated and increasing yields per unit of land. The former depends upon available arable land, available technology, costs, and accessibility.

The Panel on the World Food Supply of the President's Science Advisory Committee (1) has estimated the earth's land surface to be about 13 billion hectares, as shown in Table I. The total area of potentially arable land (about 3.2

Table I. Classification of Land by Climate and Potential Use

Climate	Hectares (millions) arable	grazing	total
Polar and subpolar	0	0	560
Cold–temperate boreal	50	190	1970
Cool temperate	910	1000	2910
Warm–temperate–subtropical	550	840	2770
Tropical	1670	1630	4950
Totals	3180	3660	13160

billion hectares) is larger than most of us realize, perhaps 24% of the total ice-free area, or more than twice the amount of land that has been cultivated at some time during the last few decades, and three times that cultivated in a given year.

Of the total 3-plus billion arable hectares, around 1 billion are cultivated each year, leaving about 2 billion uncultivated. More than half of the potentially arable land is within the tropics, and it represents an important food production possibility for Latin America. Thirty percent is in the humid tropics, 36% is in the subhumid tropics, where a season of abundant rainfall alternates with a relatively dry season, and 34% is in the semiarid or arid tropics (1).

The potential for using new lands is great, but this still does not allow us facile means of meeting future food needs if we consider that the population will be 70% greater by the year 2000 and that the costs of developing new lands will be very high, and if we recognize that we do not yet have technology for sustained high crop yields for much of this potential new area.

Perhaps only 15 to 20% of the area cultivated today is capable of maximum yields (2). Most of the research has been conducted where the climate is favorable, principally in the temperate zones (3). It has been logical to concentrate our research where it will pay large dividends, but now we must give more attention to the 80% of the lands that are less amenable to cultivation.

CROP YIELDS

While on a worldwide basis there is considerable opportunity to increase areas cultivated, this is not the case for many countries. They have no choice but to increase yields or import food.

The difference between yields at experiment stations and on farms, the gap

Table II. Ratio of High Yields to Low Yields (Based on Country Averages)[a]

Crop	1935–1939	Early 1960s
Rice	3 : 1	4 : 1
Wheat	5 : 1	10 : 1
Corn	4 : 1	6 : 1

[a]Reference 6.

between the best farm yields and national averages within countries, and between high and low national averages by countries, emphasizes the thesis that the gap between potential and real yields is very large (Table II).

Approximately 12 to 14 tons of grain per hectare seem to be the highest yields being obtained commercially today, but the world averages are around a ton or so (Table III) (2,4,5). These data show that high yields, several times national averages, are being obtained, but also indicate that the technological gap has widened (6). The question is why. The probable reason is that most of the high yields have come about because scientists in the developed countries have derived technology for favorable environments, for relatively sophisticated farmers who have the necessary inputs, under favorable economic conditions. For example, the United States planted 81 million hectares per year in cereals during the period 1948–53, with a yield of 136 million tons. Over the period 1964–65, only 62 million hectares were seeded with these crops, with a yield of 164 million tons (1).

Cummings (7), referring to an Economic Research Service, U.S.D.A. report looking ahead to 1985, wherein projections were made for potential growth in

Table III. Crop Yields

Crop	Yield (tons per ha)	Country	Reference
Wheat and soya	8 + 3	Mexico	Wellhausen (2)
Wheat and sorghum	8 + 6	Mexico	Wellhausen (2)
Wheat and rice	6 + 6	India	Wellhausen (2)
Multiple (rice equivalent)	30	Philippines	Wellhausen (2)
Sorghum (1 planting with 2 harvests)	12	Guatemala	Plant (4)
Rice	14	Theoretical	Jennings (5)

the United States, stated that corn production could be increased by almost 60%, wheat by 35%, soybeans by about 45%, cotton by 20%, and cattle production by about 60%. Most of this will have to come from increased yields and greater application of technology.

TECHNOLOGICAL PROBLEMS

As mentioned previously, there are marked differences between optimum yields that can be reached under farm conditions and the real yields currently being obtained, as shown by national averages (6). Some of the principal reasons are: lack of good seed varieties; problems in seed production and distribution of good varieties; lack of varieties that are adaptable under farm conditions, especially in mixed systems of agriculture; insects; diseases; low soil fertility and insufficient fertilizer; soil salinity; rainfall; weeds; inadequate preparation of the soil; farming steep slopes and consequent loss of fertility through erosion; date of seeding; other nontechnical factors.

Lack of Well-Adapted, High-Yielding Varieties

This is one of the principal technological problems, and in part explains the differences in yield in those areas that have received more attention and where new varieties have been adapted to fit local conditions. In contrast, the vast zones of the tropics and subtropics have been the subject of very little research, most of the improved varieties have been introduced from other regions, and they could not adapt to a new environment, principally because of problems with photoperiodism. The notable exceptions are wheat and rice, where an objective within programs of improvement was to create varieties that were not sensitive to photoperiodism, and as a result, have adapted to a wide area of the world. It is to be recommended that the same degree of effort be given to beans, corn, soybeans, sorghum, and other cereal and legume crops.

Seed Production from Improved Varieties

In the developed countries, in addition to having improved varieties, the infrastructure permits the farmer to obtain seed at reasonable cost. On the other hand, in the developing countries, the improved varieties do not exist and/or the infrastructure is deficient for the commercialization of seed; thus, the agriculturalist usually is obligated to use seeds from his own harvest. In these countries, there is little demand for improved seed and, consequently, no incentive to establish a seed distribution system by commercial enterprises, leaving the production and the distribution of seed in the hands of governmental agencies unable to cover the entire agricultural sector satisfactorily.

It should be recognized that an indispensable requisite for rapid acceleration and use of improved varieties is that they be very superior in yield and insensitive to photoperiodism. It is also important that any program to accelerate production using new varieties include a minimum package of practices already known to be effective at the local level.

Lack of Varieties Adaptable to Associated or Mixed Cropping Systems

In many countries undergoing development, the farmer frequently grows two or more crops together. He seeks in this way to minimize risks, taking into account the variation in rainfall, and his primary concern is not to obtain maximum yield of a given crop, but to ensure for himself a minimum yield. On the other hand, the research worker develops varieties to obtain maximum yields and there is very little information on the performance of new varieties when grown in association with other crops. It is only logical, if a new variety of different height or biological cycle is introduced and does not adapt well to the mixed cropping, for the farmer to reject it because its use would mean changing his farming system. Agricultural research should emphasize studies of new varieties within agricultural systems where they will actually be used in order to assure minimal risks and increased yields.

Insects

Improved plant varieties resistant to insects at the place of their selection have, upon being introduced to other regions, been unable to resist a different population of insects, and use of insecticides for their control may not be practical. Therefore, it is highly important that varieties be selected for resistance to the plagues of each region. This will require close coordination between the place where plants are being improved and the localities where they will be introduced as new varieties. In Guatemala, during the first year and a half at the new Instituto de Ciencia y Tecnología Agrícolas (ICTA), we have made major progress with the introduction of varieties from outside the country, principally from the international centers, the Center for the Improvement of Maize and Wheat (CIMMYT) in Mexico, and the Colombian International Center of Tropical Agriculture (CIAT), but the need for local adaptation to resist indigenous insects has been forcefully impressed upon us.

Plant Diseases

Plant diseases are responsible for yield losses over the entire world. Traditionally, one of the objectives of the plant breeder has been to produce resistant varieties. Much has been accomplished, but there is still much to be done. The common dry bean is a good example. In spite of the importance of the bean as food, yields have been decreasing in most areas because of disease, and in some areas have almost disappeared.

As in dealing with insects, it is necessary to identify resistant materials and incorporate them into good varieties. Collaboration of national programs with the international centers has much to offer. India and Pakistan have incorporated resistance factors into wheats from Mexico to meet local conditions. Guatemala is selecting wheats resistant to *Septoria,* but in all three cases CIMMYT furnished varieties with broad genetic bases, so the national programs could make progress rapidly. In the case of Guatemala, samples of lines resistant to *Septoria* are being returned to CIMMYT; thus, Guatemala is making a worldwide contribution because these varieties can be dispensed to other areas where *Septoria* is common.

Fertilization

We know that improved varieties have been designed to express their maximum potential yield under optimum conditions of water and plant nutrition, while many farmers of the less developed regions are using "criollo," or native varieties lacking the yield potential of the improved varieties because they have a low, but sure, yield and are not highly demanding in their requirements for fertilizer.

Also, when fertilizer use is introduced into a new area, whether for local, native varieties of plants or improved ones, there is insufficient information on fertilizer needs and, as a consequence, a general recommendation is made for a "sure" formula. This is frequently costly and in some areas is not of any benefit because one important element may be deficient, in which case all the materials are wasted. Especially in the case of nitrogen, the tendency has been to recommend optimum quantities without taking into consideration the economics of production. This problem has become even more serious during the past months because of the scarcity and high cost of fertilizer. Furthermore, the recommendations usually followed are for monoculture, and the technology for the association of crops or intercropping does not exist. There is little doubt that this aspect should be given greater emphasis in research programs.

Salinity

One means for increasing production of farm crops is irrigation, especially in those regions where new plant varieties have been brought in. It has been found that in irrigation systems in which drainage has not been planned, there is a rapid deterioration in soil quality due to the accumulation of salts, and in a short time soil productivity is diminished and rehabilitation is extremely costly. It is indispensable in the designing of irrigation projects to include plans for adequate drainage.

Rainfall

The total land area under irrigation is only a small part of that used for agriculture; most farmers depend on natural rainfall. The problem of excess rainfall is probably as great as the lack of rain. The farmer has met this problem empirically through intercropping and by farming systems we call traditional. This problem is closely related to the biological cycle, water filtration within the soil, the soil's capacity to hold water, which of course depends upon the topography, and such practices as seeding on the contour, or on raised strips. The use of fertilizers also influences the interaction of soil and water. It is easy to understand that here we are up against a series of variables for which there is very little existing information. It is important to study the many facets of the problem as a multifactorial whole.

Weeds

The weed problem is especially serious in tropical and subtropical areas. There is very little known about the effect of weeds on yields, especially the time relationship of weed population and growth, in relation to the crop. Without this information, the agriculturalist weeds or cultivates his crops when he has the time, or when he considers it necessary, and many times the damage has already occurred before the weeding is done. Considerable research effort has focused on chemicals to eliminate or control weeds, but considering the amount of labor and the unemployment problems that exist in many developing countries, emphasis should be given to hand-weeding at the appropriate time.

Soil Preparation

In the Third World, most land is prepared for farming by use of animals, or by man alone with a simple tool. These relatively slow systems do not allow the use of technology as designed by the agricultural scientist. It is important to find systems of land preparation that are adequate, in step with the local cultural practices, and that will serve in mixed cropping.

Slope of the Land

If, in addition to the conditions mentioned previously, we consider that much land is cultivated on major slopes, we can appreciate the complexity of the problem. The technology we have today has been developed for level land, principally at experiment stations.

Seeding Dates

We know that the optimum yield for each crop variety depends on seeding at the appropriate time, on the response of the plants to photoperiodism, temperature, rainfall, and other factors. Nevertheless, in a wide area of the world, planting dates are correlated only with rainfall. When the rains come late, or there is a delay in planting, reduced yields are the result. In order to solve this problem, probably what is needed are varieties that either mature faster or have a latent period that will permit them to survive without damage during dry periods. This has received practically no attention from the plant breeder.

Other Nontechnical Factors

There are many nontechnical problems that affect the use of technology. Insufficient credit, credit that is not flexible, price fluctuation, and lack of storage facilities can all increase the risk to farmers. The agricultural scientist, especially in the biological field, cannot be expected to be capable in all of these areas. He can, however, be knowledgeable about the multiple problems and be interested in working closely with other disciplines. Institutes, programs, and organizations responsible for agricultural technology need to be capable with respect to credit, pricing, and support prices in order to have the proper influence among credit, marketing, and policy groups.

ADVANCES IN TECHNOLOGY

What does science offer for continued increases in food production in the future? If we look back in agricultural history, we see that, thanks to research, there have been important breakthroughs during the present century that permitted the increased yields of today. The invention of the internal combustion engine (and, afterwards, the tractor) replaced work animals over wide areas, giving additional power to the farmer and at the same time freeing land, nearly 70 million hectares in the United States alone, that was formerly used for the feeding of work animals (8). Most of us have forgotten that the use of chemical fertilizers was a major breakthrough, without which good levels of production could not have been maintained through the years.

The creation of land grant colleges in the United States was a highly important move that solved many problems; from their laboratories and experiment stations have come improved hybrids, especially corn, that have had major impacts on agricultural production. It is interesting to speculate that the creation of the international centers such as the Rice Institute in the Philippines, the Corn and Wheat Center in Mexico, the International Centers for Tropical Agriculture in Colombia and in Nigeria, will in the future be considered as important as the establishment of the land grant colleges. We have already seen the contributions of these centers to the green revolution, with their new varieties of wheat and rice that have given the world new hope. The green revolution, largely based on these new varieties, has also stimulated governments to new programs of action, and there are already changes in agriculture. For example, different crops and sequences of crops are now being grown; in Brazil, wheat and soybean crops are grown in rotation. It is only recently that multicropping has received major attention, although it has been a common practice for many centuries in different parts of the world. Undoubtedly, the system of multiple cropping for better use of land and labor can be important.

We should be interested, not only in increasing yields, but in the nutritive value of the crops at harvest. High-lysine, high-tryptophan corn is still little used today. There are still some technical problems limiting wide distribution of corn with this gene, but there is little doubt that it will be of major importance.

Insects have been responsible for large crop losses and even famines. During recent times, attention has been given to chemicals for the control of insects, but we now find cases of resistance to insecticides, as well as unfavorable effects on the environment because of their use. Perhaps another major achievement in the control of insects will be the use of pheromones, the chemical messengers by which insects regulate growth and development. If this system is perfected, it can be of major importance in the control of insects and possibly can eliminate some species that are important pests in agriculture (1).

We know that there are thousands of plant species in the world, but only a dozen or so are used on a large scale for the feeding of man. Recently, advances in cell culture and the breaking of chromosomes have permitted the scientist to make wide crosses, for example, triticale, a cross between *Triticum* and *Secale*, which can be catalogued as the first species of plant created by man that is in current use. Triticale promises to be of special importance in marginal land areas.

STRATEGY OF SCIENTISTS

Scientists have been good technicians and poor strategists. We have tended to limit our responsibilities to science and technology, giving little attention to the use of the technology that we develop. We need to determine the pattern for research programs based on experience with farmers—not in the laboratories or the experiment stations. We should first identify problems at the farm level and solve them with the simplest technology possible. We believe that a multidisciplinary team with a production approach is needed. The final objectives of the geneticist, the entomologist, phytopathologist, economist, and others should be commonly shared. Not only should the goals be defined, but also the steps should be well planned to arrive at those goals. Plans should be made for efficient use of time, budget, and facilities. The scientists should not be diverted from the main objectives just because other facets are interesting.

An important part of the strategy should be adequate testing of technology. This should not be done only on the experiment stations, or only under favorable environments. Our technology should be subjected to stress conditions, and we should do it ourselves and not leave the work to the extension workers or the farmers. Much of this testing can be done in collaboration *with* farmers.

Tradition and convention have been responsible for institutional structures in the developing countries for the delivery of information to farmers. Research scientists have participated in a passive manner in the development of efficient systems to transfer their technology to farms, but they should be interested in the system for delivery of technology; in fact, they should be part of it. Why separate research and extension? Organize a group of scientists, give them good support, but make them responsible and evaluate them on increases in crop production.

Over the years, scientists, or scientists turned administrators, have influenced institutional structure and policy. Scientists will continue to influence policy and institutional structure if we can continue to produce. If we do not, especially under increasing demands for food, the politicians, bankers, and planners will not listen to us.

In Latin America the universities are almost always separated from the agricultural research and extension groups. Thus, there is a division between academic and technological responsibilities. Could not the university orient students more toward field agronomics? Agricultural production systems are relatively sophisticated, and it would not be necessary to lower academic standards in order to train students in applied research and give them production experience.

RELATION OF GOVERNMENTS TO AGRICULTURAL TECHNOLOGY

Governments have great influence on agricultural technology. It is not just or fair to classify governments as limiting factors, because they sponsored much of the development of agricultural technology. However, governments can bring about greater increases in use of technology and subsequent increases in production than can any other kind of organization. The green revolution in Asia is a good example. India (9) seeded 7400 acres of the high-yielding Mexican wheat in 1966 and 10 million in 1969. It can be done when there is a strong commitment to do it and the technology is adequate.

However, there is a lesson here for scientists. The governments considered the new wheat and rice "good buys." Is our technology a good buy? Governments will stimulate use of more technology when they believe that the return on the investment will be high. High returns in the view of governments are not limited to materialistic ones; part of the return can be greater capacity for feeding more people, and this has a direct social effect. Scientists can be better salesmen. Governments are made up of people who are generally not scientists. We can make governments aware of "good technological buys."

We should keep in mind that much technology is location specific. The new wheats and rices need their technology refined and adapted for specific areas. Governments can do more than they have done in the past by developing stability in flexible and dynamic programs, taking advantage of what regional and international organizations can offer, but they can move rapidly into production programs only when the technology has been tested locally and proved to be satisfactory.

Governmental administration is almost always bureaucratic, inflexible, and time-consuming. Perhaps governments have been structured in an adequate manner for general development and the welfare of citizens, but populations have been fed largely through traditional agricultural systems. However, agriculture is a biological system, dependent upon varying rainfall and a large number of individual small farmers. It appears that many governmental procedures are not organized to stimulate or manage biological systems well.

REFERENCES

1. The Panel on the World's Food Supply of the President's Science Advisory Committee, 1967, Vol. II: The World Food Problem, Superintendent of Documents, U.S. Government Printing Office, Washington, D.C.
2. Wellhausen, E. J., 1974, La situación mundial en materia de alimentos: Problemas, mejoras y prospectos para atender futuras demandas, Atalaya: Primer Coloquio Internacional, México.
3. Seaborg, G. T., 1973, Science, technology and development: A new world outlook, *Science* **181**: 13–19.
4. Plant, A. N., Final report of Contract AID/1a-408 Guatemala between Mississippi State University and the United States Agency for International Development, July 1, 1970–September 30, 1972.
5. Jennings, P. R., 1974, *Plant breeding, the green revolution and food production in the developing countries.* Donald F. Jones Memorial Lecture, Connecticut Agricultural Experiment Station, January (typed copy from CIAT).
6. Brown, L., 1965, *Increasing world food output: Problems and prospects,* Foreign Agricultural Report No. 25, United States Department of Agriculture, Economic Research Service, Foreign Regional Analysis Division, (April, 1965).
7. Cummings, R., Jr., 1974, *Food production and the energy dilemma,* Working Papers, The Rockefeller Foundation.
8. Brown, L., 1970, Human food production as a process in the biosphere, *Sci. Am.* **233** (3):160–170.
9. Brown, L., 1970, *Seeds of change,* Praeger Publishers, New York, 205 pp.

COMMENT

Ricardo Bressani · *Division of Agricultural and Food Sciences, Institute of Nutrition of Central America and Panama, Guatemala City, Guatemala.*

In terms of food and of economic development and freedom, the future of Latin America greatly depends on the success or failure of its population to understand and use efficiently the climatic and ecological differences in its various national environments, and on how well these differences can supply the kinds of foods and living conditions required by the population.

In Latin America, the climatic and ecological environment can be classified roughly as the lowlands, or *tierra caliente,* the temperate lands, or *tierra templada,* and the highlands, or *tierra fría.* Each region offers a variety of possibilities for land utilization, settlement potentials, and cropping systems. Because of this, the diversity of food and cash crops that can be produced, of breeds and species of animals that can be made productive, and of the kinds of vegetables and fruits that can be grown is quite large. However, this horn of plenty is not easily obtained because physical, social, economic, and political limitations are also large. Furthermore, agricultural research has not been given the economic backing, stability, and emphasis required to raise productivity to efficient levels.

The Latin American tropics have several advantages over temperate regions for increasing production: a large amount of solar energy, a high rate of photosynthesis, and an almost continuous growing season. Large organizations able to apply high-quality technologies have made possible the efficient production of export and industrial crops such as bananas, cotton, sugarcane, coffee, and a few others. This type of technology, however, has not yet been applied to increase the production of staple food crops, produced mainly by a large number of farmers with small or medium-sized farms. These farmers do not have capital or credit, do not control the markets, and depend on research carried out by governments, universities, or international institutions to improve their agricultural practices and increase their productivity. Increased food production for more adequate food intake and economic development, however, cannot be obtained by independent actions of individual disciplines or institutions. It is a multifaceted problem that requires a multidisciplinary, coordinated approach, not just an agricultural one. Furthermore, the solutions must be tailored for particular regions. Those proposed for all underdeveloped countries will not do because there are important differences among them.

Currently, the stated goal is usually to increase production and productivity of basic food crops as a solution to the problem of hunger. The satisfaction of hunger, however, is not, in most cases, equal to well-balanced nutrition, but is only a palliative in the present world situation. Satisfying hunger with increased

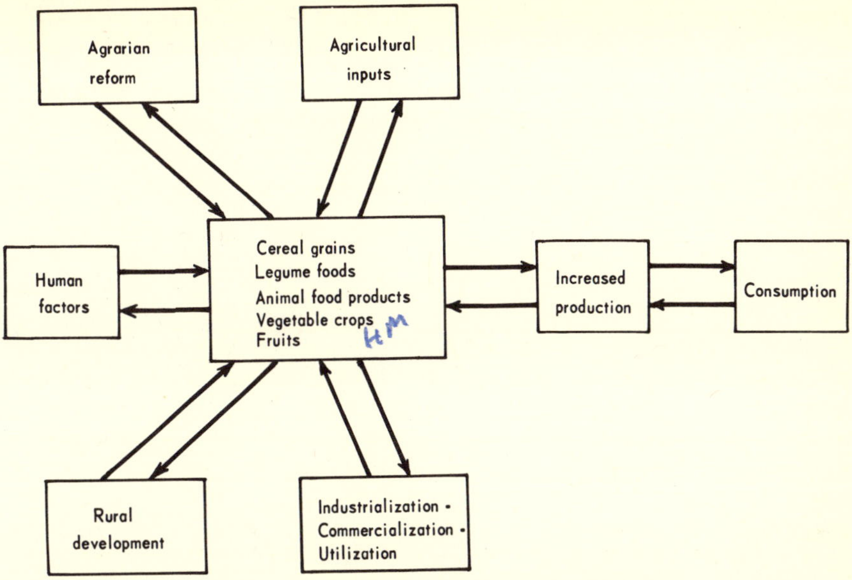

FIG. 1. Factors involved in increasing food production.

cereal grain intake does not provide the balance of nutrients required for good performance and health. This may be the only immediate solution for some regions, but the objective should be to achieve good overall nutrition, based on combining the basic food crops with adequate amounts of supplementary foods.

Dr. Waugh proposed a series of actions that, when properly developed and implemented, will result in increased production, but not necessarily in increased intake by the poor. There are other factors, seen in Figure 1, that represent constraints to both increased production and greater intake. This scheme is, of course, an oversimplification. First of all, increased food production must include greater food crops and also more animal food products, as well as vegetables and fruits. It is not enough to assume that good nutrition will result from diets composed of cereal grains and legume foods alone, even if calculations based on requirements show considerable improvement. An example is shown in Table I. In this case, baby pigs were fed a corn/bean diet, the foods consumed by most rural Guatemalan children, according to dietetic surveys. The animals were allowed to consume the diet for two-hour periods in the morning, at noon, and later in the afternoon. The results show the need to introduce higher quality protein into such a corn/bean diet, even though calculations suggest that it could meet the needs of the animals without this.

Nutrient requirements should be met with a variety of foods, and the primary objective of agriculture and agricultural research and technology should

Table I. Performance of Baby Pigs Fed Corn/Bean Diets Enriched with Various Supplements

Diet	Average food consumed, kg/8 weeks	Average weight gain, kg/8 weeks
Corn + beans (9/1)	9.97	−1.40
Opaque-2 corn + beans (9/1)	19.67	2.55
Corn + beans + skim milk	17.12	1.82

be to make this possible. Agrarian reform shown in Figure 1 is not to be taken as a political action, but as a series of agricultural policies and strategies designed to meet the overall objectives of agriculture, which are: (a) to meet the food needs of the population; (b) to meet reserve needs; (c) to meet the raw material requisites for industrialization; and (d) to meet export requirements, if this is desirable.

As important as agrarian reform is, increasing food production for the human subject is even more so. The rural farmer's life expectancy is short, probably in part because he has to subsist on a diet of cereal grains and legumes alone, and he is prone to disease. He lacks incentive and is given low-quality education and little responsibility. He cultivates the land, but does not get his fair share in return. The environment in which he is born, grows, marries, works, and rears his young does not help his performance. He spends hard working days, empty nights, long, drunken weekends, without the escape provided by diversion or entertainment, and has to satisfy his hunger with much cereal grain and a small amount of beans. Therefore, economic and social programs are needed that will increase the power of people to purchase better foods of animal and vegetable origin.

This situation must be improved as the new technology for increased production is introduced. Estimates for greater food production are often calculated on the basis of single elements, such as the number of people to be fed. In our opinion, it should also include others, such as the industrial processing of foods.

The objective is to use our skill to increase the production of those foods most suitable for all of the population, and that approach should pay attention to all factors directly related to greater availability and consumption of food.

Increased production efforts should include those activities that lead to finding varieties of the basic food grains with increased nutritional value as well as high-yield capacity. Improvement of the diet would be obtained if, for example, in a corn/bean diet, either one or both contained more protein. Some results are presented in Table II. It can be seen that the total amount of utilizable protein shown in the last column is greater when corn contains 13%

protein than when it contains 8%. If quality is also improved, still more protein is utilized.

Some calculations applied to human subjects are shown in Table III. It presents three examples: The first is the usual diet, based on foods generally eaten today, consisting of corn and beans containing 8% and 23% protein, respectively. The second shows the effect on protein utilization of consuming corn with a higher protein content; the third, protein utilization when both corn and beans have a higher protein concentration. The quality of the individual foods does not change, but when consumed together, there is a complementary amino acid effect between the two, which increases the quality of the combination beyond that of either food individually. Ideally, each should also have better protein quality, but net improvement in quality can also be obtained by consuming other complementary foods.

Increased protein may be selected by genetic means or induced by controlled application of fertilizer. Higher protein quantity and quality in corn, for example, may also be obtained by selecting for germ size. An example is shown in Table IV from actual data on the variability of germ size in corn. It may be seen that the larger germ has increases in lysine to values that approach those in opaque-2 corn. Opaque-2 corn has a larger germ than traditional corn has, which contributes to the higher protein quality provided by the endosperm.

Other means should be studied; for example, the controlled application of certain chemicals that have been shown to increase amino acid content in cereal grains and vegetable crops. These alternatives should not be discarded, because they may be simpler to use than genetically modified materials that take time to develop and adapt. The only drawback to chemically treated crops is that their quality may not be as high as that of modified plants.

Protein content and quality, however, are not the only nutrition problems. Means should be found to include, in cultivation patterns, grains of a higher energy density. Larger germ size corn is a possibility, although the increment in

Table II. Effect of the Improvement in Quality and Quantity of Protein on the Nutritive Value of a Corn/Bean Diet Fed to Rats[a]

Change in basal diet[b]	Protein in diet %	Average weight gain g/28 days	Protein efficiency ratio	Relative nutritive value	Protein utilization g %
Maize A (normal protein) (8.3%)	9.7	45	1.67	44.7	4.33
Maize B (high in protein) (13%)	12.4	56	1.52	40.7	5.05
Maize A + lys + tryp	10.0	81	2.49	66.7	6.67
Maize B + lys + tryp	12.6	119	2.45	65.6	8.26

[a]Eight animals per group.
[b]72.4% maize + 8.10% beans.

Table III. Changes in Total Protein Intakes Due Solely to Increases in the Protein Content of Basic Foods Eaten by Preschool Children

	Average intake of solid food (g)	Present protein intakes		Protein intake after increases in protein content: In maize		In maize and beans	
		Protein (%)	Total protein (g)	Protein (%)	Total protein (g)	Protein (%)	Total protein (g)
Maize	104	9	9.4	14	14.6	14	14.6
Beans	11	23	2.5	23	2.5	28	3.1
Total	115	–	12.0	–	17.1	–	17.1
Adequacy,[a] %			68.8		97.6		100.8

[a]For a child of average weight (14 kg), allowing 1.25 g protein/kg for requirement, and assuming a biological value of 100%.

Table IV. Effect of Germ Size in the Corn Kernel on Its Lysine and Tryptophan Content

	Normal corn	Large germ corn
Endosperm, % kernel	82.3	73.2
Germ, % kernel	9.8	17.1
Endosperm, g N	1.53	1.04
Germ, g N	0.29	0.55
Total N, g	1.82	1.59
Lysine, g/16 g N	3.2	3.8
Tryptophan, g/16 g N	0.67	0.74

energy may not be significant. Soybeans matching the general characteristics of common *Phaseolus vulgaris* beans may be even better in energy density. Varieties of crops should be included to increase options at the dining table.

Increased production of food crops should go together with improved nutritional quality, and nutritional quality should either be bred into the grains or added to them during processing. There are many benefits to be derived from the association of larger crops and better quality.

In conclusion, Table V shows that efficiency in land utilization depends on

Table V. Efficiency of Land Utilization through Cultivation of High-Lysine Corn for Human Consumption

	Normal	Opaque-2
Intake of corn needed for nitrogen equilibrium, g/day	547	250
Corn yield, kg/ha	3000	2700
Number of individuals in nitrogen equilibrum from 1 ha of corn	5484	10,800
Protein intake, g/day	44	28
Biological value of corn, %	46.5	82
Protein retained, g	21	23
Protein loss (feces + urine), g	23	5
Amount of corn equivalent to protein loss, g	255	55
Total amount of corn x number of individuals, kg	1398	594
Ha of land	0.47	0.22
Nutritional production efficiency of land, %	53	78

efficient protein utilization by farmers eating food with a higher nutritional value.

Human trials have shown that adults are in nitrogen equilibrium on an intake of 547 g of normal corn or 250 g of opaque-2 corn. The yields of the two types of corn have been set at 3000 and 2700 kg/ha, respectively. With these figures, calculations were made to show that 1 ha of normal corn will produce nitrogen equilibrium in 5484 men, while high-lysine corn will do so in 10,800 individuals. On the basis of the protein content and biological value as determined in human subjects, it was calculated that 23 g of protein of the 44 g ingested from normal corn were lost in feces and urine, but only 5 g were lost by the men consuming 28 g of opaque-2 corn. Converting these figures into grams of corn and number of individuals, and applying the figures to the amount of land, it is calculated that the nutritional efficiency of the land planted with opaque-2 corn is 78%, and only 53% for normal corn. A similar case can be made for mixtures of 70% corn and 30% beans, if they are supplemented with small amounts of animal protein.

These calculations show the benefits to be derived from better quality diets or basic food crops of improved quality.

11

Technological and Ecological Problems Limiting Production of Foods of Animal Origin

Pedro Solana M., Everardo González P., and Ricardo Garza T.

Instituto Nacional de Investigaciones Pecuarias
Palo Alto, México

The world food shortage, and the awareness of the danger that this problem may cause, focuses attention on the need for utilizing all the available resources in the most efficient manner, including the food potential of tropical areas. The need to increment milk and meat production in tropical regions is hindered by lack of technological information on methods for animal husbandry in the tropics. Technologies need to be developed that are efficient for the solution of the problems encountered in tropical countries. Moreover, diminished production costs can be achieved by utilizing production concepts that provide for use of available natural resources and the production of foods at the lowest possible price, even though these methods require longer periods of time. A description follows of the more common tropical climates found in Mexico, and the problems that characterize animal production in such zones, similar in conditions to many other parts of Latin America.

ECOLOGY

According to Tamayo (1), 43% of the total territory of Mexico, or 85.6 million hectares, is suitable for cattle raising because of the extensive forage areas of the plains and hills. Of the country's total area, the desert zone occupies 60.7%, the temperate zone 26.2%, and the tropical zone only 13.1%. According to Hernández (2), the tropical region of Mexico comprises two large areas: (a) the tropical humid slope near the Gulf of Mexico, with 5 million hectares of forage, mainly Guinea, Para Elephant, Buffel, and other grasses recently introduced. This zone is mainly used for raising beef cattle, but also supports large numbers of swine. Grass varieties known as "native" grasses, planted after altering the primary vegetation, are valued by cattlemen, even though the grass yield is low; (b) the tropical semiarid-to-humid zone of the Pacific slope, a transitional zone between tropical and temperate climates, where all kinds of crops may be grown. It consists of 8.7 million hectares of forages, and many vegetable and agricultural residues are utilized to feed beef cattle, goats, and swine. These two areas, although occupying only 13.1% of the land devoted to animal production, supply feed for 25% of the country's domestic animals.

Climate

In the tropical regions there are three types of climates, according to the classification system of Koeppen, modified by García (3): Climate "Af," hot and humid, with rains throughout the year; Climate "Am," hot and humid, with rains during the summer months; and Climate "Aw," hot, subhumid, with rains during the summer months.

Soils

The most abundant soils are the red and yellow laterite types, and alluvial, pink earth, and prairie soils. The majority of them are nitrogen- and phosphorus-deficient, and in some parts of Veracruz and on the Isthumus they are also deficient in potassium (4). Nitrogen, phosphorus, and sulfur applications in very rainy regions induce the growth of legumes and grasses in pastures. The essential minor elements for the growth of legumes are molybdenum, copper, and zinc (5).

CATTLE PRODUCTION ON PASTURES

Cattlemen, particularly in the beef cattle industry, rely mainly on tropical pastures for their animal feed source in Mexico. The types of vegetation in the tropics can be grouped into jungle growth, plains, mangrove swamps, and marshes. Jungles are productive once trees have been cut down, the land has been burned over, and pastures have been established. Because organic material is lost with burning, the potential of pastures for grazing animals depends on their proper management.

To evaluate the potential of a pasture for animal production, one must consider the amount and quality of the forage accessible throughout the year. Optimum production within the tropical environment can only be attained if pasture yield is maximized in quantity and quality.

The amount of available forage is linked with rainfall, and even more closely with how long the soil retains moisture and whether it contains adequate nutrients, especially nitrogen and phosphorus. The quantity factor can be easily manipulated through the introduction of improved plant species and by conservation of forages derived from the summer surplus; more important is the provision of water and nitrogen. According to Jones (6), quality is influenced mainly by the constant supply of nutrients to the soil, thus acting directly on the soil's fertility and on chemical composition of the forage, or indirectly on its botanical composition.

With fertilization of pastures, meat production per unit of land surface increases as the load capacity of the pasture is achieved. Nevertheless, Garza, Arroya, and Pérez (7) have observed that the daily average gain per animal remains constant. Under subtropical conditions, Garza, Treviño, and Chapa (8), grazing animals for 168 days on native grasses, obtained a production of 86 kg meat/ha, and doubled this yield when animals ate grass fertilized with nitrogen. When animals fed on improved forages such as Ferrer (*Cynodon dactylon* Var. Costal Cross 1) or Pangola (*Digitaria decumbens*), meat production /ha was tripled (225 kg meat/ha), and was almost five times greater after the application of 100 kg N/ha to previously infertile soil. In general, tropical pastures are used continuously and exhaustively, causing impoverishment of the land, low forage production, and invasion by weeds.

Low temperatures during the rainy season, and lower rainfall during the dry months, adversely affect forage production and animals grazing on it. Under subtropical conditions in Hueytamalco, Puebla (9), the mean meat production per animal for grazing periods of 28 days each was 15 kg in the summer, 12 kg in the rainy season, and 8 kg in the three driest months of the year. These figures correspond to those obtained for animals grazing on Ferrer grass, which proved to be the most productive, while the Estrella (*Cynodon plectostachyur*) and Gordura (*Melinis minutiflora*) were less tolerant of the low-temperature, dry months in the subtropics. Meat production amounted to 9 and 13 kg per animal during the rainy season, and 1 to 7 kg per animal in the dry season, respectively. The native grasses of the subtropics offer a production equal to or lower than that of Gordura, which is why they must be replaced by improved grasses such as Ferrer or Estrella.

In the tropical area where the hot, subhumid climate prevails, one of the problems is a dry period of six to seven months during which rains amount to only 8% of the total annual rainfall. One method of utilizing forage resources economically is to put animals on reserve pastures and provide them with a dietary supplement. Monroy (10) found that Pangola and Ferrer grasses are better able to withstand the dry months and maintain their quality than Estrella forage, thus supporting a daily weight gain of 436 g per animal, in contrast with the weight loss normally observed during this season, mainly because of lack of forage.

Supplementary feeding of grazing cattle, fertilization of pastures, and irrigation by sprinkling are beginning to be used more frequently in Mexico (11) in an effort to change from cattle raising over wide areas to more intensive systems for the fattening of greater numbers of animals for market in a shorter period. The purpose of these measures is to avoid the scarcity of meat that would otherwise occur in the future as a result of mismanagement of pastures and the lower production induced by the dry season and poor-soil forage.

Animal Production

Animal production in the tropics is generally suboptimal because of low fertility indices and the long intervals between birth and the time of adequate market weight.

Nutrition

The feeding regime of animals in tropical climates is not as intensive as it is in temperate regions. One of the main reasons is that it is impossible to produce enough cereal grains for maximum animal production in the tropics. There are good energy sources for ruminants, however, such as sugarcane, tubers with a high starch content, and byproducts of the sugar industry. Unfortunately, these are not being utilized on a large enough scale.

Not only are grains scarce in the tropics, but storing them is difficult because of high ambient temperature and humidity. Furthermore, the scarcity of cereals for direct human use throughout the world makes it illogical to base animal production in the tropics on the utilization of grains. When ruminants feed exclusively on pastures, climate affects them indirectly by determining the amount of food available to them because forage quantity and quality are influenced by rainfall and temperature. In tropical areas where a seasonal rainy period exists, a marked fluctuation in quantity and quality of forage is created, which lowers fertility and prolongs the time required to bring the animal to market weight.

In the rainy season there is so much forage that the animals cannot consume it all during its stage of optimum quality. Once it reaches maturity, this forage becomes more fibrous and has less protein and phosphorus, reducing its digestibility and acceptability by the animals. On the other hand, during the dry season, forage becomes scarce, is even less digestible because of high fiber content, and loses more of its protein and phosphorus. All of these factors together reduce the voluntary forage consumption of the animals. Tropical forages are generally insufficient to satisfy the animal requirements for trace minerals and phosphorus. Thus marginal deficiencies of these elements are frequent.

Temperature and environmental humidity also directly affect the animals' appetite. Several researchers have proved that as temperature and humidity rise, animals diminish their consumption of dry matter (12–14). This happens when the animal is unable to maintain its thermal balance; thus, some bovine species such as the Cebu, better adapted to warm climates, are affected only at temperatures above 35° C, while some European breeds reduce their voluntary consumption of feed when subjected to temperatures above 27°C (15).

The disparity in feed availability throughout the year could be counteracted with adequate programs for forage conservation and provision of supplementary minerals, protein, and energy, utilizing for this purpose agricultural and industrial by-products of the region. The adoption of these practices has been steadily increasing in tropical cattle raising, but such measures are still far from being in general use.

For swine and poultry raised by intensive or semi-intensive methods, one of the main limiting factors is the low availability of grains. There are tropical products such as yucca or mandioca (*Manihot esculenta*) and sugarcane molasses that can partially substitute for cereal grains. Yucca can be administered in fresh form (16,17), ensiled (18,19), or as flour (20,21). Sugarcane molasses can satisfactorily substitute for 20–30% of the grain in rations for swine in the growing and fattening stages, without much reduction in their weight gains (22).

As in the case of ruminants, the high environmental temperature and humidity that prevail in tropical areas during the summer reduce voluntary consumption of dry matter by monogastrics. This makes it necessary to increase the protein, mineral, and vitamin content in the rations so as to ensure an adequate intake of such nutrients during warmer weather.

Reproduction

In tropical climates, the reproductive efficiency of grazing bovine cattle is low. Calf production in Mexico fluctuates around 50% (23), and apparently is similar to that reported from other tropical countries (24). The reproduction rate is reduced both by the low pregnancy rate and by high mortality of calves during the birth to weaning period. One reason for low pregnancy rates is that cows in the tropics have fewer estrous cycles, and those in heat are less apt to conceive.

The main cause of the low reproductive efficiency of the herds is inadequate feeding. This prolongs the period between birth and the first estrous cycle, reduces the fertility of the cows, and stimulates the birth of weak, low-weight calves. The latter are easy prey to infectious and parasitic diseases common in the tropics. Bovine diseases such as vibriosis, trichomoniasis, and brucellosis can be disastrous, but they are secondary in importance to nutritional deficiencies.

We have observed that in Cebu herds raised under traditional feeding and handling systems, the estrous cycle frequently fails to return for long intervals postpartum, and may take 30 to 60, 91 to 120, and 151 to 180 days, respectively, to be reestablished. The majority of these cows lose from 50 to 120 kg during the first four months of lactation. However, the copulation frequency per conception in the cycling animals fluctuates from 1.5 to 1.8; this indicates that lack of estrus is the main cause for the long interval between births.

The copulation frequency per conception of stabled European-type dairy cattle is also adversely affected by the temperature and humidity in tropical climates (25). In the case of swine, high temperatures reduce libido and spermatogenesis in the males, and the number of embryonal deaths increases in the females, resulting in a small number of suckling pigs per litter (26).

Although the tropics are prone to a series of limiting factors for animal husbandry, they nevertheless present tremendous potential for cattle production, and the problems described above could be solved. Many cattle industries in the Mexican tropics obtain calf yields of 80% through adequate feed conservation, supplementation, selection, and sanitary and management programs.

Artificial insemination offers many advantages. On the one hand, because of the large forage production in certain seasons of the year, it is relatively easy to concentrate a greater number of cows and female calves for brief periods in small pastures located near the corrals. This facilitates detection of estrus with minimum difficulty. Traditional management of beef cattle herds in certain areas of the country, such as the State of Yucatan, is to keep cows in the corrals every morning, allowing them to graze only during the afternoon, night, and early morning hours. This obviously facilitates artificial insemination.

Genetics

The cattle of the Mexican tropics descended from animals brought by the Spaniards during the Conquest; through a natural selection process, they have adapted themselves to tropical conditions. Artificial selection on the basis of production characteristics was almost nonexistent until breeding toward the Cebu type was initiated during the 1930s. Cebu cattle of the Mexican tropics are not only adapted to tropical conditions, but also more productive.

Genetic improvement of tropical cattle must be approached through selection and utilization of the hybrid vigor of the native types crossed with Cebu cattle and other European breeds, so as to achieve interaction of productivity and adaptation to local conditions. Selection must be for improvement of reproduction, calf strength, milk production, and growth rate under the sanitary and feeding conditions of the tropical climate.

Fertility studies carried out in European breeds of cattle indicate that improvement through genetic selection alone is not possible. However, Cebu cattle retain genetic variability of the additive type that allows selection for favorable reproductive characteristics (27,28). An adequate selection program could also improve maternal ability and calf growth rates. Inadequate registries for identification and productivity of each animal handicap selection.

Management

Tropical conditions require special management measures, such as use of baths to protect against ectoparasites, and the treatment of internal parasites. It also requires that activities such as castration, dehorning, and branding of the animals be done during seasons when the fly population is low so as to reduce myiasis.

In areas susceptible to flooding, cattle must be concentrated to utilize the lower lands only during certain months of the year. The lushness of tropical vegetation implies the need to maintain weed-control programs, either by machete or through the use of herbicides, with a consequent increase in production costs. In certain areas use of herbicides is more economical, but has the disadvantage that it is not selective and thus destroys some desirable species such as wild legumes.

European dairy herds that are not crossbred with Cebus require construction of relatively costly stables. These must be well ventilated so that animals are kept in the shade practically all day; they can be allowed into open corrals only to sleep. In some cases installation of electric fans is economically justifiable (29). For crossbreeds of Cebu and European cattle, no well-defined technological guidelines exist to indicate the best form of handling such animals. In the case of improved swine breeds in the tropics, high temperature forces man to attenuate the hotness of the climate for these animals. The methods vary from water pools and sprinklers to electric fans and even air-conditioning systems.

Regarding classification of the quality of animal products, systems established in temperate countries with different socioeconomic conditions and food habits are inappropriate for the tropics. Classification norms should satisfy production and market conditions for each region to stimulate production and consumption.

Animal Health

One of the traditional factors limiting intensive development of cattle production in the tropics has been the high incidence of diseases. Many of these have not been studied in depth and no effective diagnostic or prophylactic methods are available to help control them. Countries that allocate considerable amounts of money to veterinary medical research do not suffer many of the problems characteristic of tropical zones. Lack of available funds has inhibited interest in finding means for improving animal health.

Among the major diseases, probably cattle ticks and diseases such as Babesia and anaplasmosis (gall sickness) are the most important. Although the bath system to exterminate ticks is well known and quite effective, the great investments required to carry out control or eradication programs for this parasite at national levels have not been available to date, despite different programs that have been carried out locally for years in some tropical zones in Latin America. Losses caused by this parasite are considerable; furthermore, besides transmitting diseases, they deteriorate the animals' skin and thus lower their market price (30).

Even though effective chemical products are available for the treatment of Babesia, no rapid, precise diagnostic methods are available for early detection, and it is one of the few diseases that cannot be prevented with a vaccine (31). Chemical products used for the treatment of anaplasmosis are costly and not very effective. No consistently effective vaccine is available commercially that does not cause undesirable side effects (32).

These two diseases are the greatest limiting factors for mobilizing the production of approximately a million calves in the northern zone of Mexico. Because insufficient forage is available there, calves must be exported soon after weaning, in spite of abundant pastures in the tropical area of southeast Mexico that could be utilized to feed them.

Among the infectious diseases that, up to recent times, caused great losses in Mexico was paralytic bovine rabies that crippled the animals. As a result of intensive research, Mexico now has a highly effective vaccine against this disease. At the same time, a reliable method has been developed to control the vampire bat (*Desmodus rotundus*) that transmits this disease (33).

Internal parasitism of different types induces very high annual losses in different animal species in the tropics. However, there are several effective products for their control, and this type of disease could perhaps serve as an example of a problem caused by poor dissemination of information and underutilization of an existing technology, in contrast to problems that persist because no technology exists to prevent them.

Among the more common uncontrolled parasites are pulmonary worms, *Fasciola hepatica,* and coccidiosis. Contagious diseases such as brucellosis can at times become serious problems when not diagnosed early enough to prevent their rapid transmission.

The majority of the limiting factors described could be grouped into two categories: those requiring greater knowledge, study, and research to find proper solutions, and those that remain unsolved on a national level even though methods exist for preventing them. The latter frequently is the result of a lack of infrastructure to introduce new technologies, lack of communications, and insufficient funds to build technical advisory systems. This is the main reason why it has not yet been possible to develop an efficient system for cattle production in the tropics. Isolated or disconnected attempts cannot succeed; it must be an integral part of the development process in tropical countries.

REFERENCES

1. Tamayo, J. L., 1962, *Geografía General de México,* 2a Edición, Instituto Mexicano de Investigaciones Económicas, pp. 148–175.
2. Hernández, E., 1957, *Los Pastizales Mexicanos,* Instituto Mexicano Recursos Naturales Renovables, A.C., pp. 41–46.
3. García, E., 1964, *Modificaciones al Sistema de Clasificación Climática de Koeppen,* Dffset de Larios, México.
4. Vera, R., Moreno, R., y Ortega, E., 1963–64, *Agric. Tec. Méx.* **11**: 189.
5. Hutton, E. M., 1969, *N. Z. Agric. Sci.* **3**: 142.
6. Jones, R. K. Seminar on Tropical America. Potential to Increase Beef Production, Cali, Colombia, 1975, in press.
7. Garza, R., Arroyo, D., y Pérez, A., 1970, *Tec. Pecu. Méx.* **14**: 20.
8. Garza, R., Treviño, M., y Chapa, O., 1975, *Tec. Pecu. Méx.* **25**: in press.
9. Martínez, G., 1974, XI Reunión Anual, I.N.I.P., S.A.G., México, p. 40 (Abstract).
10. Monroy, J., 1974, XI Reunión Anual, I.N.I.P., S.A.G., México, p. 41 (Abstract).
11. Garza, R., 1974, XI Reunión Anual, I.N.I.P., S.A.G., México, p. 42 (Abstract).
12. Yeates, N. T. M., 1956, *Nature* **178**: 702.
13. Wayman, O., Johnson, H. D., Marilan, C. P., and Berny, I. L., 1952, *J. Dairy Sci.* **45**: 1472.
14. Johnson, H. D., Ragsdale, A.C., Berny, I. L., Shanklin, M.D., and McLarney, S., 1963, *Missiouri Agric. Exp. Stn. Res. Bull.* No. 846.
15. Wostell, D. M., and Brody, S., 1953, *Missouri Agric. Exp. Stn. Res. Bull.* 515.
16. Maner, J. H., Buitrago, J. T., Gallo, J. T., 1967, I.C.A. Mimeo.
17. Maner, J. H., Buitrago, J. T, and Gallo, J. T., 1970. *J. Anim. Sci.* **29**: 140 (Abstract).
18. Peraza, C. C., 1970, *Exc. Nac. Méx. Vet. Zoot.,* UNAM, Mexico, Tesis profesional.
19. De Uriarte, L. A., Shimada, A.S., y Bravo, F.D., 1971, *Tec. Pecu. Méx.* **19**: 48.
20. Tehada de H. I. y Brambila, S., 1969, *Tec. Pecu. Méx.* **5**: 12–13.
21. Shimada, A. S., Peraza, C. C., y Cabello, F. F., 1971, *Tec. Pecu. Méx.* **31**: 15–16.
22. I.N.I.P., S.A.G. México, 1963, Informe Anual.
23. D.G.G. Plan Nacional Ganadero, México, 1974, Bovinos productores de carne.
24. Warwick E. I., 1967, *Factors affecting calf crop,* University of Florida Press, Gainesville, Florida, pp. 4–10.
25. Ingraham, R. H., Gillete, D. D., and Wagner, W. D., 1974, *J. Dairy Sci.* **57**: 476.
26. Robinson, D. W., 1971, XIX Congreso Mundial de Medicina Veterinaria y Zootecnia, México.
27. Deese, R. E., and Koger, M., 1967, *J. Anim. Sci.* **26**: 984.
28. Cruz, D. V., 1972, Doctoral dissertation, University of Florida, Gainesville.
29. Zepeda, J. J., Corella, E., Ruiz, D. R., y Berruecos, J. M., 1974, XI Reunión Anual, I.N.I.P., S.A.G., México.
30. Campaña Nacional Contra la Garrapata. Documento del Plan Nacional Ganadero, S.A.G., México, 1974.
31. Esparza, H., Esparza, A., y Esperón, E., 1970, La Premunición contra Anaplasmosis y Babesiosis, III Congreso Nacional de Medicina Veterinaria y Zootecnia.

32. Morales, H., y Solana, P., 1966, Determinación de los porcentajes de Infección de Anaplasmosis en México por medio de la Prueba de Aglutinación en Tubos Capilares. VI Reunión Anual C.N.I.P., S.A.G., México, D.F.
33. Surean, P., y Arellano, C., 1971. Epizootiología de la Rabio Paralítica Bovina. XIX Congreso Mundial de Medicina Veterinaria y Zootecnia, Vol. 1, pp. 28–31.

COMMENTS

Manuel E. Ruiz · *Centro Agronomico Tropical de Investigacion y Ensenanza (CATIE), Turrialba, Costa Rica.*

Data presented in this volume indicate that protein-calorie deficiency is the main cause of infant mortality and also of deficient physical growth and intellectual development, major factors limiting productive advancement in tropical countries. Compared to traditional plant proteins, animal protein is not only of higher biological value, but is also usually found in a more concentrated form, thus allowing infants to derive their protein requirements through smaller intakes of these foods.

As has been stressed in the chapter by Solana and co-workers, there are major problems in the production of high-quality animal protein in the tropics. Animals in the tropics also suffer both quantitative and qualitative deficiencies in protein. Moreover, animal production fluctuates throughout the year as a response to cyclical availability of pastures in alternating seasons of rain and drought. In addition, the genetic potential of the animals is relatively low, thus imposing a ceiling on responses to better feeding practices.

Other limitations include a lack of knowledge of farm practices appropriate for the efficient exploitation of the animal under tropical conditions, and diseases and parasites whose control is difficult if the other problems described are not solved concomitantly. A limiting factor not mentioned in the paper is that deficiencies exist in organizations created to produce and supply adequate information to the producer in the tropics. Not only are well-trained technicians too few in number, but there is also a lack of infrastructure or means for linking the professional man to the farmer.

Increasing animal protein production will require the simultaneous application of several practices in complete balance with the tropical environment. This implies considering all natural resources, their potential as food, the cultural habits of man, and his social and economic needs. In short, conditions can be improved if there is better use of animal production systems appropriately adapted to the tropical environment.*

*Tropical Training and Research Center (CATIE), 1973, Program for the development and adoption of animal production systems in the tropics, Turrialba, Costa Rica, unpublished.

Bovine production is subject to climatic changes and ecological factors to a higher degree than is swine or poultry production. Nevertheless, it has become evident in recent years that cattle production can be increased up to sixfold using pasturage alone (1). In addition to research data cited by Solana, González, and Garza, results obtained at the Tropical Training and Research Center in Turrialba, Costa Rica, are encouraging. For example, it has been found that beef production on grass alone (no supplementation) can be increased from 220 to 440 kg/ha/year by raising the number of stock from one animal (commonly practiced) to three, along with alternating grazing and fallow periods for the pastures to permit regrowth of grass.

If supplements such as sugarcane molasses are used, productivity is greatly enhanced to a maximum of 1600 kg of beef/ha/year, by feeding 3.5 kg molasses/head/day (2). The development of intensive feeding systems based on sugarcane by-products and cull banana has permitted the fattening of steers at rates similar to those obtained with corn and soybean rations in temperate climates. This is even more meaningful, considering the fact that up to 75% of the total nitrogen in the ration is supplied in the form of urea, another by-product that greatly reduces the cost of providing protein to ruminants (3).

The time has also come to look for adequate milk production systems for the hot and wet (or wet/dry) tropics. Obviously, traditional, temperate-zone-based production systems will fail in the hot tropics. This is most evident when production data are compared on a per cow basis. Here again, there is encouraging news from Turrialba. First, a new calf-raising system based on minimum milk intake (90 liters instead of 600 liters per calf), use of a nondairy by-product-based milk substitute, and grazing initiated at two weeks of age, has resulted in the production of dairy heifer replacements ready for insemination at 11 to 12 months of age at a total cost not exceeding U.S. $250 (4,5), in contrast to $450 to $700/heifer under other systems. Under intensive use of African star grass (*Cynodon plectostachyum*) and very small amounts of supplement (10% of total intake), it has been possible to produce 14,000 kg of milk/ha/year, with understandably high economic benefits (6).

Indirectly, better nutrition of the animal means more resistance to diseases and parasites. As an added bonus of the calf-rearing system developed at Turrialba, it has been found that the earlier the calf starts grazing, the more resistant it becomes to anaplasmosis.

These findings and those discussed by Solana and co-workers emphasize that, contrary to the belief that the tropics are not suitable for animal protein production, both beef and milk can be produced efficiently through the development of systems appropriate to tropical countries. It must be emphasized, however, that overall increments in animal productivity will not be achieved unless institutions and organizations are themselves improved in order to carry out the research effectively and provide the necessary technical assistance and promotion. The studies cited indicate that research can lead to highly efficient production systems for the tropics in a relatively short period of time. The limiting factor in the development of tropical agriculture will be technical assistance, unless a suitable mechanism is developed to ensure the transfer of knowledge from the experiment stations to the extension workers and the farmers themselves.

References

1. Vicente-Chandler, J., Abruña, F., Caro-Costas, R., Figarella, J., Silva, S., and Pearson, R. W., 1974, Intensive grassland management in the humid tropics of Puerto Rico, University of Puerto Rico, Agricultural Experiment Station Bulletin 233.
2. Ruiz, M. E., and Bohnout, K., 1974, El uso de subproductos in la Alimentación de bovinos en el Trópico. Tercer Cursillo Centroamericano de Ganado de Carne y Leche, EXPICA-74, Tegucigalpa, Honduras, March 10–12, 23 pp.
3. Ruiz, M. E., 1975, El uso de subproductos energéticos en la producción intensiva de carne. Cuarto Cursillo Centroamericano de Ganado de Carne y Leche. EXPICA-75, San José, Costa Rica, March 10–11, pp. 96–108.
4. Ruiz, M. E., Leal, T., Cubillos, G., Armendariz, R., and Flores, F., 1976, Crianza de terneras de lechería a diferentes edades de iniciación en pastoreo, in preparation.
5. Ruiz, M. E., Muñoz, H., Villegas, L. A., Torralba, J., and Ochoa, C., 1973, Cria de terneras de lechería a base de pastoreo y subproductos. 7° Día de Campo Ganadero, Tropical Training and Research Center (CATIE), pp. 11–13.
6. Cubillos, G., 1975, Intensive pasture utilization for milk production in the humid tropics. Ninth Annual Conference on Livestock and Poultry in Latin America, University of Florida, Institute of Food and Agricultural Sciences, Gainesville, Florida, May 5–9, pp. 29A–37A.

Marco Tulio Cabezas · *Division of Agricultural and Food Sciences, Institute of Nutrition of Central America and Panama, Guatemala City, Guatemala.*

Both Solana and Ruiz noted that beef and dairy cattle production in tropical countries is generally carried out applying extensive methods characterized by the subutilization of large forage areas, slow growth of the animals, low product yields, and poor returns on invested capital. Because of these inefficient methods of animal husbandry, the cattle industry has contributed little to the economic and nutritional progress of the tropical countries.

To improve this, cattle production systems must be intensified by applying methods appropriate to the different ecologic zones of the region. Unfortunately, too little is known in Latin America of optimum practices. Most now in use are mere copies or suboptimal adaptations of systems developed in other regions and environmental conditions that differ greatly from those in the tropics.

For example, for the formulation of animal rations, nutrient requirement standards developed in the United States and England are used in tropical countries. Little or nothing is known about the differences existing between these standards and the nutritional requirements of animals under tropical conditions.

Research by INCAP to develop an intensive beef production system with calves reveals the magnitude of such differences (1). During the first week of life, calves are artificially fed with small quantities of milk and weaned early, at five weeks of age. Thus, the calves are stimulated to consume solid foods early in life, and hence their digestive function is transformed rapidly from monogastric to ruminant. As a consequence, the animals are capable, when very young, of utilizing efficiently the fibrous foods or forages that constitute the basis of rations in the subsequent growth and fattening stages.

One month after weaning, when the animals weigh 75 to 100 kg, their daily consumption reaches 4.0 kg of dry matter per 100 kg of weight, 11 Mcal of digestible energy, and 500 g of digestible protein, and their weight increases by 0.8 and 0.9 kg per day.

According to the British nutrient requirements for animals (2), calves of the same weight need an average of 10 Mcal of digestible energy and 260 g of digestible protein per day for a daily weight gain of 1.0 kg. Using these standards, the maximum capacity of dry matter intake for animals raised in Great Britain is 3.0 kg/100 kg weight/day.

These data clearly indicate great differences in feed intake and utilization by animals under local conditions, and the inappropriateness of applying, uncritically, the nutrient requirements developed in other regions to cattle raised in the tropics. These differences may be attributed to environmental effects on feed efficiency, and on growth potential of the calves, which is possibly lower than that in countries with a temperate climate. Part of these differences could also be due to the types of food used, which vary in both quality and nutritive value according to the materials utilized in the different regions.

This is only one example of the need for local research in tropical countries in order to develop techniques for increasing the efficiency and productivity of their cattle industries.

References

1. Meléndez Guzmán, H. E., 1974, *Utilización de Urea por Terneros durante las Primeras 13 Semanas de Edad.* Thesis, University of San Carlos de Guatemala, School of Veterinary Medicine and Animal Husbandry, Guatemala, p. 52.

3. Roy, J. H. B., 1970, *The Calf, nutrition and health,* Vol. 2, 3rd ed. Iliffe Books, London, p. 164.

12

Aquatic Protein in Latin America

Georg Borgstrom

Department of Food Science and Human Nutrition
Michigan State University
East Lansing, Michigan

Data from the selected countries in Table I illustrate the large discrepancies in protein production that exist among Latin American countries, even within the same region.

Fish use in several countries, as well as in Latin America, is diverted to bolster animal production. The basic relationship of agriculture to fisheries is frequently neglected. Computation of the acreage required to produce a corresponding amount of animal protein within each country (Table II) reveals that fisheries in several Latin American countries play a far greater role than is generally recognized. The last column indicates the percentage of the aquatic protein used in the country that went into animal feeding in 1970–71 and consequently appeared only indirectly as human food.

It is not unique in the affluent world to find countries where far more fish protein serves to feed livestock instead of man, but it is crucial to Latin America, which will add 120 million more people prior to 1985, to consider the importance of fish for direct human feeding. The last column in the table underlines the significance to food science and nutrition for finding ways to channel these protein assets into a more effective use in the human diet.

UTILIZATION OPPORTUNITIES

The disproportionate waste accompanying shrimping constitutes a significant challenge to the involved nations–Mexico, the Central American republics, Brazil, Venezuela, Surinam, and some of the Caribbean islands. For each ton of

Table I. Relation of Aquatic to Other Animal Protein Intake in Selected Latin American Countries, 1970–71

	A Aquatic protein	B Animal protein	% A/B
Surinam	10.6	22.2	47.8
Jamaica	26.5	11.0	41.5
Barbados	13.5	41.2	32.8
Guyana	5.5	17.9	30.7
Dominican Republic	6.0	21.5	27.9
Trinidad	6.5	26.4	24.6
Peru	4.5	19.1	23.5
Panama	5.5	26.3	20.9
Guatemala	0.2	12.7	1.6
Argentina	1.1	62.3	1.8
Mexico	0.8	14.2	5.6
Haiti	0.3	4.7	6.4
Brazil	2.2	21.4	10.3
Venezuela	3.2	26.2	12.4
Chile	3.7	28.0	13.2
Cuba	4.2	28.6	14.7

Table II. Fish Acreage, 1970–71

Country	Million hectares	Tilled land (%)	Animal feed (%)
Jamaica	0.37	152	none
Surinam	0.032	71	none
Venezuela	2.0	62	66
Panama	0.29	52	34
Barbados	0.013	50	none
Peru	1.36	48	50
Trinidad	0.065	47	none
Chile	1.57	34	77
Dominican Republic	0.256	24	none
Cuba	1.4	18	74
Brazil	5.6	19	17
Mexico	3.7	15	80
Colombia	0.42	8	27
Ecuador	0.33	8.5	66
Nicaragua	0.04	7.5	45
Argentina	0.15	0.5	36

shrimp, 5 to 10 tons of fish are captured but thrown overboard. In addition, small-sized shrimp are discarded. This wasted catch amounts to more than 1 million tons. It corresponds to half the Latin American catch, exclusive of anchovies. Mexican efforts to regulate this by prescribing that fish in amounts equal to that of the shrimp catch must be landed have been circumvented by conversion of the fish to meal.

METHODS OF PRESERVATION

Varying degrees of effort have gone into a universal strengthening of cooling facilities, through icing on land, and by extensive investments in ice making in the marketing chains. Icing and chilling procedures apply principally to temperate and affluent regions of the globe, and especially to countries with access to appropriate technical facilities. Traditional drying, salting, and smoking procedures offer far greater opportunities to the poor nations, at lower costs for marketing, storage, and distribution. Brazil and several Caribbean islands show the value of such products in obtaining a broad, dependable spread of aquatic protein. A further good example from outside the area is offered by Indonesia.

Freezing is another procedure that has been accepted far too readily as a vehicle for expanded use of fish protein in daily food. The required infrastructure is beyond the immediate reach of the poor and hungry and is to be characterized as excessive in cost and little suited to actual needs. Even when long-distance, high-seas fishing might seem indicated, despite the heavy capital and energy demands involved, an efficient marketing of the catches for daily consumption, with regard both to time and to location, is cheaper and more effectively arranged through dried and salted items.

Minced fish, salted or canned, is increasingly becoming a highly versatile product. It can be used as such, or in various combinations, but also allows the use of a far broader range of fish species. Fish balls, a kind of counterpart to meatballs, is also a good alternative.

Dried fish has clearly demonstrated its standing in world feeding and constitutes, in several instances, a superb protein concentrate. When shredded and compressed, it is valuable in protein mixtures. Attention should be given to the mixing of dried fish into cassava flour, practiced for centuries in the humid tropics of Africa. The corresponding parts of Latin America would benefit greatly from a similar approach, to counter the extensive protein malnutrition in the cassava-growing regions.

Far more protein has been channeled through fish sausages than through any other new fish item of the postwar period. Fish sausages or similar ready-to-eat products are likely to have greater potential as a source of cheap protein than are more elaborate products. The sausages make full use of all dark meat and can be made with less accepted species. Large manufacturing plants with a daily output exceeding 300 tons operate in Japan. Japan has aided in the building of similar plants in Surinam, Brazil, and Southeast Africa.

Approximately one-fourth of the Japanese catch is converted into Kamaboko (425,000 tons), sausages (180,000 tons), and related products (134,000 tons), but, more importantly, has thereby reached broad segments of the Japanese population.

By controlling the quality of the raw material that goes into the manufacture of fish meal, the meal can be greatly improved without going the expensive and complex route of making solvent-extracted fish protein concentrate.

13

Technological and Ecological Problems Limiting the Production of Freshwater and Marine Fishes in Latin America

Henry J. Schafer

Instituto Tecnológico y de Estudios Superiores de Monterrey
Escuela de Ciencias Maritimas y Tecnologia de Alimentos Guaymas
Bahia de Bacochibampo, Guaymas, Sonora, México

Most of Latin America, with the exception of northern Mexico, Chile, Argentina, Uruguay, and the southern tip of Brazil, is located between the Tropic of Cancer and the Tropic of Capricorn. The tropical oceans have been considered to be less productive than those of the Temperate Zone because of certain environmental factors. The principal factor is the presence of a permanent thermocline in tropical waters. Surface waters are warmer throughout the year and the temperature of the water decreases gradually with increasing depth until reaching the thermocline, a zone of rapid decrease in temperature with moderate increase in depth, which, in effect, separates the colder and denser lower water mass from the warmer and less dense waters above. In temperate waters, the thermocline forms during the summer months; but during the cold season, the surface waters cool down and sink because of their increased density until the temperature in the water column becomes uniform and the thermocline disappears. Because the water column has a uniform temperature and is of equal density, surface waters and bottom waters mix, bringing to the surface nutrient-rich waters from the bottom layers. This process is called overturn, and provides a nutrient-rich environment for the phytoplankton to grow in during the following warm season (1,2).

This process does not occur in tropical waters and the nutrients in surface waters must be replenished by other means: nutrient-rich waters from river discharges and upwellings that bring nutrients from the bottom to the surface.

Fortunately, we have several important rivers emptying into the Atlantic and important upwelling zones along the Pacific coast of Latin America (3).

Phytoplankton production is very high, over 500 mg of carbon fixed per square meter of surface per day, along the Pacific coast of Panama and Costa Rica, off the Gulf of Tehuantepec, off the coast of Peru, off the Gulf of Fonseca, the Gulf of Venezuela, the north coast of Venezuela, the north coast of Guyana and Surinam, the southeast coast of Brazil between Santos and Florianópolis, the Rio de la Plata estuary, and the southeast coast of Uruguay. There are zones of high phytoplankton production, from 250 to 500 mg $C/m^2/d$, along the Pacific coast from northern Baja California to northern Chile, on the Atlantic along the southeast coasts of South America, northeastern Brazil, the Guaianas, Venezuela, the Caribbean coast of Panama, Costa Rica, Honduras, and Belize, and the Gulf of Mexico coast of Yucatán, Campeche, and Tabasco.

Zooplankton abundance is very high, over 500 mg per cubic meter on the Pacific coast of Chile, Peru, and North Baja, California; high, 201 to 500 mg/m^3, along the Pacific coast of Ecuador, Colombia, Central America and southern Mexico, and lower, 51 to 200 mg/m^3, along the rest of the Pacific coast of Mexico, and the Atlantic, Caribbean, and Gulf of Mexico coasts of Latin America (4).

Tropical waters support a much larger variety of species than temperate waters do, but the individual organisms are dispersed. In temperate waters, there are fewer species, but each is represented by many more individuals than in tropical waters. Living resources in temperate waters are more abundant and more concentrated than in tropical waters, where there is more variety but less abundance and more dispersion of the resources.

The fisheries resources in most temperate waters are fairly well known and have been studied by fisheries scientists from the developed nations exploiting them. The fisheries resources of the developing nations in Latin America have not been studied as thoroughly because of the lack of research funds and sufficient numbers of trained scientists. We still do not know enough about the magnitude of our available fisheries resources to plan their rational exploitation.

Most Latin American countries exploiting shrimp resources have fairly modern and well-equipped shrimp fishing vessels, and Peru and Chile have efficient fleets for the capture of anchovies. A few countries, like Mexico, are improving their tuna fleets and sardine fleets, and Cuba has improved its fishing fleet. Other species are being captured with small boats and relatively inefficient gear.

Most fishermen in Latin America have had little formal training, and our countries have not had a long-standing tradition in fisheries activities, unlike some countries in Europe and Asia that have been extracting a considerable portion of their food supplies from the oceans for many generations.

In many areas of Latin America, the required infrastructure for the exploitation of aquatic resources, such as adequate port facilities, roads, electric power, ice plants, processing plants, and efficient distribution channels, is lacking.

In the past, foreign species have been introduced into the lakes and other bodies of fresh water without due regard for their effects on native species. In some cases the native species have been destroyed by this practice.

Aquaculture has been practiced in Latin America on a very limited scale until recently. During the past six years, a great deal of interest has developed in establishing aquacultural practices for several important commercial species, such as oysters, shrimp, crayfish, and catfish. Scientists from the University of Miami have worked on shrimp culture in Honduras and Venezuela. The University of Arizona and the University of Sonora are conducting research on shrimp culture in Puerto Peñasco on the Gulf of California. Our institution, the School of Marine and Food Sciences of the Monterey Institute of Technology in Guaymas, Mexico, has been active since 1968 in research to develop culture of our local species of shrimp. In 1969 we succeeded in producing postlarvae of the brown shrimp, *Penaeus californiensis*, from gravid females that were collected and brought to our laboratory (5). We have conducted research on behavior, the effect of environmental conditions, and the effect of DDT on local species of shrimp, including some that were developed at our own food laboratory.

The National University of Mexico and our institution have conducted studies on environmental conditions in coastal lagoons and estuaries in the states of Sonora, Sinaloa, and Nayarit under the auspices of the Secretariat of Water Resources of the Federal Government of Mexico, with the idea of improving environmental conditions for the production of shrimp in these waters.

It seems that, at the present time, the intensive culture of shrimp is too exclusive to be economically feasible, but extensive culture programs have met with some success in Ecuador and Mexico. Large ponds have been stocked with shrimp postlarvae and juveniles in Ecuador, and these have been collected later after reaching commercial size. The Secretariat of Water Resources in Mexico has built several canals to bring fresh water and seawater into coastal lagoons and estuaries to improve environmental conditions and to facilitate the entrance of shrimp postlarvae and juveniles, with apparently satisfactory results in increasing shrimp production in some of these waters.

Oyster culture has been carried out in Chile, the states of Sinaloa and Sonora in Mexico, and Venezuela, among others, with varying degrees of success. Our institution was involved during a one-year program sponsored by the Secretariat of Water Resources in attempting to produce oyster spat under controlled environmental conditions.

Crayfish culture experiments are being conducted in Jamaica, Peru, Brazil, Panama, and Mexico, but few have resulted in successful commercial cultures at this time.

Catfish farming has been introduced on a limited scale to Colombia, Honduras, and Mexico. Our institution took part in this activity in the state of Nuevo Leon with the sponsorship of the Secretariat of Water Resources.

Trout and carp culture has been practiced in several Latin American countries for some time.

Most of the aquaculture work in Latin America has been aimed at species having high commercial value in the international market, which could eventually improve export–import balances; relatively little has been done on species that would serve to improve local nutrition.

Some of the marine fisheries resources available to us are being exploited very intensively and have reached a level at which they are being exploited at their maximum, or are being overexploited; these include shirmp, lobster, abalone, and red snapper in Mexico, anchovies in Peru, and Pacific tunas. Improving Latin American tuna fishing fleets would only allow our countries to compete more favorably for this resource and increase our share of the capture, without increasing the total capture; in the same manner, improving the Mexican shrimp fishing fleet in the Gulf of Mexico would allow us to compete more favorably with foreign fleets for this resource.

There are many other marine fisheries resources along our coasts that are not being exploited very intensively, for example, sardine and sierra mackerel in Mexico. Sardine captures increased from 19,000 metric tons in 1963 to 53,000 metric tons in 1972, and sierra mackerel catches rose from 4000 metric tons in 1963 to 10,000 metric tons in 1972 (6). We are being wasteful of some marine resources. It is estimated that 7 tons of trashfish are caught for every ton of shrimp in Mexico (7). Most of this catch is thrown overboard. If we had a way to process and utilize this fish, Mexico could almost double its yearly fisheries production. We have an average yearly shrimp catch of 40,600 metric tons which, multiplied by 7, yields an estimated 284,200 metric tons of trash fish. Our total commercial fish catch in 1972 was 302,000 metric tons. If we assume that the edible portion in trashfish, as recovered by mechanical deboning, is 50%, we could raise the amount of fish available for human consumption in Mexico by 142,100 metric tons per year. This would be equivalent to a 2.58 kg increase in the apparent per caput consumption, 74% higher than that of 1967 (6), which was 3.5 kg per person.

Most of the Peruvian anchovy catch is being processed as fish meal for animal consumption; even a reduced catch of 8 million metric tons with a protein content of 18% (8) would yield enough protein to satisfy the nutritional needs of 80 million people for one year, if we assume a daily requirement of 50 grams of animal protein per person.

To increase knowledge of Latin American fisheries resources, Mexico established a National Council for Science and Technology to provide research funds, and other countries have established similar organizations for this purpose;

unfortunately, the funds available are still very limited. During the past 12 years many Latin American universities have established schools and colleges that offer training in the exploitation of marine and freshwater resources. At this time only a few offer postgraduate training, but there is a keen interest among the more prestigious institutions to establish postgraduate programs in the near future. Training at lower educational levels is also of great importance. We can acquire efficient vessels and gear, but our fishermen need to be trained to use them. Aquaculture also needs trained personnel to be successful.

Research to determine the magnitude of our marine resources and to establish cultural practices for our local species, as well as to plan for their development and rational management, requires trained persons of the highest level, and fishing fleets and aquaculture enterprises need trained operators and support personnel. Mexico has established 30 training schools at the secondary level that combine regular courses and vocational courses in fishing and aquaculture. These schools are in their third year of operation. Additional schools at the college preparatory level, with a combined curriculum, will be established to receive secondary school graduates who wish further training.

If we are willing to provide the necessary funds for research and training, for acquisition of modern vessels and gear, and the needed infrastructure, Latin America can provide a significant contribution to improve the nutritional level of its people through the rational exploitation of its aquatic resources.

REFERENCES

1. Hardy, A., 1956, *The open sea*, Houghton Mifflin, Boston, 335 pp.
2. Sverdrup, H. U., Johnson, M. W., and Fleming, R. H., 1957, *The oceans*, Prentice-Hall, Englewood Cliffs, New Jersey, 1087 pp.
3. Harvey, H. W., 1957, *The chemistry and fertility of sea waters*, University Press, Cambridge, England, 234 pp.
4. Food and Agriculture Organization, 1972, *Atlas of the living resources of the seas*, FAO, Rome.
5. Schafer, H., 1971, *Advances in Pacific shrimp culture*, G.C.F.I. Proc. June, 1971 (23), pp. 133–138.
6. S.I.C., 1968, Estadísticas Básicas de la Actividad Pesquera Nacional, 1967, S.I.C. Dir. Gral.de Pesca e Industrias Conexas, México.
7. Borgstrom, G., 1967, *The hungry planet*, Collier Books, New York, 507 pp.
8. Food and Agriculture Organization, *Fish in nutrition*, Fishing News (Books) Ltd., London, 445 pp.

14

Food and Cash Crop Competition

Quentin M. West

Economic Research Service
United States Department of Agriculture
Washington, D.C.

Technology has transformed agriculture into one of the most modern industries in the world. In the developed nations, this technology takes on the characteristics of space-age science, with computer-controlled feeding operations, fantastically complicated field machinery, and the latest techniques of management. Even the developing nations have felt the wand of technological advance—scientifically developed grain varieties and recently introduced agricultural practices.

It seems ironic, then, that this should also be a period of extreme uncertainty in world agriculture. Severe crop shortfalls have beleaguered the developed and less developed nations alike. Weather, on which man has never imposed his will, has dealt him a severe blow in the cultivated fields, ranging from the United States to the Soviet Union, and from the African Sahel to the Indian subcontinent. This, coupled with large grain purchases on the world market by some drought-affected nations, the resultant short grain stocks, worldwide inflation, and, of course, the energy crisis, has generated a serious setback for this globe's agricultural industry.

This is highly unusual, for in the past 20 years worldwide growth in food production has been relatively steady and the rate of increase has been about equal in the developed and less developed countries. The sharp fall from this trend in 1972 and again in 1974 was indeed alarming.

In a world beset by farm production problems during the past year, Latin America stands out in a rather favorable position. Although poor weather affected several nations, the 1974 Latin American agricultural crop exceeded the

1973 crop by about 5%. Nevertheless, inflation plagues the Latin American economies, population growth continues to compromise food production gains, and import restrictions to save scarce foreign exchange are increasing.

This precarious food situation draws attention to the need in Latin America and elsewhere for increasing food production, and we certainly recognize the need for general economic growth in our nations. To fuel our economies, we need to look to the import of capital goods and, of course, this strains our foreign exchange accounts.

So, besides its obvious mandate to produce food for home consumption, agriculture has the responsibility to earn foreign exchange to pay for the imports of capital goods and raw materials for the nonagricultural sector, as well as to provide raw materials for the domestic manufacturing industry.

However, agriculture cannot stop there. It is also an important source of capital to help develop the nonagricultural sector. It must furnish employment and rising incomes for rural people if the rural sector is performing its role as a market for industrial products. It must also furnish surplus labor for the nonagricultural sector. Although vital, the last three roles occupy a relatively minor place in this presentation.

It is obvious that competition does exist between crops grown for food and those grown for other purposes. For any given plot of land, bag of fertilizer, can of pesticides, or whatever, decisions are demanded on how they will be used. But, has food been slighted? Over the long run, this may have been true. Food production may have been compromised in the interests of coffee in Brazil and Colombia, beef as an export commodity in Argentina, sugar in Cuba and its Caribbean neighbors, cotton in Mexico, bananas in Central America, and so on.

In the past decade, however, it has been a somewhat different story. Food production has advanced to more than a self-sufficiency position in Latin America. In 1968–72, the value of food produced in the region was 112% of the value of food consumed. Wheat is the only major commodity deficit, but this is more than made up for by exportable supplies of other crops. Agricultural imports are not large, about 11% of total imports in 1971 compared to 13% in 1962, but they could be much less.

In Mexico, wheat yields have tripled since the early 1950s. Colombian rice production has increased from less than 400,000 tons in the late 1950s to over a million tons in recent years. Brazil's wheat production has jumped from a little over 200,000 tons per year in the early 1960s to over 2 million tons recently. Brazil's soybeans, in part an export crop, but also an important source of domestic cooking oil, are also doing well. Production has increased from less than 200,000 tons in the late 1950s to 7 million tons in 1974. Poultry meat production in Latin America has doubled over the past decade, while egg production has increased by more than 55%.

Total food production in Latin America in 1969–73 was 30% above the production levels of 1961–65, compared to an advance of 24% for total agriculture (Table I). If we look at just the most important staple items compared to commodities principally for export or industrial purposes, we see that staple foods, with an advance of 26%, did relatively much better over the past decade than the export and industrial commodities, which showed only a 10% increase. The greatest advances in the production of staple foods relative to export and industrial commodities were in Mexico, Brazil, and the Caribbean. Of the regions shown in Table I, Central America and Panama showed the greatest percentage increase in total food production, but progress there in staple foods lagged behind that of the export and industrial commodities. Despite the advance of staple food products relative to industrial and export commodities, the production of these staple items on a per caput basis increased hardly at all for the region as a whole, and actually declined somewhat in the Andean countries and Mexico.

Among the staple food commodities, the production of corn (which in the case of Argentina is principally an export commodity), cassava, dry beans, and rice showed the greatest increases between the early 1960s and early 1970s (Table II). The relatively poorer performance of the export and industrial commodities was caused by declines in the production of coffee, flaxseed, and wool; there was a rather small increase in cotton.

Food balance data indicate that Latin American diets have been improving. For example, caloric intake rose from 100% of the minimum requirement for the whole region in 1961 to 105% in 1970. The number of countries where the average level of food consumption met minimum needs was up from 9 out of 25 to 13. Of course, there are wide variations among countries, ranging from 76% of need in Haiti to 121% in Paraguay. Moreover, the improvements made during the past decade are insufficient. It is intolerable that the average level of food consumption remains below minimal nutritional needs in half of the region's countries. Even in most countries with adequate dietary levels on the average, large proportions of the population are attempting to survive on less than adequate diets.

Despite the growing public clamor for more dependable, cheaper, higher quality food supplies, governments cannot afford to place all their agricultural resources in one basket—the food basket. Most Latin American economies are highly dependent on agricultural exports and they cannot afford to slight them if they want to continue the process of economic growth. Agriculture's most important contribution toward providing capital for the Latin American economies is probably through the earning of foreign exchange. This allows the import of capital goods to fuel the industrial sector.

Farm exports for 23 Latin American countries were up from $4.5 billion in 1962 to $6.85 billion in 1971, but over the same period their share of total exports declined from 49% to 45%. If countries highly dependent on oil and

Table I. Indices for Production for 22 Latin American Countries, Average, 1969–73[a]

Country	Total agriculture	Total food	Staple food items[b]	Selected industrial and export commodities[c]
Latin America	124	130	126	110
Mexico	131	141	127	98
Caribbean[d]	111	113	131	103
Central America and Panama	136	148	128	142
South America	121	127	125	106
Andean countries[e]	124	127	118	122
Brazil	128	139	138	98

[a] 1961–1965 = 100.
[b] Wheat, rice, corn, potatoes, cassava, and dry beans.
[c] Cocoa, sugar, coffee, tobacco, cotton, flaxseed, wool, and bananas in Jamaica, Central America, Colombia, and Ecuador.
[d] Dominician Republic, Haiti, Jamaica, Trinidad, and Tobago.
[e] Venezuela, Colombia, Ecuador, Peru, Bolivia, and Chile.

Table II. Indices of Production for Selected Commodities in Latin America, Average, 1969–73[a]

Staple food commodities		Industrial and export commodities		Other commodities	
Wheat	98	Cocoa	128	Soybeans	748
Rice	122	Sugar[b]	132	Sorghum	353
Corn	136	Coffee	87	Beef and veal	114
Potatoes	119	Tobacco	121		
Cassava	136	Cotton	103		
Dry beans	126	Flaxseed	62		
		Wool	88		
		Bananas	155		

[a]1961–1965 = 100.
[b]Includes Cuba and minor Caribbean Islands.

mineral exports (Bolivia, Chile, Trinidad, Tobago, and Venezuela) are excluded, the farm share of total exports declined from 77% in 1962 to 65% in 1971. Net agricultural exports for the region increased from $3.4 billion in 1962 to $5.2 billion in 1971. Thus, agriculture continues to be the principal provider of foreign exchange for most Latin American countries, but its exports have not kept pace with those from other sectors.

There is a continuing and growing need for farm export earnings because of the climbing costs of imported raw materials such as oil. Cost of oil for petroleum-importing nations in Latin America totaled $4.9 billion in 1974, up sharply from about $2.0 billion in 1973.

In sum, the agricultural sector in Latin America has performed a passable job in providing both food and export commodities over the past decade, but it has not come near to realizing the region's vast potential. Pressing needs for improving nutritional levels, providing foreign exchange necessary for continuing economic development, and helping to feed a world in need of ever-growing food supplies, cry out for much more of Latin America's agricultural potential to be developed effectively over the coming decade.

Looking ahead to the formulation of food and agriculture policies for the next 10 to 20 years, it is imperative that all the roles of agriculture be considered. An overemphasis on food production that resulted in a decline in agricultural exports could be self-defeating, especially in a highly urban area like Latin America. In many countries, a decline in agricultural exports would lead to shortages of foreign exchange and heavy restrictions on imports. The slowdown in imports of capital goods and raw materials would likely lead to declining rates of economic growth, with unemployment and/or lower wages in the cities. This could lead to lower nutritional standards, regardless of how much domestically grown food was available—people just would not be able to afford it.

Thus, there is a critical need in these times for expanding production of food and export and industrial crops. Population, urbanization, nutrition, and rising incomes are the major factors relating to the need for rapid growth in food production. Fortunately, this region has the land and water resources as well as the potential for yield-expanding techniques.

The Latin American population growth rate is the highest in the world, putting special demands on its food industry. The Latin American Demographic Center estimates that the region's population will grow at a rate of 2.9% a year between now and 1985; this compares to about 2.2% for the world as a whole. It appears that the total regional population of 315 million in 1974 will climb to 432 million by 1985.

Urbanization will compound the problem. People will be moving out of the subsistence economy into areas where they will have to depend upon marketed food. Each farmer will have to produce more and the food marketing system will have to carry a rapidly increasing load. The urban population in Latin America will probably increase from 56% of the total in 1970 to 67% in 1985. This means the urban population will increase 83%, or by more than 130 million in the 15-year period. Thus, marketable food supplies must increase at a rate of 4.1% a year just to remain even with the 1970 level.

The need for nutritional improvement, as noted before, is great and is compounded by changes in the demand for food products that will accompany increased incomes and rising expectations. Not only does food production need to be increased at a rate exceeding population growth in order to provide minimum caloric requirements for the region's poorest people, but rising incomes will stimulate a greatly increased demand for higher quality diets, and especially for animal proteins.

Agriculture will be required to carry a significant load in generating the foreign exchange to purchase the capital goods and raw materials needed to fuel the industrial economy.

The economic welfare of Latin American people, who are more urban than not, is highly dependent upon the growth of nonagricultural sectors. The growth of these sectors, especially manufacturing, is dependent upon imports of capital goods for new and expanding industries, and in some instances, for the raw materials, like oil or coal, that are not produced in the country.

During 1960–71, growth in manufacturing (7.1% per year) and electricity (10.9% per year) ranked highest among the various sectors in Latin America's economic growth (5.5% average). If recent favorable economic growth is to continue, these key sectors will have to continue rapid growth. To a certain degree, these sectors are dependent upon imports—machinery and other capital goods for manufacturing industries, turbines, and other equipment for electric power projects.

High prices of raw materials necessary to keep manufacturing and service sectors operating will be a problem in the future. Oil prices, for instance, are proving to be a heavy drain on foreign exchange in Brazil, Chile, Paraguay, Uruguay, Central America, and some Caribbean countries. Prices of other raw materials and basic commodities are also up—from fertilizers to coal to wheat to bauxite.

In summary, it appears to this observer that Latin American agriculture has done reasonably well in furnishing food and export commodities in recent years. If indeed a competition between these two roles for agriculture exists, it is a competition in the sense of trade-offs between these and other roles in accomplishing national goals. One role cannot be emphasized to the exclusion of another; each has its balanced and proper place.

15

Energy and Food

Malcolm Slesser

Energy Analysis Unit
Strathclyde University
Glasgow, Scotland

The Tsembaga are a New Guinea tribe who produce about 25 joules of metabolizable energy for each joule of input energy (1,2). The Americans are a highly sophisticated people using advanced technology, occupying about the same agricultural land area per caput as the Tsembaga, but who produce about 0.15 joules of metabolizable energy per joule of energy input (3). That is to say, the Tsembaga produce 166 times as much food per unit of input as do the Americans.

It is customary, of course, to regard the agriculture of developed countries as highly efficient, and so it seems, if the criterion is production per hectare or productivity per man directly employed. The American path has hidden costs, and the great abundance of food in that country is furnished, as in most developed countries, by the expenditure of very large amounts of fossil fuel energy. The problem facing the less developed countries is to decide in which direction they should go—the path taken by the Americans or that of the Tsembaga—or somewhere in between. This chapter will try to clarify the options by examining the relationships among energy, space, and food production.

ENERGY AND FOOD IN DEVELOPED COUNTRIES

Table I records some data for food production in six developed countries. Except in the case of spacious Australia, we see that, not only do they consume more energy than they produce in the form of metabolizable food, but the greater part of the energy is *not* spent on the process of growing food, but on

Table I. Energy Consumption in Food Production in Developed Countries

Country	Year	Energy to farm gate (1015 J)	Consumption, farm gate to dinner plate (1015 J)	Per year total (1015 J)	Energy ratio	Total as % national energy consumption	Source
U.S.A.	1963	2310	4125	6435	6.4	12	Hirst (3)
U.K.	1972	340	300	640	6.5	10	Blaxter[a]
Australia	1965/ 1969	87	121	208	.3	10	Gifford (2)
Israel	1969/ 1970	33	?	?	1.5	20	Stanhill (10)
Hong Kong	1971	?	?	7	?	26	Newcombe[b]
West Germany	1960	102	386	488	?	12	Estrup (11)

[a]Blaxter, K., personal communication, 1974.
[b]Newcombe, K., personal communication, 1974.

getting it from the farm gate to the dinner plate. Even so, the total energy use, although large, is but a small fraction of the total national energy budget. An exception is Hong Kong, where a large population occupies a small land area. Note, however, how large these figures are relative to energy requirement in developing countries.

In view of these facts, developed countries seeking to conserve energy are hardly likely to look at the agricultural sector, especially when the food processing and distribution sector is the bigger energy consumer. These countries, caught in the mesh of urbanization and centralization, will find it extremely difficult to reduce their energy demands for food production. Their agricultural technology will be driven by their inherited economic structure toward more, rather than less, energy-intensive systems. It is significant that the least centralized of these, Israel, shows a remarkable performance, considering its small agricultural land area.

Table II. Countries Reckoned to be Spending More than 80% of Their Energy Budget on the Food-Production System in 1967

Africa	Far East	Middle East	Americas
Ethiopia	Afghanistan	Sudan	Haiti
Kenya	Burma	U.A.R.	
Malawi	Cambodia		
Nigeria	Sri Lanka		
	Laos		
	Nepal		
	Pakistan		

Energy costs money, a fact that the oil-producing exporting countries sharply reminded the world of in the winter of 1973–74. Thus, although energy for food production may place a trifling burden on the rich, developed nations, it can place a severe burden on the more densely populated less developed ones, as in the example of India. U.S. agriculture uses more energy than the whole of the Indian economy does. Where arable land is limited, the only means of growing more food is through intensification. Table II lists a number of countries where, according to my reckoning, the energy requirements for self-sufficient food production could exceed 80% of the total energy budgets (4).

ENERGY REQUIREMENTS FOR FOOD PRODUCTION AND POPULATION

Left to themselves, natural systems cannot support high population densities. Intensification of land use demands an energy input in a manner that will be examined in detail in the next section. Look, for a moment, at the implications of increasing population on a finite area of land. Figure 1 depicts the relationship between population density, expressed as hectares of agricultural land per caput, and the computed minimum energy needed to provide both a survival diet of solely vegetable protein and the more luxurious diet of the average European. We see, for example, that at low intensities of land occupation, the energy demands are low, even for a high quality diet. Such is the situation in Australia,

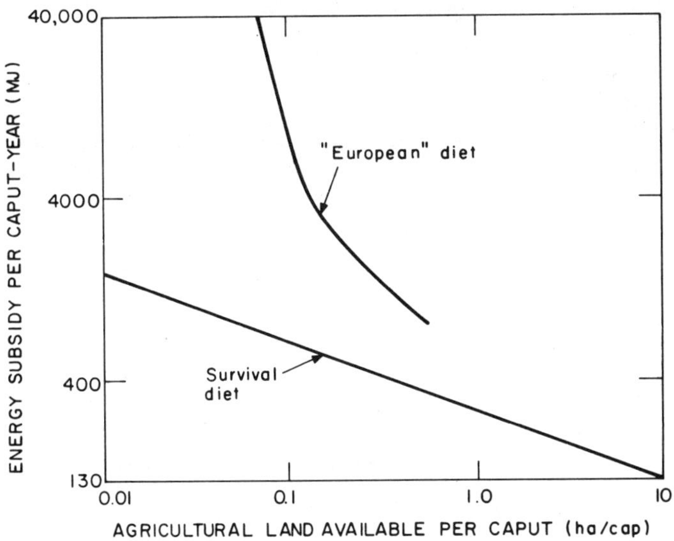

FIG. 1. Relationship between population density, expressed as hectares of agricultural land per caput, and computed minimum energy needed to provide a survival diet solely of vegetable protein in contrast to more luxurious diet of average European.

notwithstanding her developed economic system; this is reflected in the figures in Table I. By contrast, countries with occupation levels above 0.1 hectare per caput simply cannot hope to provide European levels of diet without spending prodigious amounts of energy. In fact, such countries, of which Japan is the best example, import large quantities of protein.

SYSTEMS VIEW OF FOOD PRODUCTION

Let us take a systems view of food production, as proposed in Figure 2. Into this model agricultural system, which for convenience is assumed to be one hectare in area, there fall the free goods of solar energy and rain, and the man-made inputs of fertilizers, tractors, pesticides, irrigation, and so forth. For any given agricultural system it is an easy matter to observe what inputs go into the system, and what outputs come from it. Because these inputs are many and varied, how do we express them relative to a single unit? A traditional way has been through their money value. Yet it is extremely difficult to compare money values in one part of the world with those in others. It is more convenient to relate the inputs to one physical property whose rates of exchange are fixed and well understood. Many of us who are looking at these matters have selected energy as that property.

There are many grounds for choosing energy. Berry (5), Odum (6), and many others including myself have argued that there is only one ultimate resource limitation in the world, and that is thermodynamic potential. This potential may be expressed in the thermodynamicist's language as *free energy*. For most situations, free energy is sufficiently close (usually within 10%) to the calorie value of fuels (6) to permit this well-known and understood value to be used for estimating thermodynamic potential.

For my part, I would recommend the use of energy for a further reason. Analyze the networks leading to the manufacture of any good, and it is found to

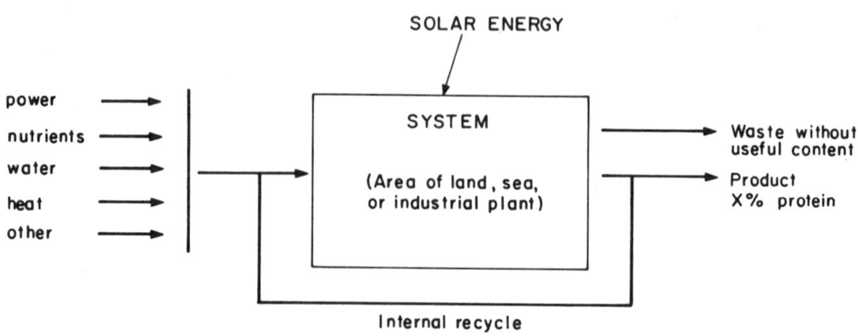

FIG. 2. Food-producing system.

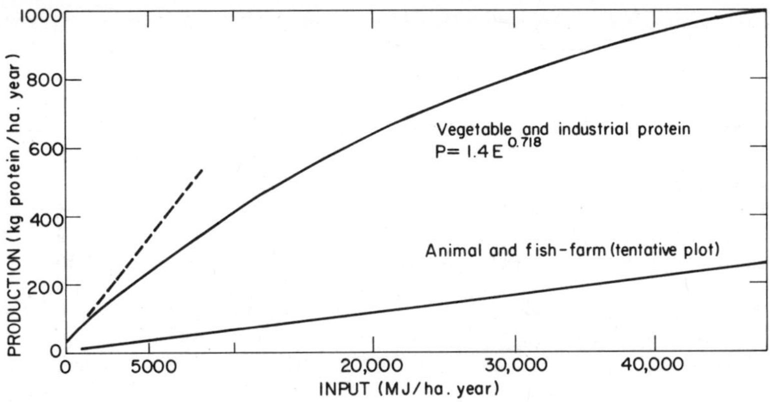

FIG. 3. 150 food-producing systems plotted in terms of their protein output per hectare vs. total inputs to the land, expressed as Mega joules energy sequestered per hectare.

be made from materials transformed by capital, labor, and energy. Analyze everything in the network, and in the last resort they are found to be transformed by labor and energy only.

Capital is merely labor and energy invested at an earlier time. Labor is renewable, and at the moment in surplus. Energy is nonrenewable, and very likely to be limited by cost and availability for many years to come. Perhaps forever.

Analysis in energy terms can be remarkably revealing. Pimentel's group at Cornell did a time series for U.S. corn production (7) and showed that as the production intensity rose, the actual energy ratio diminished. Leach (8) showed that so-called efficient British farming was actually fooling itself. For every man who works on a farm in the U.K., half a man is employed in the agricultural supply industries and six and a half are in the food-distribution industries.

In Figure 3, some 150 food-producing systems are plotted in terms of their protein output per hectare versus the total inputs to the land, expressed as Mega joules energy sequestered per hectare. The sources of the data vary from zero-input foraging cattle in the Peruvian Altiplano to some recently reported pilot plants for algae manufacture. Some assumptions, of course, had to be made in making these assessments. The energy equivalent of the physical inputs was taken from prior work (9). It was assumed that each case studied was backed by good husbandry.

There will be many conceptual objections to this plot. Genetic breeding gives higher yields? But higher yields still require greater inputs. Some crops are more productive than others? Certaintly, if one plots the metabolizable energy of the products versus the energy equivalents per hectare, a much more scattered

Table III. An Agricultural Taxonomy in Energy Terms

Examples	Energy intensity, Gjoule/hectare	Protein yields, kg/hectare
Hunter/gatherer	zero	–
Andean village (Peru)	.2	.5
Hill-sheep farming (Scotland)	.6	1–1.5
Marginal land farming	4	9
Open-range beef farming (New Zealand)	5	130
Mixed farm in developed country	12–15	500
Intensive crop production	15–20	2000
Feed lot animal production	40	300
Algae manufacture	1600	22,000

plot is found. But in terms of the protein, the relationship is much firmer, and the correlation statistically excellent.

We would not claim the last word in accuracy. Much more work needs to be done. The data for animal and fish protein are less certain. Nevertheless, the general trend seems beyond doubt. Intensification leads to diminishing returns per unit of energy input. What deductions may be made?

First, by expressing intensity of land use in energy terms, we find we may easily distinguish between marginal, developed, and highly developed agriculture (Table III), and those regions where the intensity is such that only industrial systems can function. Second, Figure 1, which arises directly from Figure 3, can be used for food policy planning. From it one may compute the minimum energy requirements of self-sufficiency at various levels of diet. Third, one may examine several routes to the same objective, and find which demands the least energy inputs.

AGRICULTURAL POLICY FOR DEVELOPING COUNTRIES

If we have proved the case that agricultural intensification calls for more and yet more energy, it follows that every nation should view its agricultural development, not only in terms of labor and land ownership policies, but in the provision of a safe and perpetual flow of energy to its agricultural sector, a sector that must embrace everything from scythes and tractors to lubricating oils and pesticides.

In the developed countries there has been a tendency to build up agricultural production by abandoning some land and intensifying use on the remainder. In a cheap energy world this was the inevitable thrust of competitive economics, in which each subsystem could optimize its own profit. In my view, the cheap energy world is gone for good. At the very best, we cannot expect to see cheaper energy sooner than 20 years after fusion reactors have proved commercially successful, a date that not even our children may witness. That date is certainly beyond the year 2010. Yet by then, present trends suggest we may have 8 billion people on this planet. For Latin America that would mean a 150% increase of its present population. The agricultural land area per caput will have fallen to 40% of its present value. The inputs will have had to triple in order to provide even the present level of food.

These are serious problems, and we should ask if there is another way of furnishing food. Figure 3 suggests there is another way. It is by reclaiming land and in giving an incentive to use those small parcels of land so typical of the Andean regions. We have set the heavy initial investment in developing new land against the lower level of inputs that the greater total area of land will permit. This process requires a conscious decision to control the intensification of existing good land to such levels, or by such means, that the marginal land will remain viable. There are many of us in Europe who wish that the European community would see it that way as well.

CONCLUSION

Energy analysis provides the key to looking into the future. Money will be the basis for how each of us individually assesses his criteria for action. Energy, I suggest, is a better yardstick for society as a whole. No country should attempt to apply the information in Figures 1 and 3 directly to its own situation. Rather, each country should set out to construct such relationships to the agriculture in its own nation. They will be surprised at the results that emerge. The methodology of energy analysis is now well worked out (6). We have a pragmatic basis for making decisions.

I have estimated that the participants of the International Biological Symposium flew some 322,000 miles by jet, which, judged on a passenger-mile basis, consumed enough energy to furnish 30,000 Guatemalans with a year's supply of corn. It is up to the participants to produce at least that much extra food from their discussions.

REFERENCES

1. Rappoport, R. A., 1967, *Pigs for the ancestors: Ritual in the ecology of a New Guinea people*, Yale University Press, New Haven, Connecticut.
2. Gifford, R. M., and Millington, R. J., 1973, Paper presented at UNESCO–Man and the Biosphere Symposium, Flinders University, Australia, May 15–18.
3. Hirst, E., 1974, Food-related energy requirements, *Science* **184**: 134–138.
4. Howell, J., and Slesser, M., 1973, An alternative approach to relative indices of development of nation states, *Technol. Forecast. Soc. Change* **5**: 253–264.

5. Berry, R. S., and Fels, M. F., 1972, The production and consumption of automobiles: An energy analysis, Report of the Illinois Institute for Environmental Quality.
6. International Federation of Institutes of Advanced Study, 1974, Workshop on Methodology of Energy Analysis, Nobel House, Stockholm.
7. Pimentel, D., 1973, Food production and the energy crisis, *Science* **182**: 443–449.
8. Leach, G., 1975, *in: The man-food equation*, Academic Press, London.
9. Leach, G., and Slesser, M., 1973, Energy equivalents of network inputs to food producing processes, Report, University of Strathclyde, Glasgow.
10. Stanhill, G., 1974, Energy and agriculture, Paper presented at the International Seminar, Heat and Mass Transfer in the Environment of Vegetation, held in Dubrovnik, Yugoslavia.
11. Estrup, G., 1974, Industrial marketing management, *Elsevier* **3**: 193.

16

Energy and Food: A Comment

David Pimentel

Department of Entomology and Sectional Ecology and Systematics
Cornell University
Ithaca, New York

I would like to add to the points raised by Slesser in Chapter 15 and summarize my own view of the critical situation that faces the world. As a result of overpopulation, energy shortages, and environmental degradation, the world is fast losing its capacity to feed itself. By 1976 the world population is expected to reach 4 billion, and, based upon projected growth rates, the world population will reach about 7 billion by the year 2000 (1). This rapid growth in world population coincides with the exponential use of fossil fuels. These have been used extremely effectively by man to manipulate and manage his environmental resources.

Energy is used for disease-control operations and to increase food production to feed mankind's growing numbers. Long before man relied heavily upon fossil energy for food production, he depended upon his own initiative as a hunter and gatherer to obtain food for himself and his family. As human numbers increased, many habitat regions could no longer support a hunting and gathering economy. A shift had to be made to a more permanent type of agriculture (2). "Slash and burn" or "cut and burn" agriculture was the first technology employed; i.e., cutting trees and brush and burning them on the land to be cultivated. This practice killed weeds and added nutrients to the soil. Crop production on the prepared land was good for 2 or 3 years, then soil nutrients were depleted. Once this happened, about 20 years were required for the forest to regrow and renew soil nutrients. Hence, about a 20-year rotation was necessary with slash and burn agriculture.

Table I. Energy Inputs in Corn Production in Mexico Using Only Manpower

Input	Quantity/ha	kcal/ha
Labor[a]	1,144 hrs	622,622
Ax + hoe[b]	16,500 kcal	16,500
Seeds[c]	10.4 kg	36,608
Total		675,730
Corn yield[a]	1,944 kg	6,842,880
kcal return/kcal input		10.13

[a]Reference 3 (See Table III in this paper for labor energy input).
[b]Ax and hoe assumed to weigh 4 kg/ha and last 5 years (20,700 kcal/kg for construction).
[c]10.4 kg X 3,520 kcal/kg = 36,608 kcal.

The slash and burn crop technology required few tools (ax and hoe) and many man-hours. For example, Lewis (3) investigated slash and burn corn culture in a part of Mexico and reported that a total of 1144 hours of labor were required to raise 1 hectare of corn (Table I). Other than manpower, the only inputs were the ax, hoe, and seeds. Similar data were obtained for corn production in Guatemala (Table II).

The yield of 1944 kg per hectare in Mexico provided about 6.8 million kilocalories. Allowing for 3000 kcal of corn per person per day, this yield was

Table II. Energy Inputs in Corn Production in Guatemala Using Only Manpower

Input	Quantity/ha	kcal/ha
Labor[a]	1,415 hrs	770,114
Ax + hoe[b]	16,500 kcal	16,500
Seeds[c]	10.4 kg	36,608
Total		823,222
Corn yield[d]	1,066 kg	3,752,320
kcal return/kcal input		4.56

[a]Corn production in San Pedro Necta, Guatemala; infertile Llano soil (reference 8). See Table III in this paper for labor energy input.
[b]Ax and hoe assumed to weigh 4 kg/ha and last 5 years (20,700 kcal/kg for construction).
[c]10.4 kg X 3,520 kcal/kg = 36,608 kcal.
[d]Reference 8.

suitable for more than six persons for one year. Obviously, an individual cannot live on corn alone and requires some additional food to meet his daily nutrient needs. The total hours per person per year to produce the food required were 190, or about five weeks of work. This was about 10% of his annual work effort.

When man started harnessing fossil fuel for crop production, agriculture was revolutionized. Great changes occurred in agricultural production and a significantly larger number of people could be supported per hectare. Despite the rapid growth of human population numbers, the use of energy has been increasing faster. For example, while it took the last 60 years for the U.S. population to double, its energy consumption has doubled just during the past 20 years. More alarming is the fact that, while world population doubled in about 30 years, its energy consumption doubled within the past decade.

Energy use in food production has been increasing faster than many other sectors of the world economy. For example, using corn as an average crop (4) we documented that energy inputs in corn production more than tripled (Table III) between 1945 and 1970. Note that the quantity of energy used to produce nitrogen fertilizer during 1970 nearly equaled all of the energy inputs for 1945. The other large inputs of energy came from machinery (420,000 kcal); fuel (797,000 kcal); drying (120,000 kcal); and electricity (310,000 kcal).

Mechanical drying of corn was one factor that increased energy input significantly during this period. This, in part, is related to one of the methods used to increase corn yields. Corn with a longer growing season collects more light energy and converts this into more corn grain. Because of the longer growing season, the corn stands in the field later in the fall and does not have an opportunity to dry. Hence, the corn has to be dried by artificial heat before it is put into storage.

The total amount of fossil energy used to grow a hectare of corn in 1970 averaged about 742 liters of fuel (7.1 million kcal) (4). An estimated 134 million hectares were planted in crops in 1970 (excluding cotton and tobacco) (5,6). With about 200 million people in the United States, this averaged about .67 hectares per caput; however, because about 20% of our crops are exported, the estimate is calculated to be about .54 hectares per caput. In terms of fuel per person for food, employing modern agricultural technology, this is the equivalent of 401 liters of fuel per person (742 liters per hectare × .54 hectares per person = 401 liters per year). If we include processing, distribution, and home cooking, the total inputs per person for the food system are estimated to be 1200 liters of fuel equivalents per person per year. Using U.S. agricultural technology to feed a world population of 4 billion on an average U.S. diet for one year would require the energy equivalents of 4800 billion liters of fuel.

To gain some idea about what the energy needs would be for a diet if U.S. agricultural technology were employed, an estimate is made of how long it would take to deplete the known world reserves of petroleum. These have been

Table III. Energy Inputs in Corn Production (All Figures in kcal) (Revised after Pimentel and Co-Workers, Reference 4)

Inputs	1945	1950	1954	1959	1964	1970
Labor[a]	31,022	23,947	22,859	19,049	14,695	11,974
Machinery[b]	446,600	617,500	741,000	864,500	1,037,400	1,037,400
Fuel[c]	1,339,800	1,521,630	1,703,460	1,789,590	1,885,290	1,971,420
Nitrogen[d]	140,800	299,200	528,000	809,600	1,144,000	2,200,000
Phosphorus[e]	25,520	35,090	41,470	57,420	63,800	111,650
Potassium[f]	13,200	24,200	44,000	74,800	101,200	147,400
Seeds for planting[g]	77,440	91,520	112,640	133,760	147,840	147,840
Irrigation[b]	103,740	128,440	148,200	170,430	187,720	187,720
Insecticides[h]	0	2,662	8,228	18,876	27,104	27,104
Herbicides[i]	0	1,452	2,662	6,776	10,406	27,104
Drying[b]	9,880	34,580	74,100	163,020	247,000	296,400
Electricity[b]	79,040	133,380	247,000	345,800	501,410	765,700
Transportation[b]	49,400	74,100	111,150	148,200	172,900	172,900
Total inputs	2,314,442	2,987,701	3,784,769	4,601,821	5,540,765	7,104,612
Corn yield (output)[j]	7,504,640	8,388,160	9,053,440	11,922,240	15,012,800	17,881,600
kcal return/kcal input	3.24	2.81	2.39	2.59	2.71	2.52

[a] It is assumed that a farm laborer consumes 21,770 kcal per week and works a 40-hour week. For 1970: (22 hours/40 hours) × 21,770 kcal = 11,974 kcal.
[b] See Table I, reference 4.
[c] Fuel, 1 liter = 9,570 kcal (reference 9).
[d] Nitrogen, 1 kg = 17,600 kcal, including production and processing (reference 10).
[e] Phosphorus, 1 kg = 3,190 kcal, including mining and processing (reference 10).
[f] Potassium, 1 kg = 2,200 kcal, including mining and processing (reference 10).
[g] Corn seed, 1 kg = 3,520 kcal (reference 11). This energy input was doubled because of the effort employed in producing hybrid seed corn.
[h] Insecticides, 1 kg = 24,200 kcal, including production and processing (similar to herbicide; see *i*).
[i] Herbicides, 1 kg = 24,200 kcal, including production and processing (reference 12).
[j] Each kg of corn was assumed to contain 3,520 kcal (reference 11).

estimated to be 86,912 billion liters (7). If we assume that 76% of raw petroleum can be converted into fuel (7), this would equal a usable reserve of 66,053 billion liters. If petroleum were the *only* source of energy and if we used *all* petroleum reserves solely to feed the world population, the 66,053 billion-liter reserve would last a mere 14 years–(66,053 billion liters/4800 billion liters = 14 years).

REFERENCES

1. National Academy of Sciences, 1971, *Rapid population growth*, NAS, Volumes I, II, Johns Hopkins Press, Baltimore, 105 pp; 690 pp.
2. Boserup, 1965, *Conditions of agricultural growth*, Aldine-Atherton, Chicago, 124 pp.
3. Lewis, O., 1951, *Life in a Mexican village: "Tepoztlán revisited,* University of Illinois Press, Urbana, 512 pp.
4. Pimentel, D., Hurd, L. E., Bellotti, A. C., Forster, M. J., Oka, I. N., Sholes, O. D., and Whitman, R. J., 1973, Food production and the energy crisis, Science **182:** 443–449.
5. U.S. Department of Agriculture, 1972, Changes in farm production and efficiency, USDA, Econ. Res. Ser. Stat. Bull. 233, Washington, D.C., 31 pp.
6. U.S. Department of Agriculture, 1968, Extent of farm pesticide use on crops in 1966, USDA, Agric. Econ. Rep. 147, Econ. Res. Ser. 23 pp.
7. Jiler, H., 1972, Commodity Yearbook, Commodity Res. Bur., Inc., New York.
8. Stadelman, R., 1940, *Maize cultivation in northwestern Guatemala*, Compiled by the Carnegie Institution of Washington, Contributions to American Anthropology and History, No. 33. Carnegie Institution of Washington Publications **523:** 83–263.
9. *Handbook of chemistry and physics*, 1972, The Chemical Rubber Co., Cleveland, Ohio, Table D-230.
10. Leach, G., and Slesser, M., 1973, *Energy equivalents of network inputs to food producing processes*, Strathclyde University, Glasgow, 38 pp.
11. U.S. Department of Agriculture, 1963, Composition of Foods, USDA Consumer and Food Economics Res. Div., ARS, USDA, Agr. Handbook No. 8, 190 pp.
12. Pimentel D., Mooney, H., and Stickel, L., 1976, Panel Report for Environmental Protection Agency, in press.

17

Balancing the Benefits and Risks of the Application of Science to Agriculture and Food Production

William J. Darby

The Nutrition Foundation, Inc.
New York and Washington, D.C.

Much as been stated in this volume concerning science and technology in relation to food production and the "strategy of science"—the essentiality of relating science to needs recognized at the grass-roots level. These societal considerations cannot be measured by production figures alone; they must be recognized in any strategy of applied science. They are benefit:cost and benefit: risk as conceived by the consumer, the producer, and the politician, not necessarily as conceived by the scientist.

What is benefit:cost? It is all the benefits and costs of a proposed action—a much broader concept than traditional cost:benefit analysis, which includes only economic considerations.

What is benefit:risk? It is that category of benefit:cost in which risk to life and health are important components of cost.

What is benefit? It is anything that contributes to an improvement in condition; risk is the chance of injury, damage, or loss.

In the analyses of benefit:cost and benefit:risk, in technology assessment of all sorts, it is obviously necessary to deal with uncertainty. Nevertheless, it should be noted that even when uncertainties, in a statistical sense, are resolved, risks to life and health are present in many individual and collective activities.

A consideration in technology assessment is public benefit versus individual (or private) risk. This consideration is inherent in vastly diverse types of decisions. For example, should we continue smallpox vaccinations? Should iodization of salt be mandatory? Should a man's home be destroyed to make way for a new, safer highway?

Societal activities that result in risks or benefits are of two categories—those in which the individual participates on a voluntary basis, and those in which the participation is involuntary; i.e., imposed by the society in which the individual lives—imposed by law, regulation, social custom, and religion.

Chauncey Starr (1), from a broad analysis of benefit:costs in sociotechnological systems, concludes that: (a) an upper guide in determining the acceptability of risk is the rate of death from disease; (b) a base guide for risk tends to be set by natural disasters; (c) societal acceptance of risk increases in a nonlinear manner with the benefits to be derived from an activity; (d) public acceptance of voluntary risks is some 1000 times greater than that of involuntary risks; (e) societal policy for the acceptance of public risks associated with sociotechnical systems should be determined by the trade-off between social benefits and personal risk.

This volume is largely devoted to the benefits, sometimes vital, sometimes nonvital, of the application of science to food production in agricultural and animal husbandry practices; in storage, preservation, distribution and use; in industrial processing and marketing, quality control, regulatory protection, and standardization. These scientific developments include public and individual benefits and risks, vital and nonvital, voluntary and involuntary, regulated or controlled and uncontrolled.

While it is reasonable to conclude that no country has maximally utilized all of the potential applications to food of new scientific technology, it is apparent that the largest abundance of food and freedom from want are in those countries where scientific technology has been most intensively developed and applied. Systems of dealing with the applications of scientific technology have been evolved, but not perfected.

The impacts of applications of science are reflected in measurable indices of health. For example, in the United States the industrialization of food production at all levels—with concomitant awareness of nutritional needs and safety—has been accompanied by a virtual disappearance from that country within this century of the classical deficiency diseases: pellagra, scurvy, rickets, endemic goiter, protein deficiency. By contrast, in many regions where food production and distribution systems are primitive, famine recurrently strikes and high death and morbidity rates continue because of pellagra, iodine-deficiency goiter, protein-calorie malnutrition, folic acid or iron deficiency anemia, vitamin A deficiency and resultant blindness. These exist in concert with severe and deadly food-borne infections.

Unwise regulatory or legislative constraints that prevent the application of science and technologic knowledge to increasing or improving food production and prevention of spoilage or losses can have disastrous world consequences.

Such risks as may result from not having the benefit of an agent should be weighed in decision-making against whatever risks, certain or uncertain, may be judged to pertain from laboratory findings in relation to any particular useful agent. What are the risks of divesting ourselves of the useful agent? Can we afford them? What are the trade-offs? Can we justify denying the benefits of use because of postulated extrapolation of experimental findings to man? Who are "we"? Scientists? I have long maintained that:

> even a broad, rationally viewed scientific perspective is insuffifcient to resolve many issues. Scientists alone cannot make decisions and enforce policy. Value judgments seldom if ever are founded on science and strict logic. They cannot be made solely on nutritional or, indeed, even toxicologic considerations. These considerations should enter into formulation of value judgments, but often do not. Value judgments made by individuals or society are composites of attitudes determined by history, by cultural experiences, by religious and ethical influences, by economic forces, and by needs. They vary with social grouping and with time. They determine the personal satisfaction of the individual and condition his way of life. It is only recently that scientific considerations have consciously entered into the making of such judgments (2).

What is the nature of the ethical problem related to food safety? The Citizens' Commission on Science, Law and the Food Supply defines it as follows (3):

> The central issue:
>
> To what extent should consumers be exposed to either known or possible added risks of various potentially toxic substances, including carcinogens, mutagens and teratogens in their foods? [To this we might add, "to shortages, increased costs, or deficiencies?"]
>
> Preliminary statements of an ethical guideline:
>
> Our guideline should reflect the proper ethics in the face of uncertainty.
>
> When faced with alternatives, we should choose that alternative whose permitted worst outcome is better than the worst outcome of any other alternative, where "worst outcome" is defined as a cumulative net balance of risks and benefits.
>
> The upper limit of the overall risk should be no greater following a change than the risk of natural disease demonstrated to be causally related to existing patterns of food use.
>
> Consumer risk is not an isolated event.
>
> Risk in food is one part of a closely-knit set of values fixed in modern man's life-style. Therefore, no useful answer to the question of acceptable risk to man can be given without taking into account the other parts of the whole life-style pattern.

The Citizens' Commission further defines the expression of the ethical problems in government regulation and the ethics of accomodation as follows:

> Government Regulation and the Ethics of Accomodation:
>
> Formation of policy decisions should rest upon the assumption that questions of policy are not solely scientific questions but are matters which also must involve society's value judgments.

> If these were solely scientific, then the scientists should propose the policy.
>
> Part of the dilemma is that scientists disagree among themselves over the meaning of some of the crucial data; such disagreements may stem from
>
> a. the scientists' lack of breadth of outlook
> b. use of an unsuitable or inappropriate model
> c. unjustified extrapolation of experimental conditions to real-life situations
> d. honest disagreement over implications of scientific data.
>
> Another part is that the conclusions that can be drawn from all available data are often uncertain.
>
> Under present circumstances, a single experiment by a single laboratory investigator can provide the basis for removing a product from the market. Scientific consensus is needed on how much experimentation is appropriate.
>
> Facts do not necessarily assess themselves; they need to be evaluated and interpreted in terms of some basic values to which our society is committed. . . .
>
> The decision of the acceptable risk should be made at two levels: (a) legislative: broad general guidelines should be defined by Congress; (b) administrative: specific decisions should be made by the appropriate administrative agency with the support of advisory boards as decribed above . . . and with the assistance of competent surveys of consumer expectations.
>
> Policy decisions should represent a consistent, coherent and rational ordering of the concerns of the four interest groups (consumers, producers, scientists and the general public . . .).
>
> In the end, the definition of acceptable risk should be hammered out in terms of clear rational principle, taking into account all the relevant interrelations and having in mind the need for periodic review and revision of regulations as new information and uses emerge.
>
> To achieve these objectives, regulatory agencies should be supported by highly competent, independent advisory boards whose members are drawn from a variety of professions and activities and whose disciplines or careers have prepared them to deal with either the special problems or the social problems.

Only within the framework of such broadly conceived deliberations can society balance the benefits and risks of the application of science to agriculture and food production. Failure to do so ultimately can lead to serious impairment of productivity and to degeneration of the nutritional health of people throughout the world.

REFERENCES

1. Starr, C., 1972, Benefit-cost studies in sociotechnical systems, *in: Perspectives on benefit-risk decision making, report of a colloquium conducted by the Committee on Public Engineering Policy, National Academy of Engineering, April 26–27, 1971*, The National Academy of Engineering, Washington, D.C., 1972, pp. 17–42.
2. Darby, W. J., 1973, Acceptable risk and practical safety. Philosophy in the decision-making process. *J. Am. Med. Assoc.* **224** (8): 1165–1168.
3. Citizens' Commission on Science, Law and the Food Supply, 1974, *A report on current ethical considerations in the determination of acceptable risk with regard to food and food additives*, 25 March, Rockefeller University, 1230 York Avenue at 66th Street, New York, New York.

COMMENT

A.E. Olszyna-Marzys · *Division of Food Control and Analysis, Institute of Nutrition of Central America and Panama, Guatemala City, Guatemala.*

The key word in the title of Darby's chapter was *balance*—balancing the benefits of the use of fertilizers, pesticides, and food additives in agriculture and food industry, without which feeding today's world population would have been clearly impossible, against risks that should be equally obvious, taking into account the fact that every chemical is potentially toxic to man or his environment. Yet, perhaps no problem that we face today has been characterized by as much imbalance of rhetoric on both sides. From organic food faddism to the DDT controversy, more extreme views have been expressed and stronger emotions stirred by otherwise reasonable and intelligent people than in almost any other field of human activity today.

The pesticide problem has constituted the noisiest part of this controversy. The "father of the green revolution," Norman Borlaug, has referred to those advocating limitation of the use of pesticides as "sentimental environmentalists," accusing them of basing their campaign on emotion, not reason.

If such attitudes persist, what hope is there of producing the proper milieu for concerted action between agricultural economists who want to produce more food at any price and the environmentalists who want to save the bald eagle from extinction, even if they see people dying from hunger in the meantime?

In the course of a project investigating various aspects of the use of insecticides in Central America a few years ago, we came across the striking fact that some Guatemalan mothers' breast milk was contaminated with persistent organochlorine pesticides, particularly DDT. The highest valid contamination figure found in the Western world prior to our study was 0.37 parts per million (1). Our results from three localities in the southern region of Guatemala are summarized in Table I. Our *lowest* result was higher than the *highest* ever found in Europe, apart from Russia, or the United States; most samples had several ppm, and two isolated cases showed around 12 ppm.

The U.S. and international permissible allowance of DDT in cow's milk is only 0.05 ppm. Samples taken very recently at other localities in Guatemala, as well as some of our preliminary results from the milk of mothers living in cotton-growing areas of El Salvador, indicate a similar order of magnitude for DDT contamination. Table II shows that cow's milk in one of the same Guatemalan localities from which mothers' milk was taken and analyzed by an identical method had a pesticide content within permissible levels. These cow's milk samples contained 40 to 50 times less residual organochlorine pesticides than the human milk samples, except for one highly contaminated sample.

What do these results mean? Nursing children living in those localities of Guatemala from which we took human milk samples consumed between 6 and

Table I. Range and Average Content of DDT in Human Milk in Three Guatemalan Localities[a]

Locality	Cotton area?	Number of samples	DDT total (ppm)				
			minimum	maximum	SD	average	± SE
La Bomba[b]	no	9	0.411	1.77	0.80	1.11	± 0.27
Cerro Colorado[c]	yes	8	1.57	6.68	1.81	3.06	± 0.64
El Rosario	yes	27	0.342	4.97	1.25	1.84	± 0.24

[a]Translated from p. 102, reference 1.
[b]Excluding one sample with 11.50 ppm of DDT.
[c]Excluding one sample with 12.21 ppm of DDT.

207 times–not a *little* more–but 6 to 207 times the acceptable daily intake (ADI) of 5 micrograms of DDT per kilo of body weight per day considered allowable by FAO/WHO.

"Yes, but what does *that* mean?" we are asked. "Have you done any morbidity and mortality studies in those localities to find a correlation between the DDT content of mothers' milk and death or illness rates?" The answer is no; all our efforts to obtain funds for such a study have so far remained fruitless. Besides, it is doubtful whether we could sufficiently isolate that effect from those of malnutrition and infection prevailing in the area to be able to attribute any higher morbidity and mortality to DDT.

One answer is that workers in factories producing DDT, and sprayers exposed to large amounts of it, and who have a DDT content in blood and fat exceeding by a hundred times or more that of average populations, have never shown any ill effects. Still, these are adults, and most are reasonably well fed. Do we really know what chronic effect it may have on a child who has consumed, during the first 10 months or so of his life, mother's milk containing a hundred times the maximum amount considered safe for adults in serious toxicological studies?

When we first presented our results, it was suggested that what we had probably shown was merely that Guatemalan children have developed a wonderful enzymatic system to cope with the insult presented by DDT. I ardently hope that is the case, because in the two years since our results have been published there has been, until very recently, practically no interest whatsoever in them. I have yet to receive any comment at all from the strong advocates of breast feeding.

The recent interest developed when the high content of DDT in Guatemalan and other Central American meat exported to the United States brought about the rejection of whole shipments at the ports of entry. The Central American cattle raisers were so alarmed that they started a concerted campaign to introduce legislation regulating the use of pesticides. Our results were then exten-

Table II. Organo-Chlorine Pesticides in Samples of Cow's Milk in La Bomba, Department of Santa Rosa, Guatemala (ppm)[a]

Sample number[b]	DDT	DDE	DDD	DDT	DDT total	HCH total	Heptachloroepoxide	Dieldrin	Endrin
LB-9	0.005	0.006	TR	0.002	0.013	0.003	0.001	0.001	–
LB-10	0.002	0.006	–	–	0.008	TR	TR	TR	TR
LB-11	0.011	0.014	0.001	0.001	0.027	TR	TR	TR	TR
LB-14	TR	0.002	–	–	0.002	–	–	–	–
LB-16	0.045	0.005	0.005	0.022	0.077	0.002	TR	TR	0.002
Range	TR–0.045	0.002–0.014	0–0.005	0–0.022	0.002–0.077	0–0.003	0–0.001	0–0.001	0–0.002
Average	0.013	0.007	0.001	0.005	0.025	0.001	TR		TR
SD	0.023	0.004	0.002	0.010	0.030	0.001			
SE	0.010	0.002	0.001	0.004	0.013	< 0.001 (0.0003)			

[a]Translated from p. 102, reference 1.
[b]Number of samples = 5.

sively used to support claims for the urgent necessity of such regulation, and it led, in April of 1974, to the introduction of comprehensive legislation in Guatemala regulating the use of pesticides, including limitations to the use of DDT. To that extent I am glad we helped a little, even if the motive for governmental action was the cattlemen's pockets and not their workers' children's health.

The main opposition to any limitation in the use of insecticdes came from the cotton growers, who use at least 70% of all pesticides. Other Central American cotton growers should look to Nicaragua and see how growers there have begun to cope successfully with this problem. In Nicaragua, the answer to decreasing cotton yields caused by resistance of pests to insecticides that exterminated their natural enemies used to be to increase the quantity, variety, and frequency of application of chemical insecticdes, from 10 sprayings per season to as many as 30 or 40. The result was still further decreases in cotton yields to show for their efforts–to such an extent that the whole industry was threatened with extinction. I am reminded of an analogous situation to which Lester Brown (2) referred; namely, that increased investment in the fishing industry has had a counterproductive effect on fish catches.

In the late 1960s, with technical guidance obtained from the University of California at Davis, a program of integrated control, based on careful biological studies, was begun, combining severely limited use of pesticides with the introduction of pest-attacking viruses, bacteria, chemisterilants, insect sex attractants, and reintroduction of natural predators. This has had the dramatic effect of tripling the yield of cotton within a few years, while reducing the amount of chemical insecticides used by a very substantial margin. At the same time, the carefully monitored DDT content of meat for export has shown a significant decrease.

The first postgraduate program in applied ecology, related mainly to the cotton-growing industry, was held recently at the National University of Nicaragua. The enthusiastic collaboration and the developing interest and understanding of the other professional's field of activity and point of view, among entomologists, biologists, agronomists, and chemists taking part in the course, both students and professors, was very encouraging and suggests that, given proper incentive and good leadership, opposing views can sometimes blend into a harmonious mix. May it not be an isolated example.

References

1. Olszyna-Marzys, A. E., de Campos, M., Farvar, M. T., and Thomas, M., 1973, Residuos de plaguicidas clorados en la leche humana en Guatemala, *Bol. Of. Sanit. Panam.* 74 (2): 93–107 (Feb.).
2. Brown, L., 1975, Man, food and environmental interrelationships, *in: Nutrition and agricultural development–Significance and potential for the tropics,* Plenum, New York, pp. 3–12.

III

Problems in the Postharvest Conservation, Processing, and Distribution of Food

18

Postharvest Losses—Impact of Their Prevention on Food Supplies, Nutrition, and Development*

H. A. B. Parpia

Food and Agriculture Industries Services, Agricultural Services Division
Food and Agriculture Organization of the United Nations
Rome, Italy

Never has so much food been produced before and never has there been so much food shortage and starvation. The need for prevention of food losses through proper handling, storage conservation, milling, and processing has received some attention at the World Food Conference as part of the immediate and long-range effort to improve food supplies. The impact that the prevention of food losses can make on food supplies, present and future, and the return this can bring by way of additional income and employment deserve greater attention. A systematic effort in this direction would not only contribute to increasing food supplies quantitatively and qualitatively, but bring greater value to the grower and better food to the consumer, and raise employment; it would also help to increase self-sufficiency and foreign exchange earnings and stimulate agroeconomic development as a whole. While much more comprehensive data are required on this subject of storage losses, there have already been a sufficient number of studies carried out to indicate the magnitude of the problem.

The figures given in Table I (1–7) are indicative of the urgent need to reduce these losses. The projected estimate for production of cereals by 1985 is 650 million tons, and that for grain legumes nearly 45 million tons. At a conservative estimate, even if 6% of the losses of these foods could be prevented through the use of appropriate technologies for storage, handling, milling, processing, and distribution, it would amount to nearly 43 million tons of food, valued at 7,140

*The views expressed in this article represent the personal opinion of the author.

Table I. Some Estimates of Losses in Different Countries

Country	Material	Loss: Percentage[a]	Loss: Value	Reference
Nigeria	Sorghum	46		(1)
	Cow pea	41		
United States	Stored grain		$ 500 million	
	Packed food		150 million	(2)
	All crops		3500 million	
India	All grains			
	Field loss	25		
	Storage loss	15		
	Handling & processing loss	7		(3)
	Other losses	3		
Germany	Harvested grain		DM 71.4 million	(4)
Sierra Leone	Rice	41		(5)
	Maize	14		(6)
Tropical Africa	All crops (storage and handling)	30		(7)

[a]These percentages refer to postharvest losses unless otherwise stated. Although the figures refer to specific crops in most cases, they are sufficiently indicative to lay emphasis on the problem of food losses.

million dollars annually, considering an average price of cereals to be $150 and $300 per ton for grain legumes. If this estimate is correct, then even an expenditure of 2 billion dollars per year over the next five years to achieve this objective would be justified.

The United Nations Secretary-General, in his Strategy Statement on Action to Avert the Protein Crisis in Developing Countries, stressed that it would be irrational to concentrate only on producing more food while ignoring the sizable preventable losses due to insects, rodents, birds, molds, and, in some countries, monkeys, both in the field and at various postharvest stages. He urged a determined and well-financed campaign against food losses, which could more than eliminate food deficits in many countries (8). Moreover, the return from investments to prevent losses would bring greater benefits, at a much faster pace, than perhaps any other single effort.

MAGNITUDE OF RODENT INFESTATION LOSSES

Among the agents responsible for loss of food in the field and during storage, rodents appear to take the largest toll. The potential for the reproduction of rats represents a staggering figure. They breed at the age of 3 to 4 months and continue to do so up to the age of 18 months. The period of gestation is 21–25 days. The females come into heat about every 5 days and can breed within a day after giving birth. A female averages 3 to 5 litters of 8 to 10 young ones each. Many of them die, but in one year a pair can often produce 60–70 offspring that survive to maturity. It is fortunate that ecological conditions are not suitable for the survival of the entire rodent progeny, otherwise man might have been displaced from the earth. With increases in food production, the conditions for their survival are becoming more favorable, and therefore adequate measures are required for their control. There are a few surveys on losses caused by rodents both in the field and during storage of food grains, but the extent of damage that rodents can do is illustrated by some outstanding examples.

An emergency had to be declared on the island of Mindanao in the Philippines in 1953 when close to 70% of the crop was destroyed by rodents. A similar emergency was declared on the island of Madagascar in 1965 when 80% of the crop was destroyed by rodents. The studies carried out by Ramakrishna and co-workers (Tamil Nadu Agriculture University, Colmbatore, India, personal communication) have indicated that between 46 and 78% of a crop can be destroyed by rats. This damage can be done at different stages of growth, whether as freshly sown seed, seedlings, or half-blades, as well as during storage.

In a comprehensive study carried out in a single food grain warehouse in Calcutta, the population densities achieved by the lesser bandicoot rat were observed. The mean population estimated during an 11-month period was 190.7 rats, with a mean density of 0.8 rats per square meter (9). The adult female bandicoot rat averages 11.3 pregnancies per year and produces 69.9 young annually. Six adult rats eat daily enough food for one man. In India, with a rat population of up to 2,400 million, the losses are tremendous.

Control of rodents can be achieved by using the well-known technique of gaseous fumigation of burrows, combined with the newer method of liquid fumigation, specially suited for the varieties of rats that erect barriers in their burrows. Baiting should also be done simultaneously with the use of rodenticides such as norbromide, zinc phosphide, or barium carbonate incorporated into a low-protein bait. Safe methods for the employment of baits under rural conditions have been worked out so that no harm is done to children or farm animals. Physical methods of rodent control, such as trapping, are also quite successful. For effective control, a combination of such methods has to be worked out under different circumstances, based on a sound knowledge of rodent behavior.

Similarly, control of rodents in grain warehouses can be carried out with certain structural improvements to make them rodent-proof. A 10 cm rat guard skirting along a warehouse above ground level successfully prevents rodent entry. Where old warehouses are in use, they can also be made rat-proof by means of introducing a 15-cm polished band of cement on the surface of the wall at a height of about 1.5–2 meters around the whole building, and by separating the steps from the main structure by 50 cm. In addition to the use of well-accepted techniques for baiting, poisoning, fumigation of burrows, and other methods, it is possible to make the jute storage bags rodent-repellent by treating them with a composition of chemicals containing malathion in heavy oil.

INSECT INFESTATION CONTROL

Depending upon the type of food grain and the conditions of storage, the losses due to insect infestation vary between 10 and 40% (Table I). Nearly 40 to 70% of food grains are produced, consumed, and stored in rural areas under very unsatisfactory conditions. The climate for insect infestation in tropical countries is ideal and losses caused by insect infestation can be very high. The pulse beetle, for example, passes through eight overlapping generations in one year. The progeny of 40 eggs can reduce the weight of the infested grain by 49% in just six months, besides contaminating it with metabolites like uric acid. Chick peas with 15% kernel damage gave a milling yield, during their splitting, as low as 65%, as against 82% when insect damage to the grain was 2% (Table II) (10). Similarly, in the case of groundnuts, insect infestation results in reduction of viability, an increase in fatty acids, and lower oil extraction yields (Table III).

A number of techniques have been developed in different parts of the world for control of insect infestation during storage in tropical climates. Many of them have proved very successful. Mention may be made of the "Durofume process," which consists of fumigation of stacks of bagged food grain by a mixture of ethylene dibromide and methyl bromide; this effectively destroys both adult and immature insects. The mixture penetrates well because of its vapor pressure at warm temperatures. It is necessary to vary the percentage of ethylene dibromide and methyl bromide according to the food grains to be treated. One application per year is adequate to maintain the grains insect-free for over nine months. This treatment also keeps the microbial count low. The

Table II. Effect of Insect Infestation on Yield of Milled Chickpea (*Cicer arietinum*)[a]

Condition	% kernel damage	% yield
Uninfested	2	82
Infested by insects	15	65

[a]Reference 1.

Table III. Changes Effected by Storage and by Insects in Groundnut Kernels in 6 Months[a]

Insect responsible for damage	Kernel damage %	Viability %	Fat acidity as oleic acid %	Yield of oil %
T. castaneum	53.3	27.4	3.7	46.6
O. surinamensis	69.5	16.0	4.2	46.2
N. rufipes	71.9	25.6	3.8	46.5
Insect-free	–	88.2	1.6	49.2

[a]Source: *Food Science* (India) *6:* 30, 1957 (February).

cost of chemicals and application per ton of food grain is about U.S. $0.15. Reinfestation of the bags can be prevented by using pretreated bags with a special formulation developed for the purpose. It consists of a high viscosity, oil-based composition of chemicals that are insect-repellent. If malathion is included in the bag treatment as described earlier, even rodents are repelled.

Some of the safe and effective methods of infestation control worked out for rural areas follow.

1. Improvement in the traditional underground as well as overground structures could be achieved by using a heavy-gauge polyethylene film lining cemented with a coating of bituminized mud-plaster to prevent the moisture migration generally responsible for the growth of fungi.

2. Activated clay containing meta-hydrogen halloysite can be mixed in food grains to the extent of 0.5 to 1%. It removes the fatty layer from the surface of insects, which then die of dehydration. This treatment also keeps the food grains free from further infestation.

3. The addition of a 0.2% tricalcium phosphate mixture containing pyridoxine and glucose to food grains inhibits the growth of insects. Consumption of this mixture in small quantities by insects completely upsets their metabolism and metamorphosis. Besides being an insecticide, tricalcium phosphate serves as calcium and phosphorus enrichment for the grain (11).

4. Ethylene dibromide adsorbed on compressed paper or cardboard in the form of small tablets strip-packaged in laminated aluminum foil has proved successful in rural and household storage of food grains. These are also very effective in protecting seed material.

5. After disinfestation of food grains in jute bags has been carried out, it is necessary to take measures for preventing reinfestation. For this, a formulation known as Durobase 3, consisting of lindane, DDT, and malathion (rodent repellent) has been worked out. It has proved very effective when sprayed on stacks of food grain bags.

Table IV. Effect of Insect Infestation on the Chemical Composition of Kaffircorn, Wheat, Chickpea,[a] and Pigeon Pea Dhal (Period of Infestation, 2 Months)[b]

Material		Moisture %	Kernel damage %	Bulk density %	Frass %	Insects/ 100 g	FFA mg KOH/ 100 g	Uric acid Total mg/100 g	Uric acid Apparent mg/100 g	Uric acid True mg/100 g	Fungi colonies/g	Thiamine μg/g
Kaffircorn												
Jowar	Initial	9.71	0.0	0.76	0.0831	4	22.00	2.00	1.31	0.69	400	3.2
S. oryza	Control	11.38	1.0	0.63	0.2314	63	28.21	4.19	3.16	1.03	700	3.1
	Infested	13.29	23.0	0.63	0.6417	193	40.63	7.00	4.39	2.61	3100	2.7
Wheat	Initial	8.73	0.0	0.77	0.0473	0	21.61	1.93	0.60	0.33	200	5.0
S. oryza	Control	9.43	0.0	0.77	0.1713	0	27.64	2.43	1.10	1.33	800	5.0
	Infested	11.24	12.0	0.77	0.4171	156	33.80	2.71	1.10	1.61	3400	4.2
Chickpea												
B. G. Dhal	Initial	10.94	0.0	0.77	0.0933	0	76.17	1.32	0.91	9.41	300	5.5
Rhizopertha	Control	12.67	0.0	0.70	0.2743	4	87.62	2.29	1.37	0.92	700	5.4
and *Tribolium*	Infested	13.52	10.0	0.70	0.6891	30	104.70	6.48	4.39	2.09	2700	4.6
Pigeon pea												
R. G. Dhal	Initial	12.27	0.0	0.79	0.0847	0	69.43	4.43	3.91	0.52	300	4.3
Rhizopertha	Control	12.94	0.0	0.70	0.1313	3	74.66	9.88	5.51	4.37	800	4.2
and *Tribolium*	Infested	13.04	9.0	0.70	0.3394	255	89.65	11.23	6.83	4.40	3300	3.9

[a] *Cicer arietenum*.
[b] Source: Personal correspondence with Dr. M. Swaminathan and Mr. S. K. Majumder, Central Food Technological Research Institute, Mysore, India.

In rural areas where the percentage of literacy is low, there is great advantage in using activated clay and tricalcium phosphate as pesticides, as these grain protectants are nontoxic and safe.

A certain amount of precaution becomes necessary when ethylene dibromide tablets are used, however. Several other insecticides, such as aluminum phosphide tablets, have been used successfully, but they present a hazard because their toxic effects on humans are not easily detectable. Moreover, aluminum phosphide in permissible dosages is not very effective against certain insects, including *Sithophilus oryzae,* which happens to be the main infesting organism of rice.

Adverse effects of insect infestation on some foods are given in Tables IV and V, based on personal correspondence with Dr. M. Swaminathan of the Central Food Technological Research Institute, Mysore, India, and reference (12). These data show a reduction, not only in protein efficiency, but also in other nutrients and acceptability. Insect infestation also creates very favorable conditions for moisture absorption, which encourages fungal growth.

IMPROVEMENTS IN RICE-PROCESSING TECHNOLOGY

Inadequate technology used in the milling and processing of food grains and improper maintenance of equipment cause quite high losses. Many developing countries use outdated rice-milling equipment, maintained in an unsatisfactory manner in most cases. Many of the mills are so small that they cannot produce adequate quantities of by-products such as rice bran, which could be utilized efficiently. Table VI, based on studies in India, shows that it should be possible to raise the milling yield by 1.5–3.5%. If the rice-milling industry is modernized, even at the present level of rice production, many countries should be able to overcome almost half of their rice shortage.

Table V. Uric Acid Content, Kernel Damage, and Acceptability of Market Samples of Soft Wheat[a]

Number of samples tested	Uric acid range (mg/100 g)	Kernel damage, %		Organoleptic score[b] range
		Minimum	Maximum	
31	0–1	0	3.5	9–6
35	1.1–5	0	10.4	7–6
16	5.1–10	2.7	10.8	6–5
3	10.1–15	9.4	18.5	5–3

[a]Reference 12.
[b]Organoleptic scores of chapati (unleavened bread). Samples with scores higher than 4 are acceptable.

Table VI. Average Milling Yields of Rice from Paddy in Conventional and Modern Mills

Type of mills	Raw		Parboiled	
	Total rice %	Head rice %	Total rice %	Head rice %
Modern rubber roller mills	72.5	55	73.5	70
Conventional disc sheller mills	71.0	50	73.0	68
Engelberg type "huller" mills	69.0	45	72.0	66

Most developing countries are very short of fats and oils as well as cattle feed, and rice bran is an excellent potential source for all of these. If the rice mills are large enough, or if several can be grouped together to obtain at least 10 tons of bran per day, this would make it possible to set up an economical unit for solvent extraction of the oil. If the bran is extracted soon after milling, there is no problem of hydrolytic rancidity, which develops early during storage because of lipase activity or microbial contamination.

Whenever a number of small mills are located at long distances from the solvent extraction plants, the lipase can be inactivated by suitable treatment. Rice bran contains 15–18% fat that could help to meet the urgent need for calories in the Indian diet. Furthermore, extracted rice bran containing about 15% protein could be used efficiently for the manufacture of composite cattle feed to produce additional animal food for human consumption.

PARBOILING

Over 50% of the 40 million tons of rice produced in India, and almost the entire rice production of Bangladesh, is consumed in parboiled form. The traditional processing consists of soaking paddy for two to three days, followed by steaming, drying, and milling. This has the advantage of fixing the vitamins present in the peripheral bran layers into the kernel. The traditional practice, however, has several disadvantages in that the product develops an off-odor from microbial fermentation and also results in production of mycotoxins. While several sophisticated processes of parboiling exist, a simpler process has been developed that consists of soaking paddy at 70°C for four to five hours, steaming, and mechanically drying. This not only speeds up the process, but yields a product of high quality. If larger quantities of rice were parboiled, it would not only improve the nutritional quality of the rice diets through making more vitamins of the B group available in the rice, but also reduce considerably the breakage during milling. By this means beriberi can be eliminated without vitamin fortification (13). Modern techniques of parboiling also eliminate the need for sun-drying and the losses caused by birds during this process.

LEGUMES

Grain legumes are an important source of protein in most developing countries. Because they are rich in lysine, they provide a valuable supplement to the cereal diet. However, the traditional milling (husking and splitting) techniques are not only inefficient, but result in breakage and powdering losses. An improved process has now been developed that involves conditioning of the skin for easy removal and employs the pearling technique to prevent breakage. Table VII shows the improvement in yields of various legumes. Were this method adopted, about 1.5 million tons could be added to the food supplies of India alone.

WHEAT

Although wheat (15) is the largest of the world cereal crops, it has been mainly confined to more advanced countries. Its production in developing countries is, however, increasing. Urbanization is causing widespread use of bread. The wheat supply would go farther, both quantitatively and qualitatively, if milling of flour were restricted to about 85% extraction, as was done in the United Kingdom during World War II.

LOSSES IN PERISHABLE FOODS

An underdeveloped economy and consequent technological backwardness are also reflected in the fruit and vegetable processing industry. In the United States over 50%, and in the United Kingdom nearly 40%, of the fruits and

Table VII. Milling Losses of Grain Legumes in India[a]

	Yield by	
Legumes	Traditional method, %[b]	Improved method, %
Chickpea *(Cicer arietinum)*	75	85
Pigeon pea *(Cajanus cajan)*	72	87
Green gram *(Phaseolus radiatus)*	65	85
Black gram *(Phaseolus mungo)*	71	85

[a]Husking and splitting.
[b]Bench scale results.

vegetables produced are processed into various products, while in India barely 0.4% of the total production of fruits and vegetables is processed. The situation in a number of other developing countries is not very different.

It is estimated that close to 30% of fruits and vegetables are wasted at various postharvest stages because of defective handling, packaging, transport, and distribution; there are few ventilated or refrigerated vehicles in use. If this wastage can be reduced to even half, the diet will be improved substantially, both qualitatively and quantitatively (14). Conditions for optimum refrigerated storage have already been worked out for most fruits and vegetables, and the information has been supplied to the industry. The main difficulty, however, lies with the transport and marketing system, a further indication that technology cannot succeed in isolation from other socioeconomic conditions.

The losses in fish handling, storage, and transport are also quite high. A simple technology that can assist even small-scale fishing operations has been worked out. A newly developed insulated, reusable basket, based on traditional packaging materials (bamboo and reeds), is helping to increase the distribution of fish along the coast for up to 40 km by use of bicycles; originally, fish could only be sold within a radius of 12–16 km from the sea. The basket can also be transported for distances of 400 km in trucks and on the tops of buses (16).

Improved techniques for sun-drying of fish have been standardized. After proper cleaning and treatment with sorbic acid, the shelf life of dehydrated fish has increased from three to nine months. Such products also have good markets in several countries of Southeast Asia.

SOCIALLY ORIENTED TECHNOLOGIES: THEIR SELECTION, TRANSFER, DEVELOPMENT, AND UTILIZATION

In many respects, development of the less advanced countries has heretofore been conceived as an extension, or transplant, of existing and even obsolete technologies from advanced countries. It is obvious that this has not produced the desired results, as is clearly indicated by the widening gaps in income and overall economic development. What is needed by these countries is perhaps something quite different.

Science is universal, but this is not necessarily true for technology. Unless science, technology, and society interact in an effective manner, the problems will not be solved. Only about 2% of the world's expenditure for science and technology research and development is invested in developing countries. There is a need, not only to increase this amount, but to utilize the limited resources in a manner that will produce optimum socioeconomic improvement.

Technology selection, transfer, development, and utilization require a clear policy to be made with the active participation of the scientists involved in agricultural, food science, and nutrition research, and the establishment of a system to implement it. For this purpose, agricultural production, storage, handling, milling, processing, and distribution have to be considered an integrated system to meet food and nutrition requirements, and thereby stimulate agroeconomic development. To fulfill this objective, a proper infrastructure must be developed to cover the following:

a. Establish a proper mechanism for identification of the problem in order to fulfill the socioeconomic objectives.

b. Create a sound information service to provide the required information *in a usable form.*

c. Examine critically the existing traditional art-technologies, and select those for conversion into modern science technologies that would produce a real impact.

d. Investigate critically modern technologies that, after adequate adaptive research to make them socioeconomically useful, can be utilized by the industry in a country.

e. Development appropriate level modern science-based technologies.

f. Maintain a constant vigilance over existing technologies to prevent obsolescence in terms of changing conditions.

g. Advise the industry and government on planning so as to include the research and development component at an appropriate stage in the plan for sound technoeconomic progress.

h. Maintain constant improvement of staff competence in terms of their knowledge of specialized subjects on the one hand, and their social awareness on the other.

i. Exchange of first-hand experience among research institutions can help to stimulate work and improve quality. *Such experiences among institutes in developing countries,* working under similar conditions socially, economically, climatologically, and geographically, can be of special significance in the field of food and agricultural research institutes.

j. Mobility of personnel among research institutions, industry, universities, and certain departments of the government, including planning bodies, should be encouraged.

k. In developing countries, the ability of industry to bear the risks of new technologies is very limited. Therefore, the risk factor must be minimized in prototype and pilot plants to prove the economic feasibility of new processes.

l. Where product testing and marketing are required, the institute should run a pilot plant for interested entrepreneurs and assist them in gaining sufficient confidence. Once this is accomplished, the institute should help them to set up a commercial operation, even lending services of institute staff for a fixed period when deemed necessary.

m. Where consultant services are not available, a special organization or a division of the institute should be set up for undertaking such work to create turnkey plants on a performance guarantee basis.

The scientific community has a vital role to play at national, regional, and international levels. There is need for the existing scientific and technical organizations concerned to have a fresh look at the picture in the light of the recommendations of the World Food Conference and provide the necessary leadership. The prevention of food losses, both qualitative and quantitative, through a sound program of agroindustrial development, deserves high priority in developing countries in view of the impact it can make on improving their food supplies and economy.

REFERENCES

1. Colon. Res. Publ., 1952, No. 12, p. 40.
2. Metcalf, C. L., and Flint, W. P., 1962, *Destructive and useful insects: Their habits and control,* 4th ed., revised by R. L. Metcalf, McGraw-Hill, New York, 1087 pp.
3. Central Food Technological Research Institute, Res. & Ind. Conf. CSIR, New Delhi, 1965.
4. Frey, W., 1951, Flaugblatt, Biol. Bundesanstalt. Nr. 05, 8.
5. Colon. Res. Stud., 1959, No. 28, 52.
6. Tech. Rep. W. Afr., 1962, Stores Prod. Res. Unit, No. 13.
7. Food and Agriculture Organization, 1964, Information Bull. 24.
8. Strategy Statement on Action to Avert the Protein Crisis in Developing Countries, 1971, Report of the Panel of Experts on the Protein Problem Confronting Developing Countries, United Nations Headquarters, 3–7 May (1971), ST/ECA/144 E/5018/Rev. 1.
9. Spillett, J. J., 1968, *The ecology of the lesser bandicoot rat in Calcutta,* Thesis presented at The Johns Hopkins University, Baltimore, Maryland.
10. Milner, M. (ed.). 1972, *Nutritional improvement of food legumes by breeding,* Proceedings of a Symposium Sponsored by the Protein Advisory Group of the United Nations, held at the Food and Agriculture Organization, 3–5 July, Rome, p. 286.
11. Majumder, S. K., and Bano, A., 1964, Toxicity of calcium phosphate to some pests of stored grain, *Nature* (London) **202** (4939 A): 1359–1360.
12. *Proceedings of the First International Congress of Nutrition,* London, 1962 (J. M. Leitch, ed.), Gordon and Breach, New York, 1965, Vol. 3, p. 91.
13. Rice in India: The Techno-Economic Review, Central Food Technological Research Institute, Mysore, 1966.
14. Report of the Study Group on Food Losses and Their Prevention of the National Nutrition Advisory Committee, Government of India, 1967, p. 14 (Unpublished).
15. Food and Agriculture Organization Production Yearbook, Vol. 20, 1966, Rome.
16. Central Food Technological Research Institute Annual Report, 1965, Mysore, India.

19

Control of Postharvest Losses Caused by Fungi in Food and Feed Grains

C. M. Christensen

Department of Plant Pathology
University of Minnesota
St. Paul, Minnesota

and

H. H. Kaufmann

Grain Research Laboratory
Cargill, Inc.
Minneapolis, Minnesota

The major causes of postharvest losses in stored grains are rodents, insects, mites, and fungi. Damage caused by rodents, insects, and mites has long been recognized, and effective methods have been developed to control these pests. That fungi also cause spoilage has been realized only in the last few decades, and although a great deal of information has been accumulated on the nature, cause, and prevention of these losses, this is not widely appreciated.

To some extent, the hazards of spoilage in stored food grains increase with the amount stored in any given lot. However, relatively small amounts of grain, e.g., 100 to 200 kg, sufficient for a small family from one harvest season to another, may suffer the same degree of spoilage and for the same reasons and from the same processes, as grain stored in silos or warehouses holding thousands, or tens of thousands, of tons. Presumably, if food grains are to be produced and stored in the developing countries in amounts sufficient to serve the needs of the increasing urban populations, they will have to be stored in large warehouses, not in family-size containers. Modern techniques enable us to keep any quantity of grain, if it is in good condition when received, safely stored for months or years and, moreover, enable us to detect any slowly developing spoilage long before it becomes serious, and thus allow us to avoid the heavy losses that have been common in the past and that still occur, even in the developed countries, when the practices and principles of good grain storage are disregarded.

MOISTURE CONTENT

Satisfactory grain storage requires that those in charge of the grain know at all times whether any of the grain in a given bulk or warehouse has a moisture content high enough to permit storage fungi to grow and cause damage. It is impossible to emphasize this too strongly: Some cases of spoilage occur because those in charge of the grain knowingly risk high storage hazards. Most cases of severe spoilage have occurred because those in charge of the grain did not determine its moisture content.

For various reasons, the moisture content of stored grain may differ considerably from that shown in the records. These are given in detail by Christensen and Kaufmann (1–3). The most important reasons are as follows:

1. The moisture content of a representative sample of a given lot, regardless of how well it is measured, cannot indicate the range in moisture content within the lot, and may give a false idea of the storage risk of that lot. If any portion of the lot has a moisture content high enough to permit storage molds to grow, they will grow, regardless of the average moisture content of the sample. This should be obvious, but to many of those in charge of stored grain it evidently is not.

To determine the range in moisture content in a given bulk of grain, several samples should be taken shortly after the grain is stored and each sample tested separately for moisture content. Samples also should be withdrawn periodically during the storage life of the grain and tested for moisture content and other characteristics, as described below. The accuracy of the moisture meter should be checked occasionally by having samples oven-dried—both men and machines sometimes err.

2. If different temperatures prevail in different portions of the bulk, moisture will be transferred from the warmer to the cooler portions, the rapidity of the transfer depending on the moisture content of the grain and the magnitude of the temperature difference.

3. Openings of one sort or another in the storage structure may also permit water to enter. Respiration of insects, mites, and fungi produces water, so that once spoilage gets underway it is self-perpetuating and, usually, self-accelerating.

A program of regular inspection, sampling, and testing will detect these hazards before damage has a chance to become severe. As a matter or principle, anyone in charge of stored grain should always suspect that, somewhere in the

Table I. Minimum Relative Humidity for the Growth of Common Storage Fungi at Their Optimum Temperature for Growth (26°–30°C)

Fungus	Minimum relative humidity %
Aspergillus halophilicus	68
A. restrictus, Sporendonema	70
A. glaucus	73
A. candidus, A. ochraceus	80
A. flavus	85
Penicillium, depending on species	80–90

grain mass, conditions are not as good as they appear to be. Wariness, not complacency, is the watchword.

The minimum relative humidities for the growth of various common storage fungi responsible for spoilage are given in Table I, and the moisture contents of various grains and seeds in equilibrium with the same relative humidities are given in Table II.

MONITORING OF TEMPERATURE IN STORED GRAIN

As stated in the beginning, most processes that result in spoilage in stored grains are accompanied by a rise in temperature. Also, differences in temperature between one portion of the grain and another result in transfer of moisture from the warmer to the cooler portion, and this results in increased danger of spoilage. For these reasons, monitoring of temperatures throughout any amount of stored grain helps the overseers to detect incipient spoilage before it becomes serious.

Table II. Percent Moisture Content of Various Grains and Seeds in Equilibrium with Different Relative Humidities at 25°–30°C

Humidity	Wheat, corn, sorghum	Rice		Soybeans	Sunflower	
		Rough	Polished		Seeds	Meats
65	12.5–13.5	12.5	14.0	11.5	8.5	5.0
70	13.5–14.5	13.5	15.0	12.5	9.5	6.0
75	14.5–15.5	14.5	15.5	13.5	10.5	7.0
80	15.5–16.5	15.0	16.5	16.0	11.5	8.0
85	18.0–18.5	16.5	17.5	18.0	13.5	9.0

Thermocouples are attached to cables that extend from top to bottom of the bins, at intervals of about 6 feet, or 2 meters, apart on each cable, which should be from 20 to 25 feet apart, so that there will be one thermocouple per 2000–3500 cubic feet of grain. Relatively dry grain is an excellent insulator, one-third as good as cork, and so a "hot spot" may develop without being immediately detectable by a temperature rise at the nearest thermocouple. However, no extensive spoilage will develop without some temperature rise being detectable.

Any temperature rise of more than a few degrees C is almost certain to mean that advanced spoilage is under way in that portion of the grain where the temperature rise is occurring. In stored malting barley, for example, any detectable rise in temperature, even as little as 1° C, is regarded as possible trouble to be investigated and taken care of at once, whereas there have been examples of overseers in charge of hundreds of thousands of bushels of maize or soybeans not becoming at all alarmed at consistent small rises in temperature from day to day or week to week, and sometimes, as a result, have suffered heavy losses that could have been avoided easily had they only heeded the warning given by the temperature-monitoring system.

A case in point: In the fall of 1973, a grain firm in the high plains of west Texas, where storage conditions are not at all severe because of the low humidity throughout much of the summer and low temperature during most of the winter, stored approximately a million bushels of maize. Much of the maize had moisture contents above 18% when loaded into the bins, giving it very high storage risk. When the grain was unloaded in late January, most of it was so spoiled that it could not be marketed. The firm had no temperature-detection system of any sort in the bins (the managers "did not believe in them") and had taken no samples from the bins at any time. The spoilage was their own fault.

Temperature-detection cables are a vital part of good grain storage; they have been in use for more than 50 years, and their value has been recognized throughout the world wherever grain is stored in bulk. As is true with other aids to good grain storage, the mere installation of a temperature-monitoring system does not in itself prevent spoilage, but the information that such a system provides to an intelligent and alert warehouseman can enable him to detect trouble in its incipient stages, and so avert serious loss.

AERATION

The major function of aerating stored grain is to bring about a uniform and moderately low temperature throughout the grain mass. The uniform temperature reduces the transfer of moisture from one place to another in the grain, and a moderately low (5–10°C) temperature reduces the growth rate of storage fungi if the grain has a high enough moisture content to permit them to grow. A moisture content of 14% in soybeans, for example, will permit a moderately rapid invasion by fungi at a temperature of 30°C. Yet, we stored many samples of soybeans with moisture contents of 14.0–14.3% (these were Grade No. 2 soybeans being loaded onto ships for export) at 5–8°C, and after four years they still were in excellent condition, sound and bright, and had not been invaded in even the slightest degree by fungi during storage.

Grain-infesting insects become inactive below about 15°C, and although both mites and some fungi can develop slowly down to a temperature of 0–5°C, they will not cause any appreciable damage within a year's time in grain that was sound when stored, even if it had a moisture content in equilibrium with a relative humidity of 75–80%—a high enough moisture content so that, at a temperature of 25°C, extensive spoilage would develop in a few months.

As an example, at Toluca, Mexico, which is at an altitude of about 2500 meters, the climate is relatively moist, but cool. Corn and wheat are stored there, in bulk and in bags, for a year or more without damage and with a minimum of care. In the hot, and sometimes humid, valleys a short distance away, storage problems are always severe. Even in the relatively hot and humid climate of San Juan, Puerto Rico, however, large quantities of maize and wheat (one firm, ConAgra, has several bins of 500,000 bushel capacity) are maintained at high quality by a combination of: (1) storing only grains of known high quality; (2) fumigation and sanitation to keep the populations of grain-infesting insects and mites, and of rodents, low; (3) an excellent temperature-monitoring system; (4) aeration during periods when the temperature is below 25°C and the relative humidity is below 75%; (5) a program of sampling and testing to enable them to know, at all times, the condition of the grain throughout the bins. They are applying all of the modern techniques of good grain storage. Compare this with the case described above, in Texas, where the same techniques, although equally available, were not used.

To achieve the greatest benefit from aeration, the grain must be relatively free of foreign material, or "fines." (In U.S. Grain Standards, foreign material in maize is defined as that which will pass through a 12/64-inch round-hole sieve). Even if maize contains only 2–3% fines when it is loaded into a bin or tank from an overhead spout, these fines collect in a cone in the center—the so-called spout line—that may be made up of 50–60% fines, packed solid. Air forced through the grain passes around, rather than through, this cone of compact material, and it is there that spoilage usually gets under way first.

The usual rate of aeration to achieve a uniform temperature throughout the grain is on the order of 0.1 cubic feet of air per minute per bushel of grain. At this rate, a uniform temperature is achieved throughout the grain in about 100 to 120 hours. This rate of aeration does not dry the grain appreciably, even if the air forced through it is of low relative humidity. For appreciable drying to occur, an aeration rate of 2–6 or more cu ft/bu/min is required—that is, from 20 to 60 times or more the rate used to achieve a uniform temperature. Once the uniform temperature is attained, aeration can be discontinued until such time as the temperature, as indicated by the monitoring system, rises in one portion or another.

SAMPLING AND TESTING

Taking samples of stored grain and examining and testing them to determine their condition is basically not any different from many other kinds of sampling. For many years, the United States has had regular plant disease surveys of its growing crops to determine what diseases were developing where, so that defensive measures could be taken against them. Similarly, surveys report diseases in livestock and in the human population to detect outbreaks of disease in their early stages, so that measures can be taken to suppress them.

The case with stored grains is not different. We now know, without question, the major causes of grain spoilage. We can detect the presence of these agents in various ways, and can measure their increase long before they cause serious damage. We also know which moisture contents and temperatures permit these causers of spoilage to develop. This knowledge enables us, by examination and testing of samples taken from a given bulk or lot, to evaluate rather precisely the current condition and future storability of that lot. This measurement and evaluation require some laboratory facilities and a modicum of mycological expertise, as well as sufficient experience to establish categories of condition and storability, but the approach is basically simple. That it works is shown by the fact that it has been in successful use by several grain firms in the United States for more than 20 years, and by some in Mexico for more than 10.

Briefly, the procedure is as follows: Samples of approximately 0.5 kg are taken from as many different portions of the bulk as desired (a vacu-probe permits taking samples from almost any depth of any mass of grain or other granular material). Each sample is put into a separate moisture-proof container and sent to the laboratory. There the samples are tested for moisture content, examined for obvious damage, and 100 kernels are surface-disinfected, placed on an agar medium designed to reveal storage fungi, incubated for three days at 30° C, and the number and kinds of fungi present are recorded. Sufficient background experience has been accumulated to indicate that, if a given percentage of surface-disinfected kernels yield one or another of the possible fungi, there will be a given degree of storage risk. These storage fungi are relatively few in number, and are so easily recognized that any moderately intelligent person can, after a few hours training, identify them with certainty. Nothing particularly esoteric is involved.

As stated by Burrell (4): "In cool or temperate climates a well-planned and well-managed aeration system can greatly reduce the damage by insects, mites, and fungi, the chief hazards to quality in stored grains and seeds. Even in warm climates, selective ventilation can effectively limit damage caused by these agents, and so can be of tremendous value in preserving quality. The prevention of moisture transfer, through maintenance of a uniform temperature throughout the bulk, greatly reduces the chance of development of hidden or unexpected local areas of deterioration within the bulk. Unquestionably, the development of effective aeration systems has been a major contribution of modern engineering technology to grain storage. Combined with the use of temperature detection systems and a program of regular sampling and testing, it has revolutionized grain-storage practices and has brought these far along the road from a somewhat chancy art to at least a moderately exact science."

In sum, the principles and practices of good grain storage are known, and where they are applied, storage losses are minimal, even in environments of high storage risk. They often are not applied and, as a result, heavy grain losses are occasionally experienced during storage and transit, even in the developed countries. Some research will be required to adapt to specific sites in the developing countries the practices of sanitation, fumigation, aeration, regular measurement of temperature and moisture content, and routine sampling to evaluate condition and storability. This will require more attention to the problem than the developing countries have devoted to it thus far.

REFERENCES

1. Christensen, C. M., and Kaufmann, H. H., 1968, Maintenance of Quality in Stored Grains and Seeds, Agricultural Extension Service, University of Minnesota, Extension Folder 226.
2. Christensen, C. M., and Kaufmann, H. H., 1969, *Grain storage–The role of fungi in quality loss,* University of Minnesota Press, St. Paul, pp. 36–49.
3. Christensen, C. M., and Kaufman, H. H., 1974, Microflora, *in: Storage of cereal grains and their products,* C. M. Christensen (ed.), Amer. Assoc. Cereal Chemists, St. Paul, Minnesota, pp. 170–172.
4. Burrell, N. J., 1974, Aeration, *in: Storage of cereal grains and their products,* C. M. Christensen (ed.), Amer. Assoc. Cereal Chemists, St. Paul, Minnesota, p. 478.

20

Food Processing Problems and Potential

Joseph H. Hulse

International Development Research Centre
Ottawa, Canada

The English verb *to process* is derived from the Latin *procedure,* which means "to go on or to move from one place to another." Only in the late 19th century did the verb *to process* acquire the connotation of subjecting a material or substance to a treatment that would cause it to change its form or properties.

Essentially, what English-speaking people mean when they talk of food processing is transformation—the changing of food material from one form to another—or conservation—the protection of the food from decay or loss. Consequently, the French words *transformation,* which means literally "to change from one form to another," and *conservation,* which is derived from the Latin verb *conservare,* meaning "to keep from harm, decay, or loss" are more meaningful than the English word *processing.*

Among those whose business it is, *food processing* and *food technology* are used almost synonymously. In the original Greek, *technology* probably meant a discourse on the fine or applied arts. Today, out of a wide choice of dictionary definitions, *technology* might reasonably be defined as "the science of the industrial arts," or even "the artful use of science."

In spite of a considerable investment in food research over the last 100 years, we know more about *how* to transform and conserve than *why* the processes of transformation and conservation take place. In fact, most of the progress made has consisted of mechanizing methods of transformation and conservation that were traditionally performed by hand.

The oldest of all known food processes—the milling of cereal grains into flour and the transformation of the resultant flour into bread—has changed little in basic principle during 6000 years. The ancient Egyptians used grinding, sieving, and aspiration to separate the white endosperm flour from the seed coats and embryo of the wheat grain. Only during the past 20 years have we witnessed the first fundamental change in the bread-making procedure, in which "mechanical development" has replaced several hours of fermentation in order to bring about desirable changes in the dough structure.

From its earliest beginnings, food processing has been, and in large measure still is, based upon empiricism, in contrast to the electronics and chemical industries, which have been created out of demonstrable scientific principles.

At the risk of generalizing in extremis, I would propose that scientific principles can be more readily transferred and transplanted than technologies. The difficulty of transferring technologies between countries widely different in cultural heritage and economic development is the root cause of many of the difficulties and frustrations that less developed nations have experienced in trying to establish viable food processing industries.

In proposing this generalization, it is recognized that greater differences in economic, social, and technical development are to be found among the so-called less developed nations than between some of the less developed and those classed as developed. India includes among its citizens a far larger number of university graduates in food and related sciences than are found in a great many so-called developed countries. The government of India supports what is probably the largest food research institute in the world. The universities of Egypt were teaching science related to food and agriculture long before the first university was established in North America. Nevertheless, either from choice or because of the manner in which bilateral and multilateral aid programs have been regulated and administered, many of the food processing research and development programs, even in the most advanced of the less developed countries, have been guided, and often directed, by technologists and technological philosophies imported from the developed world.

Industrial food research in the developed economies of North America and Europe is predominantly concerned with first, the creation of new products and processes, and second, with quality control, or what has recently come to be called "quality assurance." Both product and process research and development are aimed primarily at saving labor. The continuously growing spectrum of "convenience foods" in the form of canned and frozen precooked meals, and the prepared mixes for soups, sauces, bread, cakes, and desserts, have one purpose: to reduce the work load of the industrial cook and the housewife in their respective kitchens. An "improved" process by which to manufacture any one of the 10,000 or more items sold in North American grocery stores generally means a process that generates a larger number of product units per man-hour of labor.

Every manufactured food product must meet certain standards of quality and identity, some of which are defined by the manufacturer and others imposed by government regulatory agencies. In common with factory and transportation workers, laboratory scientists and technicians are comparatively expensive to employ. Consequently, laboratory technicians are being replaced by a range of analytical instruments of ever increasing complexity, but requiring comparatively little human effort per unit of output.

Throughout the economically developed countries one finds a large number of institutes of food research, some of which are owned by single corporate enterprises, some by groups of industries having a common interest, some operated jointly by industry and government, and some by federal or state governments. While each has its own characteristics, determined by specific purpose, almost all have certain essential common features. These include product and process development laboratories and pilot plants where the latest labor-saving product or device is invented and tested before being put into production. In addition, there are the highly instrumentalized analytical, physical, and microbiological laboratories where the standards of product identity and quality and process control are defined and put into operation.

To many technologists of the developed world, a research and development institute such as this has become a sine qua non to a progressive food industry. In seeking planned development of their indigenous food processing industries, many governments of less developed countries, by choice or perforce, have turned to expatriate advisers and foreign donors for guidance. Not a few of these advisers appear to have dodged the issue of helping the poorer countries to examine realistically, comprehensively, and pragmatically the immediate and urgent needs of existing indigenous food processing industries, and the nature and scale of transformation and conservation facilities that would best suit the countries' needs and resources. Instead, the foreign advisers chose the simpler path of prescribing a food research institute typical of those found in their own more developed economies. Thus, instead of carefully compiling and analyzing the problems existing, they took the easier course of designing buildings and drawing up catalogues of imagined essential equipment.

Where such research institutions were equipped through multilateral or bilateral aid, the recipient governments were often pressed to select all of the equipment early in the life of the project. As a result, many of these institutions were equipped before any detailed program of necessary research had been defined. Under such unfortunate circumstances, projects tend to be selected and justified by the nature of the equipment provided rather than by the immediate needs of the indigenous food and agricultural economies. This "cart before the horse" approach continues to plague and constrain many of the food research institutions in the developing countries. In addition, and perhaps more seriously, it strongly inclines their food scientists and technologists to remain attached to their laboratory and pilot plant equipment rather than to go out and address themselves to the many serious difficulties of the existing food conservation and distribution systems.

It is remarkable that in spite of the many difficulties they have faced, not the least of which has been a shortage of foreign exchange and technical skill with which to maintain their equipment and essential resources, many of the food research institutes in the less developed countries have given valuable service to their countries' industries and economies. Nevertheless, in a number of cases a more relevant and worthwhile service could have been provided with much less elaborate physical facilities and expense.

Research institutes are costly to maintain; their equipment has to be repaired and replaced. In general, the more complex the equipment, the more it will cost to maintain it. Where it is deemed essential to provide technical equipment of foreign manufacture, the original donors are strongly urged to make a long-term commitment to its repair and maintenance. Such donors are, however, even more strongly urged not to press upon developing nations equipment and technological systems irrelevant to their needs and capabilities.

It is to be hoped, in the future, that multilateral and bilateral donors will see fit to grant to the scientists of the less developed countries a much greater degree of responsibility for both formulating and managing their own programs of research and development. If the scientists and technologists of the developing countries are allowed to make their own mistakes, for the most part the mistakes will be no more disastrous than many of those made by so-called foreign experts.

The education and training of food scientists and technologists in relation to the needs of the less developed countries is a subject too complex to be treated comprehensively here. One could cite many instances, particularly in postgraduate research programs in developed countries, of students from less developed countries being given training ill-suited to their needs.

In several projects financed by the International Development Research Centre (IDRC), it has been possible for graduate students in agriculture to receive theoretical training at a Canadian university and return to their home countries to carry out their practical thesis research on a problem directly related to their own urgent national needs. One would hope to see more food science and technology students from Africa, Asia, and Latin America receive training in fundamental principles in universities of the developed world before returning to their own countries to carry out their thesis research on applied problems of relevance and consequence. As is suggested later, even more valuable would be international centers of research and training established to serve the needs of several developing countries within the same regions.

A number of developing countries have sought to import processing technologies through licensing agreements with food processing companies in developed countries. The difficulties of transplanting a total technological system, or a component of such a system, into an unfamiliar and often uncongenial environment are not easily surmounted. In addition, the direct cost of technology transfer may prove exceedingly burdensome to the recipient countries.

The direct costs of technology transfer include the right to use patents, licenses, manufacturing and marketing know-how, trademarks, advertising materials, and technical support services.

A United Nations Conference on Trade and Development study in 1971 estimated that, for all less developed countries during 1968, the direct costs of technology transfer amounted to $1.5 billion in foreign exchange, and that direct transfer costs to the less developed countries are increasing at the rate of roughly 20% per annum (1). If this trend can be extrapolated in constant dollars, the result will be a net foreign exchange debit to the less developed countries of nearly $9 billion by 1980 (Figure 1). Such direct transfer costs have been calculated to be roughly equivalent to 5% of net imports, and 2½ times the total domestic expenditure on research and development in all of the less developed countries.

Governments of developing countries that enter into such technology transfer agreements may also find themselves shouldering a heavy burden of indirect costs. These may include the deliberate overpricing of raw materials, capital goods, and equipment sold by the parent company in a developed country to its subsidiaries or licensees in less developed countries. Such deliberate overpricing is one means by which the parent company seeks to repatriate its foreign investment; for the developing country it represents a very heavy drain on foreign exchange.

It is not unusual for such licensing contracts to include restrictive clauses. In a study of the five countries of the Andean pact, more than 70% of licensing contracts were found to contain restrictive export clauses. About 73% of such contracts between food and beverage and related companies in the Andean Pact countries prevented exports of the products they manufactured (2).

The list of cases in which governments of the poorer nations have been persuaded, on the basis of advice given by foreign experts, to purchase and

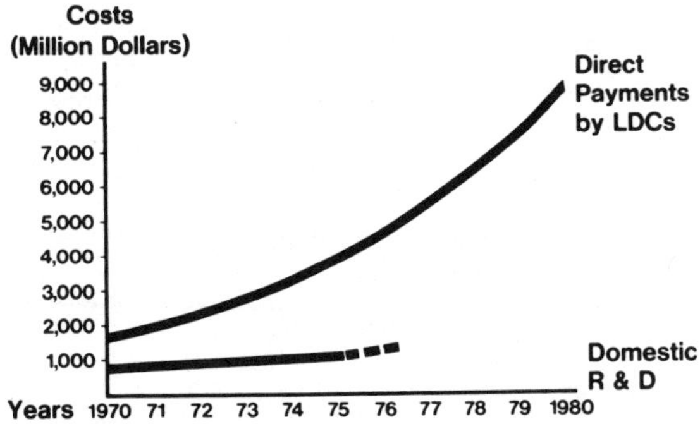

FIG. 1. Projection of costs of domestic R & D and direct payments by LDCs for transfer of technology 1970–1980.

install large food processing factories and complexes provides a sorry litany of misadventure and misfortune. At least two African countries have bought large-scale tomato processing equipment from overseas. In one instance it was subsequently discovered that the country could not possibly produce, in the quantity needed, the quality of tomatoes required to make tomato paste; in the second, because of inadequate quality control, an entire year's production of canned tomato products was destroyed through swelling and leaking. In both Africa and Asia one finds pineapple canning plants that cannot operate economically because there are not enough pineapples available.

Several Asian countries have imported rice processing facilities totally unsuited to their economic and physical environment and resources. In another Asian country one can observe beautiful cultured oysters being spoiled by an unsatisfactory smoking and canning system.

One cannot believe that all of the faulty advice that led to these misadventures was given maliciously or mischievously. These examples emphasize, however, how urgent it is for the developing countries to acquire the technical skills and experience needed to define and develop the food conservation and transformation systems suitable to their own economies.

Probably the greatest obstacle to technological development in the less developed countries is the shortage of relevant knowledge and experience. The poor nations of the world represent more than 70% of the earth's population. They produce less than 45% of the world's food crops, and receive less than 20% of the world's cash income. In terms of what it costs, 70% of the research in the world is carried out in the United States, 20% in other rich nations, and less than 2% in all of the poor nations combined (Figures 2 and 3) (3).

In most less developed countries, overall expenditures on research and development are small. Considering the relative economic importance of agriculture, there is an extraordinarily low investment in food and agricultural research.

Foreign companies of the developed world hold almost 90% of all the patents registered in the developing countries, and there is little evidence to suggest that the proportion of patent ownership is changing significantly.

So far, this paper has addressed itself in a broad generalization to the problems that relate to the introduction or expansion of food processing

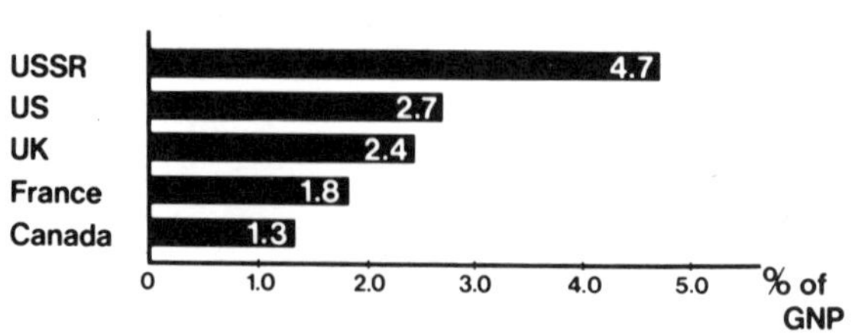

FIG. 2. R & D in developed countries.

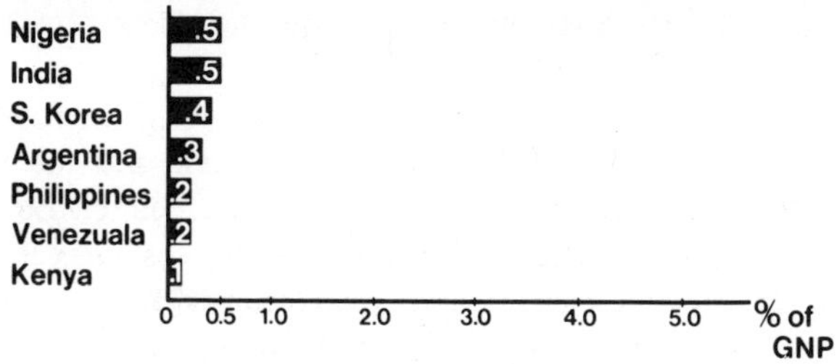

FIG. 3. R & D in developing countries.

industries in less developed countries. The variability within these generalizations is indeed great if, for example, one considers the differences in technical and economic development between the more advanced nations of Latin America and the countries of the Sahelian zone of Africa. It is virtually impossible to propose, for such extremes, a universally appropriate food processing policy or a formula by which food processing systems can be successfully established and maintained. Nevertheless, it can be stated as a general truth that efficient food transformation and conservation systems can bring about a more uniform distribution of basic agricultural products, an increase in and a diversification of rural employment, and an incentive to increased agricultural production by providing a more constant and stable market demand. Efficient food industries contribute to economic stability through the stabilization of agricultural production, prices, and markets.

A recent study in the Sahel by an IDRC team indicated that food grain production in that unfortunate region could, and would, be significantly increased if adequate means existed for marketing grains grown in excess of farmers' subsistence requirements (4).

If they are to avoid a continuous and disastrous drain upon their meager foreign currency resources, it is essential that the less developed countries increase food production. Over the past 10 years their food production has been increasing, on average, at the rate of about 2.7% per annum. Over the same period food demand in these countries has been increasing by 3.5% per annum. During the past 20 years the continents of Africa, Asia, and Latin America have changed from sufficiency to deficiency in their production of edible food grains, and their imports of grains from North America and Australia have increased from 26 million tons to 92 million tons per annum.

Having admitted the impossibility of prescribing a universally applicable formula for food industry development among the less developed countries, I would urge, particularly to the least developed, that the highest priority be given to the conservation of their indigenous food crops. It is essential that they reduce to an absolute minimum the enormous losses that occur from the time of harvest to the time the food is delivered to the consumer. In the absence of more efficient systems of conservation and distribution, the hideous specter of hunger and malnutrition will grow larger year by year.

International agricultural research centers such as the International Maize and Wheat Improvement Centre (CIMMYT) in Mexico and the International Rice Research Institute (IRRI) in the Philippines have demonstrated that high-yielding cereal cultivars and efficient multiple cropping systems can significantly increase the yields of edible cereal grains, food legumes, and root crops per unit area of land per unit of time. There is limited value in increasing agricultural productivity if more than 30% of the crops produced are consumed by rodents, insects, mold fungi, and other predators. Conservation and transformation processes are required to increase the efficiency with which crops are harvested, threshed, dried, processed, packaged, stored, and transported with minimum loss from the regions and seasons of abundance to those of scarcity.

In many less developed countries the consumption of food products such as bread and alimentary pastes, derived from imported wheat, is steadily increasing. At the same time the production, per caput, of traditional crops is declining. For example, data from the FAO Production Yearbook (5) indicate that since 1950 per caput production of legumes has steadily fallen throughout Asia: chickpea from 6 to 3 kg, soybean from 1.2 to 0.9 kg, and lentils from 0.6 to 0.4 kg. By appropriate and comparatively simple processing technologies, food legumes and tropical cereal grains such as sorghum and millets can be transformed to a wide variety of attractive foods and included as ingredients of bread, pastas, biscuits, and infant foods.

The basic principles by which to conserve and transform these and other tropical food crops are known, but relevant technological systems appropriate to the capacities of many less developed countries have yet to be elaborated. It is within these countries themselves that the technological systems of transformation should be devised, tested, and adapted into food processing industries. However, few if any of these countries can establish, within their own boundaries, all of the facilities for research, development, training and demonstration, and manufacture necessary to create the food conservation, transformation, distribution, and marketing facilities of the scale and kind required. Nor do I believe that the less developed countries can, or should, rely upon the established technologies and the technological advisers of the developed countries. I do believe, however, that the developing nations can create the technological systems they need *if* they will seek to do so cooperatively.

Groups of developing nations can solve many common technological problems when they are given the opportunity and the resources to cooperate among themselves. One could cite many examples of successful technological cooperation among developing countries. The first example, the Canada Mysore Project, began in 1963. Through the leadership of the Government of India and the Central Food and Technological Research Institute (CFTRI), with financial support from Canada, a training program was provided at CFTRI for all the nations of Southeast Asia. During the subsequent 10 years, more than 800 Asian scientists received training in food conservation and transformation in courses ranging from a few weeks to two years in duration. A recent survey of all those who attended such courses produced the following interesting results: Close to 200 former students responded, and over 90% indicated that the courses had been relevant and helpful to their subsequent careers.

The second example is more recent and also involves Asian scientists, many of whom received training at one or another of the Mysore courses. It was proposed by an Asian food technologist that IDRC should make possible the formation of an Asian working group on food science and technology, a group that would, among its own members, define the problems of common concern and the means by which they could work cooperatively to solve these problems. At the first meeting representatives from nine Asian nations decided that the highest priority should be given to improving the postharvest technologies related to rice, with particular emphasis upon those that could be employed by the small farmer and the small-to-medium rice processing mills. As a first step, with IDRC support, a training course was provided by the University of the Philippines, where the managers of small rice mills and other persons directly interested received an intensive five-week program of training. Subsequently, six of the nations involved defined a program of interdependent research and demonstration projects, each to be undertaken by a different Asian country, and each of interest to the whole group of rice-producing nations. The overall program will be guided and directed by a committee of policy makers and technologists on which each of the participating countries will be represented.

The second priority, the processing and preservation of fish by techniques and systems applicable and economically feasible throughout Asia, was formulated at a meeting held in Bangkok during October, 1974.

The third priority, the processing of food legumes, will be studied, and it is hoped that a network of projects will be defined at a meeting to be held early in 1975. In addition, another group met in Asia and outlined a cooperative program of cassava processing, particularly as it concerns the processing of cassava for animal feeds, to be used both within the region and for export to more developed economies.

The Asian scientists and technologists have produced a Directory of Food Technology (6) covering most of the food research going on in the various countries of the region. This will be brought up to date from time to time, and the information has been so arranged that it can be processed by computer. Through the facilities of CFTRI at Mysore, an abstract service covering food technology publications directly relevant to the region has also been set in motion.

We in IDRC should like to encourage similar cooperative initiatives in other regions of the less developed world. It is unlikely that every less developed country, particularly the poorest, can afford the luxury of a large, expensively equipped, food research institute. It should, however, be possible, with effective cooperation among nations having similar environments and similar problems, to establish regional institutes for research and training in food processing analogous to the international agricultural research centers such as CIMMYT and IRRI, who are providing such a magnificent service for farmers throughout the world. International regional applied research centers could provide new technologies appropriate to the technical, economic, and physical climates of their constituent countries—technologies to be adapted by the national institutions to the needs of their own agricultural and industrial systems.

Regionally integrated programs of research and training can help the least developed nations to acquire the indigenous scientific capability necessary to select and manage the technological systems best suited to their needs. In the absence of an adequate indigenous scientific capability, governments of the less developed countries risk being led repeatedly into unwise technical choices and into attempting costly and inappropriate technological transfers.

There is a further consideration in this matter of realizing the full potential of food processing industries in the less industrialized nations. In many of them the small, locally owned industries find it too expensive to establish any kind of research facility within their own corporate structures. Consequently, the responsibility for food research and development is often assumed entirely by national governments. It is my firm belief that, even in developed countries, there is a comparatively low adoption rate by food processing industries of technological developments financed entirely by government agencies. Unless the existing food industries make some contribution, however small, to the cost of the research program and are granted a significant voice in guiding and directing that program, the benefit these industries will derive from such research is likely to be very limited. Consequently, I would recommend that national programs of food research, demonstration, and training be joint government–industry undertakings.

I would also urge that in the conceiving and implementing of food industry research and development programs, governments and scientists of the less developed countries seek to adopt a flexible and imaginative approach. The classical research institute composed of expensively equipped laboratories is not an inevitable necessity. A number of countries have found they can provide a more useful service to their food industries by employing mobile laboratories for research demonstration and quality control. These ensure that the scientists do their work in close proximity to, not in isolation from, the industries they are intended to serve.

Also, it is often advantageous to insist that every research scientist spend at least one year working in a food processing factory before being admitted to a national industrial research institute. It is doubtful if any scientist can adequately serve an industry if he or she has not worked in that industry and learned at first hand the problems by which its progress is constrained.

In summary, an efficient system of conservation, transformation, and distribution is an essential component of every nation's food and agricultural economy. Although most of the underlying scientific principles are universally applicable, many of the technological food and training systems that adequately serve food industries in *developed* nations are inappropriate to the economies of the *less developed.*

In order to select and to put into operation the food conservation and transformation technologies best suited to the needs of the less developed nations, several steps must be encouraged.

1. These nations should develop their indigenous scientific capabilities and technological experience by embarking upon their own programs of applied research and development, and concentrate upon the improved protection and utilization of the crops they already produce.

2. They should establish their applied research facilities through cooperation between government scientific institutions and existing food processing industries, and these industries should be required to make a financial contribution to the research program and be granted a significant voice in devising and directing the program.

3. They should cooperate, among themselves, to form mutually supporting and complementary networks of research and development for their common interests and, where necessary, create regional international centers for applied research, development, and training in order to economize upon their available resources and to spread the responsibility most effectively.

4. The multilateral agencies, bilateral donors, and foundations who support international development in food and agriculture should also encourage such initiatives as have been suggested by providing the necessary financial resources without seeking to direct the programs to be undertaken.

It is essential that the scientists and technologists of the developing world be permitted, and indeed encouraged, to guide their own technological destinies. In our experience they are eminently capable of doing so.

REFERENCES

1. United Nations Conference on Trade and Development, Report by the UNCTAD Secretariat, Transfer of Technology. United Nations Conference on Trade and Development, Third Session, Santiago, Chile, April 13, 1972. TD/106, November 10, 1971, p. 17.
2. Junta del Acuerdo de Cartagena, Policies relating to technology of the countries of the

Andean Pact: Their foundations, United Nations Conference on Trade and Development, Third Session, Santiago, Chile, April 13, 1972. TD/107, December 29, 1971, pp. 13–14.
3. United Nations Educational, Scientific and Cultural Organization. Statistical Yearbook 1972, United Nations Educational, Scientific and Cultural Organization, Paris, 1973, pp. 658–665.
4. Forrest, R. S., Petersen, T. A., Hogue, J. J., and Steckle, J., 1975, *The post-harvest food grain industry in semi-arid Africa,* The International Development Research Centre, Ottawa, (February, 1975).
5. Food and Agriculture Organization, 1971, Production Yearbook 1970, Volume 24, FAO, Rome.
6. *Directory of Food Science and Technology in Southeast Asia,* Revised Edition, Compiled by E. V. Araullo, International Development Research Centre, Ottawa, 1975.

COMMENTS

Antonio Bacigalupo · *Universidad Nacional Agraria, Lima, Peru.*

Hulse brings into focus some of the successes and failures inherent in most of the systems of foreign aid exported to developing countries. My remarks will only attempt to reinforce and complement some of his ideas from the viewpoint of developing countries. I have selected 10 of the problems that, in my opinion, are the most important, as well as four courses of action that could spark the food processing potential of most Latin American countries.

The worst problems of the food processing industry in Latin America are these:

1. *Local food processing industries have limited perspectives.* It is not uncommon to see industries that know little, or at least do little, for such basic related activities as agricultural food production and national and economic social needs. Concentration on short-range projects has often slowed down long-range actions. For instance, food industries have been based on imported foods instead of on local production of indigenous foods. This has led, quite naturally, to a limited view of the potential role and importance of the food industry as a dynamic force in national development, and as an instrument of social and nutritional improvement.

2. *Local industry does not support research or technological development.* In general, the local food industry gives little or no support to food research; it prefers to buy patents and processes from abroad. This explains why many excellent local food resources such as potatoes, beans, quinua, cañihua, and sweet potatoes are neither industrialized nor processed by modern technology.

3. *The local food industry is often not efficient and well adapted to local resources and conditions.* Many food industries suffer from inefficiency because of antiquated equipment, uneconomically small operating capacity, or unneces-

sarily sophisticated equipment—all of which increase the production costs. As a consequence, it is not rare to find such industries seeking economic subsidies from the consumer or the government.

Lack of an adequate infrastructure in a country, such as roads, storage capacity warehouses, and engineering firms, contributes to the overall inefficiency of the food industry. Moreover, environmental resources such as solar energy and hydroelectric energy have not been used to develop economical local technology.

4. *Food research of governments and universities is extremely limited and often unrelated to the problems of the industry.* Research efforts are frequently scattered over too wide an area to be effective, change direction too often, and relate to what is fashionable rather than to the needs of the country or the food industry. It is often easier to obtain funds to repeat experiments carried out in developed countries than to adapt existing technology to local conditions. There is still little academic or governmental enthusiasm for improving traditional technologies.

5. *Expanding government bureaucracies have little interest in the development and growth of the food industry.* This is an important factor and is associated with the belief that food research is not essential and does not increase productivity.

6. *Research often remains inconclusive and unapplied.* Because the industry is not prepared to utilize work of the laboratory or pilot plant, research frequently ends where it is begun.

7. *Food research is carried out in piecemeal fashion, disconnected from related activities.* The food technologist forgets that the food he processes is to nourish human beings, create new jobs, and contribute to national wellbeing. He has paid exclusive attention to the economic impact of food and its flavor, texture, and the like.

8. *Food technologists have little access to government decision-making.* In national decision-making, food technologists have little influence compared with politicians, economists, and national planners. They must be criticized for not speaking up for the potential contributions of food science and technology.

9. *When the technologist does speak out, the public does not hear or understand what he has to say.* It is difficult for technologists to understand one another's specialties and much harder for the general public to grasp the unnecessarily mysterious jargon used by most of us.

10. *The local food technologist does not receive sufficient credit when he does something useful.* Unfortunately, the food technologist is rarely recognized in his own country. Many assume that the technologists from underdeveloped countries, regardless of their preparation, must also be underdeveloped.

To solve some of the above problems confronting the application of food technology in Latin America, I would propose the following:

1. *Develop an adequate research infrastructure;* i.e., develop and test fully promising food processing developments.

2. *Develop better research methodologies to change from producing theoretical solutions to practical ones.*

3. *Improve the handling of foods and management of feeding systems.*

4. *Foster more participation of food technologists in policy-making decisions.* The contributors to this volume know what can be accomplished by the application of food technology, which can make important contributions to solving national and world food problems. Applied science and technology is an essential link between the forces of science and those of politics.

Javier Pérez Villaseñor · *Departmento de Biotecnología, Universidad Autónoma Metropolitana-Unidad Iztapalapa, México 13, D.F.*

In discussing Hulse's chapter, I wish to emphasize some general principles and make a few specific comments.

Role of Science and Technology

It is generally recognized that development at the national level can be effectively catalyzed by sound implementation of science and technology. In general, the rich and affluent countries have used science and technology for their development and the very impoverished countries have not. A policy on science and technology for national development should have at least the following objectives to be effective:

1. Identify problems and contribute effectively to solutions that are soundly based scientifically, technically, and economically.
2. Develop and strengthen the economy of the country.
3. Promote the development of new technological initiatives.
4. Above all, every effort of a sound policy must be oriented to improve mankind's lot on a permanent, just basis.

While it is true that progress toward these objectives will help to break the technological backwardness–lack of opportunities–malnutrition–poverty cycle, it is not less true that they are difficult to reach. Nevertheless, each country must make every effort to speed up its progress and raise its self-reliance in order to avoid more human suffering.

It has been stated that science is pursued for the sake of knowledge and insight and therefore science is natural and universal. Technology is then essentially applied science. It can be said that science is "know why" and technology is "know how" and consequently, technology transfer means the successful "show how" to manufacture something new or better.

How to Achieve Successful Technology Transfer

How does one efficiently utilize the scarce resources available in the less developed countries to build scientifically, technically, and economically sound food industries that, among their many functions, should provide work for the unemployed hand laborer, improve nutritional standards, raise the balance of trade by exporting finished and semifinished products instead of exporting raw materials, and, above all, create the mystique to raise both self-image and self-confidence of the country in its human resources? It is obvious that many requirements have to be met.

Awareness of the Problem

Among the people making the policies, economists and planners alike, there should be a clear awareness of scientific and technological progress that can be linked to national plans for development, with specific objectives of improving the productivity of industry and fostering its growth.

Research and Development Centers

New research and development centers, or reinforcement of the existing ones, if at all possible, should be promoted to carry on the following objectives:

1. Survey and identify technoeconomic problems that require solution in the area of food conservation and processing.

2. Select, modify, and transfer appropriate technologies for an economically sound food industry, adequate for its particular environment.

3. Undertake research based on available scientific information for developing, modifying, and upgrading food processing in order to raise efficiency and productivity so that they can compete successfully on the world market.

4. Provide industrial consultants and extension work on the basis of available information, to make better use of the existing and imported technologies for manufacture of high-quality products. At the same time, assistance to the industry should be provided in preparing project reports and carrying out feasibility studies to prove the worth of selected or newly developed technologies, and in particular, assistance should be given to small- and medium-scale industries that are in great need of this type of guidance.

5. Set up pilot plant facilities where new technologies, or imported ones, can be tested before actually going into operation, in order to decrease the risk of failure for small- and medium-scale industries.

6. Assist the government in establishing a sound policy for technology transfer regarding what technologies to import, when to do so, and on what

terms. All of these actions lead to a very important question: Who is going to carry on this work? Obviously, this responsibility rests on the shoulders of nationals with the proper education and training.

Education and Training

The objective here is to create and foster the development of the needed human resources, at the various levels of the pyramid, that will secure the active participation of committed, well-qualified personnel who are oriented to identify and solve problems. To build up the necessary reserves of personnel, students may be sent abroad to study, but while away they should be kept in touch with the people and needs of their own countries. This would help to prevent them from becoming uprooted, or becoming foreigners in their own countries once they return.

New curricula, at both the graduate and undergraduate levels, should be established in the so-called less developed countries. These curricula should be designed to take into account the specific needs and opportunities within a country, because experience has proved that these problems are not solved best by copying foreign curricula and approaches. In designing the curriculum, one should also include the necessary courses on economics and management in order to improve indigenous entrepreneurship, which is so much needed by the less developed countries to foster the growth of their own industries.

Specific Comments

Hulse's presentation clearly shows his knowledge of the situation prevailing in many of the developing countries, and my comments are meant to complement some of his concepts.

Food Research

Because one finds a well-to-do minority and a vast underprivileged majority in the less developed countries, food research and technology must be reoriented in order to satisfy both groups, with greater emphasis on improving products for the less privileged whose purchasing power is so low that most, if not all, of the processed foods are out of their reach. To improve their nutritional status, local technologies should be developed to enable them to make better use of the little purchasing power they have. These "home and industry applied technologies" should make a substantial improvement in the nutritional quality of food, should be inexpensive, should not change the methods of preparing such food nor alter its characteristics, and lastly, the ingredients should be widely available. Following this concept, for example, we have studied the enrichment of the

Mexican tortilla by cooking raw mixtures of corn and whole soybeans with great success.

Information and Documentation

In reviewing what has been done on a given subject, one should make a thorough evaluation of the state of the art and become acquainted, not only with the work published in widely known scientific journals from developed countries, but also with journals from less developed countries, which do publish extremely useful data, for example, the Indian Journal of Food Science, or Tecnologia de Alimentos from Mexico. I have found that, many times, because they share characteristics of underdevelopment, these countries' technologies are better suited to other developing countries.

Technology Transfer

With regard to technology transfer, less developed countries should be helped to increase their awareness of both the positive and the negative impact of technology transfer in suppressing or restricting the development of the "indigenous structure of science and technology" that is so necessary. While importation of skills can promote the development of a country, the indiscriminate importation of technology can undermine the country's economy by imposing a perpetual drain on its foreign exchange resources and introducing unfair competition with local industry. In the long run, it may have a devastating effect insofar as it demoralizes the local entrepreneurs and their development of expertise. Moreover, it is clear that uncontrolled foreign collaboration often displaces the native scientists and engineers. Before a country buys technology from abroad, it is absolutely necessary for it to assess carefully the impact of such importation on its economy and employment potential.

Juan J. Schildknecht · *Alimentos, S.A., Guatemala City, Guatemala.*

One of the means to combat malnutrition will continue to be of utmost importance for the solution of this problem: the preparation of vegetable mixtures of high protein content derived from the combination of cereals, legumes, and oilseeds, and their by-products. Developing countries are in great need of low-cost foods of high nutritional value for the poor sectors who represent the majority of the population. For the manufacture of foods of this type to be economically feasible, the raw material utilized must usually be predominantly local.

"Raw materials" and "ingredients" are different. Maize, for example, in its original state is a raw material. After undergoing a cleaning and milling process that eventually results in removal of hulls, black tips, and germ, it is transformed into semolina, or flour, and thus becomes an ingredient to be used in the preparation of a formula.

A food product must comply satisfactorily with: (1) the acceptability and tolerance tests at individual levels; (2) evaluation of its nutritive value in humans; and (3) acceptability, judged by the results of marketing trials carried out with representative samples of the population. Once all specifications concerning its chemical, physical, and organoleptic characteristics have been fulfilled, a flow chart is prepared to select the equipment and accessories required for the processing of the product.

The technology for processing rice or milling wheat into flour does not represent a major problem, because the processes involved have been thoroughly understood for a long time. Furthermore, as years go by and experience accumulates, they are constantly improved, new installations are set up, and many of the existing ones are being remodeled. On the other hand, the raw materials used and the final products have been, and continue to be, carefully studied and are already well known. The situation changes, however, when the purpose is to manufacture new foods that require the utilization of mixtures of ingredients and of raw materials that have been little or not at all utilized for human consumption.

For example, if maize is used as one of the ingredients, ample technology is now available because for the past 10 years there has been a great demand for products obtained by the dry milling process. This has brought about the installation of many new mills, mainly on the African continent. However, if sorghum or millet is used, the technology available is less advanced. The same is true for processing cottonseed and other cereal grains, and for legumes and oilseeds not now in general use for human consumption.

When a combined flow chart for the processing of raw materials into ingredients is established, the need will be evident for introducing changes and modifications in order to adapt the system as easily as possible to each of the materials to be processed. If, after formulating the ingredients, they are subjected to partial or total cooking in order to offer the public a convenience food requiring little cooking, it is logical to expect additional technological problems.

To manufacture food incorporating flours of unusual origin, it may be impossible to import technology from highly developed countries without adaptation. This is because one is dealing with food products tailor-made to suit the culture and food habits of a specific country. Therefore, technology has to be developed and adjusted by manufacturers within the countries where the products will be used, with the assistance of research and nutrition institutes.

These are our experiences with the installation of the new Alimentos S.A. plant in Guatemala for the manufacture of Incaparina and other food products.

As pointed out by Hulse, food processing has been, and continues to be, empirically done and on a large scale. His suggestion that research scientists undergo apprenticeship in food industries prior to their admission to a research institution is important. Experience can be attained only with practice, and sundry small details can be learned only when facing the daily problems that industry encounters, none of which can be found in textbooks.

IV

Social and Economic Problems Limiting Food Supplies and Consumption

21

Food Distribution — Limitations on Supplies and Consumption

J. C. Abbott

Food and Agriculture Organization of the United Nations
Rome, Italy

This chapter examines the factors in food distribution that result in unsatisfactory levels of consumption for large parts of the world's population.

ECONOMIC PRINCIPLES GOVERNING FOOD DISTRIBUTION

Production and marketing of food is undertaken to meet evident market demands. It is not difficult to establish that world demand for food is unsatisfied at present prices, and that it will expand rapidly over the next 20 years from population increase alone, without allowing for any rise in per caput income in the developing countries. It is more difficult to determine how far nutritional demand is likely to be effective economically.

Effective demand is limited by price at any current prevailing consumer income/production cost equilibrium. Thus the outstanding change in food demand on a world level that began before the Second World War has been the shift from grains to pulses to animal protein foods in the richer countries as incomes have risen. Animal protein consumption has risen sharply in Japan, for example, in reflection of expanding consumer income, and demand for the traditional soy products has fallen back. Average meat consumption per person in Japan increased by almost 60% between 1969 and 1972.

This has not only attracted meat supplies away from the low income countries, it has drawn cereal, oilseed, and protein ingredients for livestock feed away from them, too. In the developing countries in 1969–71 consumption of cereals averaged about 230 kg per person; almost all of this was consumed directly. In such countries as Canada and the United States, however, total annual cereal consumption is over 800 kg per caput, of which only about 90 kg are consumed directly. The balance is fed to livestock. The 370 million tons of grain used annually for livestock feed in these countries in 1969–71 was greater than the total human consumption of cereals in China and India together.

Food Exports at the Cost of Domestic Consumers

Large-scale shipments of potential protein food supplies such as oilseeds, oilcake, and fishmeal also proceed from the developing countries to meet the market demand in Europe, North America, and Japan for concentrated livestock feed. The developing countries are constrained by economic necessities to export whatever portion of their production will find a more remunerative market in the developed countries. Little foreign exchange is available to pay for food movements in the opposite direction. Processed and other specialty foods are imported in small quantities for those few consumers who can afford them. Where food imports are needed on a large scale they are necessarily the cheapest available, or what can be obtained on concessional terms.

There are some countries where livestock and meat are exported, while large segments of the population remain on very low protein diets because they cannot afford to buy more of the meat produced in their own country. Such "perverse" movements are generally founded, however, on solid economics. Beef has been exported from Guatemala while a large part of the domestic population could hardly buy any because the price was too high. The incentive provided by the export market led to a doubling of beef production. Restricting exports by government intervention would not mean, however, that this extra production would then be available for the home market. It would soon decline for lack of effective demand. More than 100,000 tons of rice are exported annually from Nepal, yet in the mountain villages people are said to be starving. To divert exports to them the government has both to forgo exchange earnings and to provide subsidies that will bring down the price to a level they can afford. It has not the means to do this except on a very small scale. Also, China exports substantial quantities of meat, while the protein intake of its own population remains among the lowest in the world.

ACHIEVING A MORE EQUAL FOOD DISTRIBUTION

Various ways are open to governments whereby they can adjust food distribution along socially desirable lines. In Europe the peak of achievement in this direction probably came during the last World War. Rationing of major food items coupled with special distribution programs and subsidies gave the population of England, for example, a healthier diet, on the average, than it had before or has had since.

Policies introduced for this purpose subsequently have approached their goal by seeking to reduce disparities in purchasing power, by evening out peaks and troughs in supplies due to natural causes and uncertain incentives to producers, by promoting improvements in freely operating food distribution systems, and, eventually, by direct adjustment of the pricing and distribution process for strategic food products.

Redistribution of Consumer Incomes

It has already been noted that low food consumption is largely a response to low spending power. Redistributing incomes to raise the lowest level can be expected to have a direct effect on the proportion of the food supply going to the former lower income groups.

Preliminary analyses of a number of Latin American countries show that a moderate change in income distribution would result, given the circumstances of those countries, in a direct rise of some 9 to 9.5% in total food demand over 1970–80, or about 13 to 14% in the case of a "drastic" change in income distribution. A drastic change in income distribution has been carried through in Cuba, for example. Many foods have to be rationed there because incomes and prices no longer constitute a barrier to consumption for many of the people.

Incentives to Producers

However successful a government may be in reducing disparities in consumer incomes, it cannot afford to reduce the incentive for production. There has been a tendency for this to occur in some of the countries where sharp income redistribution programs have been carried through.

Production potentials can be more fully realized only if the producers have adequate incentives and supporting services. For instance, the price policies for farm products need to be formulated and implemented in such a way as to fix prices at incentive levels and to ensure that such prices are actually received by farmers. "Incentive level" also implies that the prices of farm products maintain a realistic relation to the prices of farm inputs.

For many years the government of India pursued price policies motivated primarily by concern to keep down the price of basic foods to consumers in the politically sensitive big cities. The effect was to reduce incentives for agricultural production. Pursued over a period of time, such a price policy diverts investment into other areas of economic activity and so reduces the capacity of agriculture to respond quickly, even when food shortages are reflected in higher prices at the farm gate.

Most Latin American countries have recognized the need to provide adequate price incentives to farmers and have set up specific marketing institutions to implement them. INDECA in Guatemala is one example; in Colombia it is

EDEMA, in Costa Rica the National Production Council. To be effective they must be able to announce at the beginning of the production season a floor price that farmers will receive, and be able to implement this by setting up machinery to ensure that the farmers actually get this price. In practice, their performance is uneven.

Supply and Price Stabilization

These agencies are also commonly used to operate supply stabilization programs that will cushion the effect on consumers of periodic shortages resulting from circumstances beyond man's control, such as droughts, floods, and earthquakes. Many governments have set up national stabilization and food reserve systems, but when the crisis comes they are often not strong enough to protect the people who are most vulnerable to price rises resulting from shortages—the lower income consumer. To cushion the effect of a very short crop a national stabilization agency must have stocks it has carried over from a previous year of ample harvests, or be able to draw upon supplies held available elsewhere. The implementation of supply and price stabilization for basic grain programs able to cope with all eventualities imposes heavy demands on the resources of most developing countries. Their problems include lack of information on existing marketing channels and movements, and on stocks and prospects; lack of skilled, reliable personnel; and inadequate capital.

Traditional Food Supply Systems

The urban poor suffer from the everyday shortcomings of the food-marketing channels on which they depend for their supplies. Approximately half the amount of money spent by Latin American consumers on food pays for marketing services; only half is received by the farmers, livestock raisers, and fishermen from whom the food originated.

The wide gap between the price paid by consumers and that received by the farmer is due partly to reductions in weight and volume occurring during the marketing process. Part of the farmer's output is eliminated en route because it would not meet consumers' standards, or because it has deteriorated in quality. Some of the losses result from poor management in harvesting; insect, rodent, and fungus damage in storage; packing in inadequate containers; rough handling; and delays during transport. Wastage of some fruit and vegetables in distribution can well reach 30% or more. Many of the agricultural products containing the most food value are highly perishable, and their marketing calls for specific handling, treatment, and storage arrangements, especially in tropical climates.

The role of a marketing system in bringing a valuable product in good condition to consumers, and promoting consumption, is outstanding in the case of fish. Integrated large-scale organization of fishing and marketing is rare in developing countries. The long-standing absence of a marketing system for fish, either fresh or dried, lies behind what might seem a striking nutritional anomaly—the massive exports of fishmeal from Peru while large numbers of its 12 million people remained on a low-protein diet. Because there was no system of bringing acceptable fish to the inland population, especially in the Sierra, there was little familiarity with fish—except for salted sardines in limited quantity—as a normal ingredient of the diet. There is still a carry-over effect on consumption when people from the Sierra move to Lima and come within easy access of fresh fish at relatively low prices.

A comparable situation prevails in the areas adjacent to the various ports in developing countries such as Egypt, India, Pakistan, and Guatemala, where profitable industries exporting frozen shrimp and prawns have grown up in recent years, and in Mexico, exporting sardines. Inadequate internal marketing arrangements interrelated with lack of consumer interest have effectively limited domestic utilization.

Marketing services involving transport, labor, materials, and risk have always to be paid for, but some marketing costs include extra margins obtained as a result of local monopoly, not only by private intermediaries, but also by workers' unions and municipal enterprises that do not allow free opportunity for competition. Urban food distribution in Latin America is still largely based on the traditional retail structure of small-scale groceries and large numbers of specialized retailers in public markets. Most of these retailers have a small sales turnover; the efficiency of their operations is low and their selling prices are comparatively high.

Improving Urban Food Supply Systems

There is an urgent need for improving most urban food distribution systems. Major approaches include:

1. construction of new wholesale markets and supply centers designed and sited to avoid traffic congestion and facilitate the use of better handling methods and organization;
2. promotion of vertical linkages between enterprises along the marketing channel to reduce costs due to small-scale, independent operation and uncertainties regarding supplies and outlets—these linkages may be achieved by direct integration of successive enterprises or by voluntary groupings;
3. public provision of services to support those engaged in food distribution, including short and longer term credit on convenient terms, technical and business advisory services, price and outlook information services;
4. provision of practically oriented training facilities adapted to the requirements of the managers and staff of food distribution enterprises.

These approaches are being pursued with varying degrees of determination in the different cities of Latin America, Africa, and Asia. New wholesale markets and food supply centers are being set up in many cities to avoid traffic congestion and simplify handling. FAO has been asked to advise on the planning of new wholesale markets for Beirut, Buenos Aires, Dar-es-Salaam, Mexico City, Teheran, and Sao Paulo, to quote only a few examples. Case studies and technical conferences on the organization of integrated channels from farm to city consumer have attracted wide interest (1,2). New integrated organizations are having their effect on services to consumers. The linking of a retail chain in Recife with a rice mill in the Sao Francisco Valley area of Brazil led to a 15% reduction in the price of rice to consumers in Recife.

Government Initiatives

There is still a long way to go, however, before governments are fully convinced that they can help farmers and consumers by providing supporting services to commercial food distribution systems. Too often their intervention is short-lived and misguided in nature. Recognizing that retail prices prevailing on free markets are too high in relation to many consumers' incomes, governments have been inclined to impose retail price controls. The implications of such measures are frequently not thought through fully. Only too often the effect is to create a black market at the retail level and discourage further production on the farm. Initiatives have been taken by some governments to set up their own enterprises intended to offer food at lower prices than those set by independent retailers. In practice it has often been found difficult for them to operate even within the margins of existing channels.

Governments have felt obliged to take such measures because commercial enterprise did not come forward fast enough with outlets designed to serve the lower income groups of consumers. There is a tendency for the first of the new integrated enterprises, sparked by a natural interest in profit, to be directed mainly toward consumers of the medium and higher income levels. The services offered by the supermarket or self-service grocery chain are those of convenience in buying a large number of items at one place, prepared ready for consumption, with prices clearly marked. Because of the range of products handled under one management, basic foods can be offered at low prices and the managers make up their profit margins on products sold to higher income consumers and on nonfood items. However, it is probable that supermarkets still appeal most to those consumers who are able to buy a considerable amount of food at one time and want to do it quickly. The lower income consumer has much less appreciation of this kind of service: He has neither the cash nor refrigerated storage facilities to buy large quantities at one time. On the contrary, he may have to buy small quantities on credit—a facility generally only available from the small retailer who knows him personally, and whose services involve higher total distribution margins.

To balance this tendency, some governments have joined with commercial enterprises to promote the interests of lower income consumers. The Nutritional Supply Programme (PAN) in Bogotá has been initiated by the Bogotá Supply Corporation (CORABASTOS), a government-supported but autonomous food marketing improvement agency, to help traditional small- and medium-scale food retailers to increase the efficiency of their operations and to assure a continuous supply of basic food items at low prices to the consumer. In 1972, sales through PAN amounted to U.S. $2.6 million, or 0.7% of total food sales in Bogotá. The average margin of the affiliated retailers was 12% and their prices were about 15% lower than those of other stores. Another notable Latin American example is Companía Nacional de Subsisténcias Populares (CONASUPO). It operates some 800 self-service stores in the lower income areas of Mexico City. Their sales, featuring basic foods and reconstituted milk, amount to about 15% of total food sales. Charging lower prices than other retail outlets, they are able to influence substantially the overall price level for basic foods. Some government subsidies are involved.

Two-Price Systems

A more specific solution to the problem of paying enough to producers to keep supplies coming forward, yet ensure that lower income consumers can purchase their needs, lies in some sort of two-price system. If an average retail price of $100 per ton of some product is needed to maintain an adequate level of production, then a socially oriented marketing system might sell 60% of the total supply at $120 per ton and 40% to lower income consumers at $80 per ton. The total amount of money obtained to pay for production and marketing is the same, but by welfare criteria, a more efficient distribution has been secured. The lower income group has been enabled to buy what it needs. Consumers with higher incomes have been asked to pay more, but they have more money available and, with a more varied dietary intake, generally attach less importance to purchases of basic foods. Requirements for implementing such systems are: (1) A large part of the supplies of the basic food concerned must come into the hands of a single assembly and wholesaling agency committed to operating the program; and (2) there must be some means of distinguishing the lower from higher income consumers at the retail level.

The starting point is usually the public agency that operates a national supply and price stabilization program for basic grains. At the retail level it must either maintain its own outlets or sell through shops contracted to apply agency prices. Consumers can be distinguished explicitly by ration cards, or approximately by location of retail outlets or timing of sales in some situations.

Commercial exponents of "market segmentation," as it is called in professional circles, have other more sophisticated devices based on packaging, branding, and style of promotion. In the United States lower income families have been given stamps that, when presented to certain retailers, count as part of the price and so reduce the payment required.

A two-price system has been operating in India for rice and wheat through "fair price shops" over many years now. These shops receive wheat, for example, from the government procurement system for Rs 1.25 per kg. They sell 2 kgs to each consumer at around Rs 1.28–1.30 on presentation of a ration card. Taking into account the value of the sack itself, their margin of profit is about 5%. About half the quantity marketed goes through this channel; the balance is sold on the free market at prices ranging from about the same to 60% higher according to quality, location, and season. Through a similar program in Sri Lanka, consumers with an income below the minimum taxation level receive 2 kgs of rice per week free. Some 30 to 40% of the total supply is distributed in this way, originating for the most part as imports. The Sri Lanka program involves a very large government subsidy and may not be feasible, or desirable, in many other countries.

A way of applying the same principle to milk in one African city was to sell at a lower price, early in the morning, from bulk vehicles standing in the street in low income districts. Milk in containers was delivered to other areas for sale at higher prices by authorized retailers. The provision of milk, protein-fortified foods, and complete meals in schools, either free or at very low prices, is another well-known way of reaching at least the school children of lower income families.

Elements of such programs are to be found in many Latin American countries. To implement such measures calls for major inputs of capital, organizing ability, and consistent government support. That they are feasible is clear, provided there are the means and the will.

The ability of some countries to implement such programs is restricted by the limited resources at their disposal. It would be a worthy objective of international collaboration to assist them in such socially desirable programs.

In summary, food is produced and distributed in response to economic demand and incentives. It is important that governments keep these principles in the forefront of their planning; otherwise they may take measures intended to help consumers, but that in practice will prove contrary to their longer run interests. Positive steps to improve food distribution include price incentives to producers, supply and price stabilization measures, support to rationing programs, and vertical linkage of enterprises making up urban food supply systems, and introduction of two-price programs. Where the lower income consumers far outnumber those able to pay higher prices, international support may be needed to enable national governments to implement these programs effectively.

REFERENCES

1. Food and Agriculture Organization, 1972, *Planning and operation of wholesale markets in Latin America,* Report on the Technical Conference on Planning and Operation of Wholesale Markets, held in Brasilia, F.D., Brazil, 18–22 October, 1971, FAO, Rome.
2. Food and Agriculture Organization, 1973, *Development of food marketing systems for large urban areas,* Report of the Technical Conference on the Development of Food Marketing Systems in Large Urban Areas in Latin America, Buenos Aires, Argentina, 8–17 May, 1973, FAO, Rome.

COMMENTS

George C. Warner · *US/AID, Lima, Peru.*

Centralization of food distribution as a means of reducing food costs requires capital and may reduce employment. It is important to evaluate the alternative benefits of using such capital elsewhere, evaluate the effects of the unemployment created, and compare the costs and benefits.

In regard to food costs and prices, it would be useful if more reference could be made to percent of income spent for foods rather than simply the percent of price reduction (or increase) expected from a particular intervention. In an inflationary period the price figure may not reflect ability to purchase and use food.

Lastly, I fear an overkill is in progress in efforts to divert grains from animal to direct human consumption. Cattle in less developed countries are often raised on pasture that, for various reasons, is not suited for grain production. Finishing lots feed cattle corncobs and stalks, molasses, cottonseed meal, and related high-fiber wastes that complement food production for human use rather than compete with it. We must continue to use the marvelous capacity of ruminants to provide us with protein.

Juan del Canto · *Division of Applied Nutrition, Institute of Nutrition of Central America and Panama, Guatemala City, Guatemala.*

The discussion on the distribution of food mentioned rationing associated with wars, natural disasters, and intervention programs. In developing countries of Latin America and other regions, rationing by price is more common. It is less noticeable, but affects the majority of the low-income population. It is very efficient in limiting the possibilities for obtaining food in those countries in which the distribution of wealth and income leaves the majority at a subsistence level.

Neither supermarkets full of various foods nor phrases like "Today everything is available" are necessarily good indicators of efficient food distribution. Under some circumstances the situation may actually be worse than in war or disaster situations when few foods are visible in the supermarkets, but food is distributed more equitably by rationing of available food to all individuals regardless of income.

22

Population Trends and Policies in Latin America

Hildebrando Araica A.

Ministry of Health
Department of Population and Planning
Panama, Panama

The countries that constitute Latin America* have undergone a series of changes of varying character and intensity since World War II. Convulsions of social and economic origin have seen the birth of the first Socialist state, and have been linked to many violent changes in political power that have put social institutions to very hard tests. A state of economic dependency tends to intensify multiple social problems, particularly those related to food supplies and consumption, and has determined changes in social and political attitudes that have led to new approaches, strategies, and programs for solving food problems. Cooperative international action has played an important role as both promoter and coordinator. The Economic Commission for Latin America (ECLA) has assumed the task of creating a social conscience in our hemisphere regarding the origin and character of the main economic difficulties to be faced. The analyses and projections of economic and social development were the first significant steps taken by our countries. This fundamental action was followed by joint efforts toward import substitution, development planning, industrialization, promotion of economic integration through common markets, and studies of income distribution. As Prebisch pointed out in 1970 (1), this joint effort has taken place within the context of direct foreign investments that strongly influence indigenous economic development. These investments constitute a

*The term *Latin America* herein applies to all of the Spanish-speaking countries south of Rio Bravo, including Brazil and, in the Caribbean area, Cuba, the Dominican Republic, and Haiti.

material expression of the dependency mentioned earlier, and have tended to delay national technologic development. They have also absorbed national enterprises that were relatively advanced technologically because of local difficulties in obtaining credit, or because foreign executives are more interested in monetary returns than they are in encouraging our economic development, leading to strangulation from without, because of debt payments to foreign investors.

Aside from these considerations, the transference of national enterprises to foreign control awakens acute concern when important decisions for national life are made from outside our own countries. This is also true for existing enterprises that have for a long time been exploiting natural resources. A very significant evolution has started whereby through negotiations a country tries to reach agreements that will permit it to achieve national control, either immediately or within a reasonable period of time.

Another concern is the advance of foreign investment into the banking system of a country and the transference to foreign hands of banking establishments already in existence. The foreign banking branch has a specific and limited function in foreign investment or foreign trade operations, but its expansion to other activities can create unnecessary problems. There is some far-seeing legislation in this field, and perhaps the strictest is that of the United States, in regard not only to transfer of funds, but even to the establishment of foreign banks (1).

In spite of the various problems arising from unfair exchange relationships at the international level, inflation, unemployment, limited export capacity, and scarcity of capital, Latin America has made significant social progress in such areas as education, health, and housing conditions. However, enormous deficits still exist in these areas and serious obstacles limit access of the whole population to the benefits of the development process. Associated with the unsolved problems of Latin American economic underdevelopment is the appearance of social, economic, and political problems due to urbanization. Slums or marginal urban sectors are not a recent phenomenon for the main Latin American cities, but they have grown rapidly in the postwar period (2). The rural population has migrated to the cities in the hope of sharing in urban economic development, but our metropolises have not been able to absorb their own increasing labor forces, much less the rural migrants. The latter live a hard life in misery belts and neglected slums, and their dissatisfaction and impatience emphasize that there is no room for complacence in Latin America (3).

It is within this framework that an accelerated demographic expansion of a magnitude never known before by humanity has occurred in Latin America. This paper reviews and analyzes population policies in Latin America in response to this phenomenon.

THE POSTWAR POPULATION OF LATIN AMERICA

When World War II ended, little was really known about the dynamics, distribution, and composition of the populations of the Latin American countries. In nine, the last census information pertained to years prior to 1940, and in four others no census had been taken for 25 years. It was imperative to know the magnitude, growth rate, and characteristics of the population. The need for such knowledge grew out of the numbers of war refugees and displaced persons seeking new places to settle. The governments of less developed countries were asked to assess their capability for assimilating these people, from the standpoint of natural resources and agricultural production. The 1950 Census Program of the Americas was the hemisphere's response to the need for a minimal degree of comparability of results based on common tabulations and concepts. This effort, never undertaken before, was a landmark in technical cooperation and understanding among the Latin American nations. All but two of them conducted a census of human resources in the middle of the present century (4).

Thanks to the 1950 Census Program of the Americas, there was gradual improvement in sampling research and in the assembling of vital statistics, and further census efforts in 1960 and 1970 have provided basic demographic documentation on the postwar Latin American population. The estimates of the Economic Commission for Latin America for 1950 and 1960 indicated that the population of the Latin American Republics increased 31.7% during that decade, or from 155.6 to 204.9 million. This increase, amounting to an annual rate of 2.8%, makes Latin America the most rapidly growing region in the world, clearly more than Oceania (26.9%) and Southwest Asia (28.3%) (5). Latin American Demography Center projections show the population of Latin America continuing to grow at the 2.8% rate annually during the decade between 1960 and 1970, especially in the Middle American subgroup composed of the countries of the Central American Isthmus, Panama and Mexico (6). In this area, the population grew at an annual rate of 3.3%, followed by the tropical countries of South America, with 2.9%, and the Caribbean region with 2.4%. The temperate countries of South America registered the lowest demographic growth rate, at 1.8%.

Prior to World War II, Latin America had been growing at the rate of 2% per year, and the growth rates did not differ much among its subregions. Apparently, the discoveries of medical science and progress in public health services had not extended to Latin America, perhaps because of the economic crisis of the 1930s and the Second World War. Demographic acceleration from 1950 to 1970 suggests the rapidity with which medical and sanitary advances had an effect in Latin America once they were applied.

Mortality

Many Latin American countries had mortality rates surpassing 20 per 1000 in the years preceding the war, and an average life expectancy at birth of around 40 years. Spectacular decreases in mortality occurred during the years 1950 to 1955, and fell to 10 per 1000 in the 5 years from 1965 to 1970. Life expectancy at birth rose to 52 years in the period between 1950 and 1955, and reached 60 years in the span between 1965 and 1970. The differences in mortality among the Latin American countries continued to diminish, reaching only a 6-year difference between the highest and lowest life expectancies. It should be stressed that deaths due to infectious and parasitic disease, so closely related to malnutrition and inadequate environmental conditions, accounted for 14% of the total deaths in 1950, reaching alarmingly high levels in Guatemala, Honduras, Bolivia, Paraguay, and Nicaragua. Even by 1968 the situation had not improved in Guatemala, Nicaragua, and several other countries, but death rates were lower in Cuba, Argentina, and Uruguay.

Fertility

All indicators classify Latin America as a high-fertility region. Before World War II its gross birth rate probably varied from 40 to 45 per 1000. For the 1950–1955 period, when more and better information became available, the birth rate was estimated to be 41 per 1000; the lowest value, 27 per 1000, was found in temperate South America, while Middle America and tropical South America had maximum values of 46 and 45 per 1000, respectively.

In the 1960s notable changes occurred in the knowledge of contraceptive methods and attitudes concerning procreation. This was partly a consequence of direct or indirect foreign influences that are reflected in the decrease in fertility rates observed in the years 1965–1970, and they have fallen even more rapidly since. In these years, birth rates in Latin America fell to 37 per 1000, and only Middle America exceeded the 40-per-1000 level. The countries of temperate South America recorded the lowest birth rates (24 per 1000), with tropical South America reaching a birth rate of 39 per 1000.

As a consequence of the high fertility rates that characterized the majority of the Latin American countries, in 1970 it still had the demographic profile of a very young region; 43% of its population was less than 15 years of age, and only around 4% were 65 years or older. The high dependency load is evident. In Latin America the ratio of dependency load has a value of 87, while in Africa it rises to 90, reaching its lowest value in the Soviet Union and Europe, where it is only 57. As may be assumed from the fertility data, the highest percentages of the young and dependent population are observed in Middle America and in the countries of tropical South America.

Recently, attention to urban growth of Latin America has been accentuated, because when cities receive an influx from rural areas they absorb a great proportion of the population growth of the rural sectors. Between 1950 and 1960, the population of Latin America increased by 50 million, but only a third of this increase occurred in the rural areas, in spite of the fact that more people lived there than in the cities (7). In fact, in that decade the urban population increased 56%, while the rural gained barely 17%. In 1970 the urban surpassed the rural population. The degrees of urbanization of the subregions were as follows: temperate South America, 74.2%; Middle America, 55.6%; tropical South America, 50.6%; and the Caribbean, 38.8%. In contrast, in 1970 Oceania was 75% urbanized, while in Asia the figure was only 21%.

According to Cardona and Simmons (8): "With respect to the historic experience of Europe and North America, the urbanization levels in Latin America are very high compared to its industrialization levels. Partly as a consequence of these factors, unemployment and underemployment rates in Latin America are extremely high. Furthermore, the industrial growth that is taking place in the region is relatively intensive, and this is the reason why it absorbs only a small number of laborers. While the greater part of European and North American laborers headed towards the cities in search of more secure and better-paid jobs, Latin American laborers apparently go to the cities because of the absence of any type of work in the rural areas." This phenomenon does not show any signs of decreasing, and explains the exceptional growth of cities with one million or more inhabitants that, in 1970, had already absorbed 33% of the total population, a percentage surpassed only by North America.

PERSPECTIVES FOR THE POPULATION OF LATIN AMERICA

The high potential of demographic growth, intrinsic to the young population structure, together with the fertility levels observed, make one foresee that the Latin American population will have risen to more than 600 million inhabitants by the end of the 20th century. This is not a prediction, because one cannot foretell exactly what will happen to fertility, mortality, and international migrations. It is a hypothesis based on currently available data. The 1973 United Nations population projections for Latin America are shown in Table I, including the Caribbean Islands, Belize, French Guiana, and Surinam (9).

From the figures in Table I it can be deduced that at the end of this century, Latin America as a whole will have diminished its rate of increase to 2.4% per year. Nevertheless, there seem to be reasons to suppose that the demographic increment will diminish more than the projections, although it is not easy to foresee what influence more general and intensive use of contraceptive methods of high efficacy will have on the fertility rates.

The International Strategy for the Second Decade of the United Nations

Table I. Projected Latin American Population from 1975 to the Year 2000 (Millions)

Year	Total	Caribbean	Middle America	Temperate South America	Tropical South America
1975	326	28	79	39	180
1980	374	32	93	42	207
1985	429	36	109	45	239
1990	490	40	128	48	274
1995	554	44	149	50	311
2000	626	49	173	53	351

Development Program assumes a possible demographic growth rate of 2.5% per year in the present decade. It would seem logical that if this goal, and the economic and social objectives that determine it, are reached, it will decrease even more in what remains of the century (10). It is worth emphasizing that the preconquest population of the tropical countries of South America was probably similar to that of North America and that the latter has surpassed it because of massive migration. Before the turn of the century, Latin America's population will surpass that of North America.

As may be observed in Table II, rather a moderate decrease in fertility is

Table II. Projected Gross Reproduction Rates (Percent) and Years of Life Expectancy at Birth in Latin America: 1970–2000

Subregion	1970–1975	1975–1980	1980–1985	1985–1990	1990–1995	1995–2000
Latin America						
Fertility rate	2.57	2.45	2.32	2.18	2.04	1.90
Life expectancy	61.9	64.0	65.9	67.6	69.4	70.6
The Caribbean						
Fertility rate	2.37	2.21	2.05	1.93	1.81	1.70
Life expectancy	64.0	65.6	67.0	68.2	69.3	70.3
Middle America						
Fertility rate	3.11	3.00	2.83	2.70	2.51	2.33
Life expectancy	61.7	64.0	65.7	67.3	68.6	69.9
Temperate South America						
Fertility rate	1.50	1.43	1.36	1.30	1.24	1.18
Life expectancy	67.3	68.8	69.8	70.5	71.2	71.7
Tropical South America						
Fertility rate	2.63	2.48	2.32	2.16	2.00	1.84
Life expectancy	60.6	62.8	65.0	67.1	69.0	70.8

foreseen for Latin America as a whole. Actually, there is reason to expect more pronounced decreases. The decrease expected for the tropical countries of South America was achieved, for example by Trinidad and Tobago, in only 11 years, and Puerto Rico reached this target in approximately 10 years, as projected for the Caribbean (11). Any changes in the fertility hypotheses will imply important changes in the age composition of populations. Dependence relations could decrease gradually from the 87% level seen in 1970 to 72% by the end of the century. For comparison, United Nations projections indicate that the African continent will maintain itself at about the 90% dependency rate. Europe will not vary significantly either; its levels will stay close to 55%. The analysis of the structure by age and sex is of obvious interest in development plans, because economic, social, cultural, and political functions have a demographic frame. These functions are influenced by different population groups, for example, the school population, the economically active sector, and females of reproductive age.

Kindergarten children (< 4 years old) will increase from 46 million in 1979 to 85 million in the year 2000. A tremendous effort awaits Latin America in the training of enough teachers and building the necessary number of schools to cope with this demand, as well as to overcome existing deficits.

Other problems will be serious unemployment and underemployment, scarcity of capital, and an exceptional increase in the 15–64-year-old group. According to the projections, this population group, which now amounts to 152 million, will increase to 362 million by the end of the century. The size of this group is of major importance, not only because of its need for economically productive work, but also because it contains the women of reproductive age. The population of retirement age—from 65 years on—will also almost triple by the end of the century, when it is expected to reach 29 million.

The 100% growth in the school-age population from 1970 to the year 2000 in Latin America compares with 140% in Africa and only 1% in Europe. In Latin America kindergarten-age children will increase 82% during the period 1970–2000, while in Africa the increase will be 126%, and in Europe only 4%. Evidently, pressures and investment needs will be altogether different in these regions.

These demographic changes will bring about transformations in employment, food marketing, transportation, public education, and industrial structure and will accelerate urbanization processes in the remaining years of the 20th century. The United Nations projects 470 million human beings in cities by the year 2000. In temperate South America, practically 9 out of 10 of its inhabitants will live in urban sectors, and the infrastructure costs for housing, transportation, water, sewage and industrial waste disposal, and public safety will absorb increasing proportions of the national income.

The perspectives point to the fact that the population of Latin America, which in 1970 represented 7.8% of the total world population, will represent

10% of the total in the year 2000. As the hypotheses for fertility projections reveal, it is impossible to visualize how Latin American fertility could drop to mere replacement levels before the end of the present century. Demographic inertia, the force inherent in the age composition of the population necessary to extend the increment, will cause important increases beyond the year 2000 before the Latin American population reaches zero growth. According to present United Nations calculations, Latin America will reach the replacement level between the years 2035 and 2040, and cease growing around the year 2125, when its population will have increased to 1.3 billion, at which time it would be expected to stabilize birth and mortality rates at a level of about 13 per 1000. Based on other hypotheses, Tomás Frejka has estimated that Latin America's growth potential will arrive at totals of 824 million or even 1.7 billion inhabitants in the year 2150 (12).

POPULATION POLICIES IN LATIN AMERICA

The complex political, economic, and social context under which the phenomenal Latin American demographic growth has occurred during the post-war years has created problems. The interrelationships of these problems with social disorganization, inequitable trade relationships, and neglected human resources generate the need for policies, programs, and actions that will provide progress, justice, ecologic, and demographic changes. Latin America's demographic inertia demands development planning.

It is generally accepted that economic development has great influence on fertility, mortality, and migration, and constitutes a very important factor in determining demographic behavior. In addition, there is almost unanimous consensus that when economic development has a broad social basis, it gives rise to a considerable reduction in fertility. But, what is the nature of the inverse relationship? Many persons believe that under equal circumstances, a country with an accelerated demographic growth will encounter more difficulty in reaching economic development than another one with lower population growth rates. However, there is a wide variety of opinion, from the one that high population growth rates made economic development impossible, to one suggesting that such rates, whether high or low, are a component of the development process, with very little importance, or none at all, for the process itself. Others simply state that accelerated population growth contributes to economic development (13). This statement summarizes the different positions taken in regard to population growth. In fact, it implies a "population theory" that attempts to explain the factors determining demographic increment. Even in academic circles, political preconceptions as well as pure reason determine attitudes toward population.

In general, Latin American countries look at demographic dynamics and the distribution of their populations within an ample frame of considerations regarding economic and social changes. Moreover, in a region relatively devoid of demographic information, where at best the planning process is in an adolescent stage, it would be utopian to expect economic and social development plans with integrated demographic policies and clearly defined goals and the means of carrying them out. There is still a long way to go in this field. At the Latin American Population Conference held in Mexico City in 1970, Carmen A. Miró posed the following questions with respect to population policy: What? Why? How? (14). Any population policy that is not simply family planning would be a conglomerate of goals to be reached in relation to the size, composition, distribution, and rate of changes in the population. The decisions regarding such policy should be taken by the public sector, as part of real economic and social development plans. Population policy must be strongly developed and executed, because it is unthinkable to leave the achievement of specific population goals to chance. A population policy must be adopted to integrate demographic, social, and economic goals with development plans.

Experience with population policies in Latin America demonstrates that this is a field where there is little precision and much confusion at the decision level, partly because of lack of knowledge about demographic realities, and very little perception of population problems as such. Only four of the countries of this region recognize the existence of any population problem in the demographic content of the economic and social plans. The population in these four adds to an approximate total of 33 million inhabitants (15).

It is therefore quite impossible to discuss a Latin American population policy, much less one concerned with limiting demographic growth in all of the countries. Much can be learned from the Preparatory Latin American Meeting of the World Population Conference held in April, 1974 in San José, Costa Rica and the subsequent Latin American participation in the World Population Conference held in Bucharest the following August. Although discussion of demographic policies was accorded importance, they were considered in the context of economic, social, cultural, and political interrelationships. Particular emphasis was placed on the fact that the population policy—as part of the economic and social development programs—is mainly a national matter that each country must discuss, formulate, and decide upon in accordance with its cultural characteristics and its basic situation and perspectives. Thus, it was stressed that in some Latin American areas such policy should consist in speeding up the population growth, if possible with immigration assistance, to derive full advantage from their great resources potential (16). The possibility that in certain countries, urban or rural settlement programs could be carried out for the purpose of obtaining a gradual redistribution of the population, was pointed out. It was also emphasized that population policies cannot be designed without taking into account, and possibly modifying, existing policies in the fields of education, health, housing, environmental sanitation, and general social policy.

The statements of the Delegations of Brazil, Argentina, Cuba, and Mexico were outstanding for their diversity. Brazil rejected any proposition directed at reducing demographic growth, on the basis of the scarcity-of-resources argument. It was pointed out that no such scarcity existed, and that crises were apparent and many times the consequence of political measures within some states, while in other instances the roots of problems were of technologic origin. Reference was made to information from the United States of America that confirmed how difficult it would be to draw conclusions from the past regarding the relationship between resources and demographic growth.

The reciprocal implications between population and income were caustically simplified by pointing out that if Brazil's population were reduced to one person and the internal products were maintained at the present level, such an individual would be the wealthiest in the world. It would be quite dubious that he would feel happy living alone in an area of 8.5 million kilometers. The Delegation stressed the fact that it would be wise to detain growth to only a unit, because reduction to zero of the denominator would increase *nobody's* fortune to the infinite, converting him into the wealthiest and perhaps the happiest *no being* of the world.

Argentina, on the other hand, criticized the wastage of resources in the more developed countries, particularly of foods, and pointed out that in its country the people should benefit from its now empty, immense, wealthy spaces. Thus, Argentina would encourage big families and promote international policies oriented toward bringing immigrants to its territory, particularly from Latin America; it would also legalize the status of its illegal immigrants and would try to gain back its emigrants. Its goal is to reach the XXI Century with a population of 50 million inhabitants instead of the 35 million foreseen in the demographic projections, if no significant changes occur in the variables that determine population change. The idea is that Argentina will grow demographically to be more self-sufficient.

Cuba considers that underdevelopment problems do not derive from demographic growth or from urban concentration. The decrease in Cuban fertility rates, stated the Delegation, is a consequence of the participation of women in the economic sector, of improved and more extensive education programs, and of the substantial improvements achieved in rural life. With respect to urbanization, it was pointed out how decentralization of productive activities has influenced the nature of urban concentrations in the country. Emphasis was placed on modernization of rural housing, elimination of unemployment and illiteracy, establishment of schools in rural areas, and universal education. To cope with its problems, Cuba had not concentrated on contraception, but rather on development tasks geared toward improving the lot of the neglected majority in the more essential aspects of education and health. In the latter field, malaria, poliomyelitis, diphtheria, and tetanus neonatorum had been eradicated, and all forms of infantile tuberculosis were practically nil.

Mexico, in presenting its General Population Law, which basically is a migration law although it includes basic features designed to influence the development of other demographic variables, gave major emphasis to the need for those countries to legislate their population status freely, without foreign pressure, and with their own economic development as the fundamental objective.

Peru rejected neo-Malthusianism, insisting that countries promoting family planning should be providing more stable economic aid to the less developed countries. It denied the thesis that malnutrition, deficient housing conditions, and unemployment are caused by a high demographic growth rate. The Peruvian delegate also stressed its country's resolution to defend and utilize its own natural resources.

Some countries, burdened by very serious population problems, proposed measures to reduce the rate of demographic increase; others with less serious population density also declared themselves in favor of a slower pace of demographic growth. However, the common note was the recognition of the nations' sovereignty to decide their own policies within their own economic and social development frames.

Finally, it should be added that the Latin American countries, along with the rest of the world with the exception of the Holy See, joined in the consensus, adopted in Bucharest, for a Population Plan of Action. The development of this plan obviously involves the implementation of demographic research and action geared to execute those parts relevant to population policies and characteristics of each country.

The Plan of Action covered such matters as morbidity and mortality, procreation and formation of the family, demographic growth, population distribution and internal migration, international migration, and population structure, with special reference to sex and age. It recognized the heterogeneity of the prevailing situations in the different regions and countries, proclaimed the sovereignty of decisions, and underlined respect for human rights in the determination and execution of policy. It also clarified that cooperation of the industrialized countries in population matters does not replace or reduce the need for economic cooperation with less developed countries, and emphasized that population policies should be designed and executed within the broad context of economic and social development.

REFERENCES

1. Prebisch, R., 1970, Transformación y Desarrollo: La Gran Tarea de América Latina, Instituto Latinoamericano de Planificación Económico y Social (ILPES), Santiago de Chile, p. 111.

2. Comisión Económica para América Latina, 1963, *El Desarrollo Social de América Latina en la Post-Guerra,* Documento E/CN. 12/660 del décimo período de sesiones celebrado en Mar del Plata, Argentina, Mayo, p. 69.
3. Prebisch, R., 1970, Transformación y Desarrollo: La Gran Tarea de América Latina, Instituto Latinoamericano de Planificación Económico y Social (ILPES), Santiago de Chile, p. 14.
4. Instituto Interamericano de Estadística, 1953, *Relato del Censo de las Américas de 1950,* Washington, D.C., p. 2.
5. Carleton, R. O., 1966, Crecimiento de la Población y Fecundidad Diferencial en América Latina, Centro Latino Americano de Demografía (CELADE) Santiago de Chile, p. 7, Published by Unión Internacional para el Estudio Científico de la Población.
6. Centro Latino Americano de Demografía, 1972, *Boletín Demográfico* No. 10, Año V, Santiago de Chile, CELADE, pp. 4–5.
7. Carleton, R. O., 1966, Crecimiento de la Población y Fecundidad Diferencial en América Latina, Centro Latino Americano de Demografía (CELADE) Santiago de Chile, p. 21.
8. Cardona, R., and Simmons, A., 1974, Hacia un Modelo General de la Migración Interna en América Latina, Selecciones de Población del Population Reference Bureau, Oficina Regional para América Latina, Bogotá, Colombia, p. 1.
9. Naciones Unidas, 1974, Perspectivas de la Población Mundial y Regional, Documento E/CONF.60/CBP 15, de la Conferencia Mundial de Población, Bucharest, Rumania, p. 8.
10. Comisión Económica para América Latina, 1971, *América Latina y el Segundo Decenio de las Naciones Unidas para el Desarrollo,* Documento E/CN.12/869 del décimo cuarto período de sesiones, Santiago de Chile, p. 23.
11. Office of Population Research, 1972, Princeton University, *Population Index* 38 (2): 236.
12. Marks, J., 1974, Proyecciones de la Población Mundial: Rutas Alternativas para el Crecimiento Cero, *Boletín de Población,* Publication of the Population Reference Bureau, Bogotá, Colombia, p. 28.
13. Stamper, M. B., 1973, La Política de Población en la Planificación para el Desarrollo, *Informe sobre Población/Planificación Familiar,* No. 13, p. 3.
14. Miró, C. A., 1970, Política de Población: Qué? Por qué? Para qué? Como?, *in: Actas de la Conferencia Regional Latinoamericana de Población, Mexico, D.F.,* pp. 276–281.
15. Stamper, M. B., 1973, La Política de Población en la Planificación para el Desarrollo, *Informe sobre Población/Planificación Familiar,* No. 13, p. 12.
16. Comisión Económica para América Latina, 1974, *Informe de la Reunión Latinoamericana Preparatoria de la Conferencia Mundial de Población, San José, Costa Rica,* Documento ST/ECLA/CONF.48/L. 7/Rev. 1, pp. 8–9.

COMMENTS

Eduardo E. Arriaga · *Data Evaluation Branch, International Statistical Programs Center, U.S. Bureau of the Census, Washington, D.C.*

There is a tendency to misunderstand world population policy. It is often stated that only recently has there been an attempt to conduct some population policies through the family planning program. A common error is to consider that any population policy should tend to reduce fertility.

First, Latin America has had one of the most effective population policies of the world and, second, family planning is only an instrument of the population policy. Latin America had a population policy without precedence in the world during the period 1930 to 1960. Mortality reduction was well achieved. The decline in mortality in Latin America in 30 years was similar to the decline in western Europe during 100 years (1). The decline in Latin America was due to application or diffusion of health knowledge (2). It was in 1960, when the population census results were known, that the rapid population growth in Latin America became of concern to those international organizations that were helping to reduce mortality. Planners of the public health programs had forgotten about the other demographic variable: fertility. The result was the demographic imbalance in population growth and age structure.

In the last decade, some effort has been concentrated on programs for reducing fertility. Nevertheless, the result in general has been insignificant, with the exception of a few countries such as Costa Rica and Chile. The future is uncertain because it is easier to reduce mortality than fertility. Nevertheless, there is a need for planning population policies integrated with the social and economic development programs of these countries (3–5). Such programs should take into account the actual population, natural resources, social conditions, and development possibilities. Taken into consideration must be the effect of natural increase and age structure of population on the economic development of a nation, how fertility affects the income distribution of the society, and the crucial problems of labor force, concentration of people in cities, water supply, traffic congestion, educational problems, rural conditions, and other population problems.

Some of the imbalances created by the continuous and uncontrolled population growth in Latin America and in the world, particularly in relation to food production, need emphasis. The world is becoming more urbanized every day. This has created an imbalance in the recycling of natural substances. When the world population was relatively small and dispersed in rural areas, the waste of agricultural and human products was returned immediately to the soil. Because the world was not densely populated and population was growing slowly, there was enough time for those substances to return to their natural state. Today, on the contrary, agricultural products are transported to the cities. This means that we are transporting to the cities chemical substances as well as part of the soil of the rural areas, transformed into food. These agricultural products are consumed in the cities and their waste does not go back to the rural areas. Thus the natural cycle has been broken, but what is even worse, urban populations are polluting water, air, and earth.

We still do not have any satisfactory solution for the problem. Not only are we making soil in rural areas poorer—hence the urgent need to use fertilizers—but in addition we are contributing to the erosion of rural areas and the pollution of the world. If we were able to analyze this process for another planet, we would think it destructive; for ourselves, we call it progress.

Ten years ago we thought that new techniques would solve the problem of famine. During the last 10 years, around 800 million people have been added to the world—persons who have to be fed and who have produced a more crucial problem of hunger. But still we are ingenuous, hoping that technical discoveries will solve the world hunger problem. How that will happen is hard to know, but an increase in food production (if it is possible) without policies for controlling and stopping human overpopulation will only postpone for a short time the problem of feeding the newcomers. There is no doubt that we are already too many. The complete answer is not in an increased amount of food; it is not in better income distribution; it is not in better international collaboration. These are necessary and desirable, but only partial, temporary, and insufficient for long-range human well-being. The only permanent solution is, without doubt, population control.

References

1. Arriaga, E. E., and Davis, K., 1969, The pattern of mortality change in Latin America, *Demography* 6 (3): 223–242.
2. Arriaga, E. E., 1970, *Mortality decline and its demographic effects in Latin America,* Population Monograph Series No. 6, Institute of International Studies, University of California, Berkeley.
3. Arriaga, E. E., 1970, The nature and effects of Latin America's non-Western trend in fertility, *Demography* 7 (4): 483–501.
4. Arriaga, E. E., 1970, Necesidad de politicas de poblacion en America Latina, *Demographia y Economia* (Mexico) **VI** (1): 79–97.
5. Arriaga, E. E., 1975, Population and economic planning: A macro analysis, International Statistical Programs Center, Bureau of the Census, Washington, D.C.

Carlos Tejada · *Director, Institute of Nutrition of Central America and Panama, Guatemala City, Guatemala.*

I am in agreement with Araica's views on population trends. Both he and Arriaga have approached this subject from the standpoint of its relation to economic and social development. It is equally important to relate it to health, nutrition, and food problems.

Araica's discussion is in two parts. The first deals with the postwar population dynamics in Latin America. These data need not be discussed further, but they do help predict the future. The second part, dealing with population policies in Latin America, a topic of much controversy, is based on the following premises:

1. Population policy is not a synonym for family planning.
2. Population policy must be formulated by the public sector and incorporated within the economic and social plans.
3. Population policies have not yet been adopted in Latin America with the exception of four countries.
4. Population policy must be national and decided in accordance with the present situation, future perspectives, and individual cultural characteristics of each country.

I fully agree with these four concepts and would only like to develop further the first point, relating to family planning. From a nutrition and health point of view, this constitutes a service that must be made available to all families. This is true regardless of the effects on demographic trends, which are difficult to demonstrate on a short-term basis. In this manner the greater intervals between births lower the mother–child risk and the nutrition of the family unit is improved by an increase of per caput food availability.

Isolated family planning programs of the vertical type have not had any substantial effect on the birth rate. On the other hand, the effective demand for this type of service is very low when families have not yet reached a better standard of living, whereby they would be in a position to consider the importance of family planning. In other words, family planning programs must be considered as a means to improve the quality of life, not just as a measure for birth control.

Araica's data raise a series of questions and point out actions that must be implemented as soon as possible. The figures in his first table are not hypothetical and are not subject to great change; they are the result of the structural characteristics and tendencies of the present Latin American population. Although actions geared toward modifying the different demographic variables are under way, the population of Latin America, by the year 2000, will have doubled, bringing the total to approximately 626 million inhabitants, to whom we must offer better living conditions than exist at present. This represents a challenge to the present generation. Population growth in Middle America, including Mexico, will be proportionately greatest. Its present population of 79 million is expected to reach 173 million in the year 2000.

As Araica emphasized, the population dynamics in Latin America reflect the underdevelopment that prevails in the majority of the countries of this continent, which is greatly exacerbated by the demographic problem. Therefore, it is necessary that, within their own development policies, the countries define a clear and explicit demographic policy. According to the recommendations of the World Population Conference in Bucharest, this should include goals to reduce population growth, morbidity, and mortality, and to improve the status of the family and of women, and to minimize the maldistribution of populations.

As stressed by the Pan American Health Organization in its last quadrennial report (1970–1973), it is necessary that development be modified and measured, not by the gross national product and similar indicators devoid of a real distributive justice, but more from the viewpoint of the welfare of persons, families, and societies and the better distribution of national income and resources. Consequently, within the components of the development policy, food and nutrition policies should accompany demographic policies.

These demographic and food and nutrition policies should take into account those factors related to the availability, adequate consumption, and biologic utilization of food, and the dynamics and characteristics of the population to be fed. It is our function to present the problems to those with the power of decision, to motivate them to define and establish sound policies, and to give them the guidance and collaboration required for implementation of these policies.

Dale D. Harpstead · *Department of Crop and Soil Sciences, Michigan State University, East Lansing, Michigan.*

Any projection we make relative to population growth is, in the final analysis, also a food availability curve. The only real point open to argument is the quality of life we wish to build into the projections.

23

Cultural Interaction and Child Nutrition (Toward a Curvilinear Compromise?)

Derrick B. Jelliffe and E. F. Patrice Jelliffe

Population, Family and International Health Division
School of Public Health
University of California
Los Angeles, California

Cultural factors can affect dietary intakes in many ways, including the production and use of foods for the feeding of young children and pregnant and lactating women (1). Knowledge of the culture helps to explain the local pattern of nutrition and health, assists in establishing rapport with the community, and facilitates the introduction of nutrition-related programs (2,3). To be able to relate to the culture is a prime requirement for the community worker. A rough system of classifying customs into nutritionally beneficial, harmful, neutral, and uncertain has been suggested (1,4) so that appropriate programs may be chosen.

In the past, much of the attention has often been given to the effects of indigenous cultural practices, especially those strikingly different from Western methods and considered harmful. Questions of the interplay between cultural attitudes and philosophies are also of great interest. While interactions between different cultures have occurred throughout history, these were usually relatively slow, via diffusion by travelers and traders, or through military conquest. By contrast, the impact of so-called Western technological culture ("Westernism") has been extremely rapid, recent, and dramatic. In the nutritional field, the outcomes of such interactions have often been adverse. Examples are such alterations in food habits as the increased use of sugar, white flour, carbonated soft drinks, alcohol, tea, and displacement of breast feeding of infants by bottle feeding.

WESTERNISM–A LINEAR CULTURE

So-called Western culture has roots in many other past civilizations, but in its modern form arose in parallel with, and as a product of, the Industrial Revolution. This new Westernism can be categorized as *linear,* and characteristically can be thought of as striving to be direct, efficient, quantitative, rapid, impatient, and technology-based. It was until recently also ebullient, assured, forceful, and aggressive. However, recent limitations, unexpected side effects, and failures have led, in some quarters, to an overreactive hostility to science inconceivable 10 years ago.

Visible examples of Western linear culture include road systems–freeways compared with ancient, winding streets; the square concrete box architecture of modern cities; and calligraphy changed from medieval elegance to the perpendicular linearity of present-day typescript.

In medicine, the tremendous scientific advances during the second half of the last century in the fields of bacteriology (and consequent aseptic surgery and chemotherapy), radiology, and so on, were all part of the unfolding Western linear culture. These spectacular successes led to modern medicine's being hospital-laboratory-curative in emphasis, and training of the health staff, including medical students, became hospital-based, with exaggerated prestige and weight given to the laboratory.

In fact, what is now termed *medicine* was early recognized as only *one* of several available health systems in the Western world. Originally, it was differentiated by the label *allopathic* (or reactive) medicine, and, indeed, this approach was and still is its forte–instances include reactive responses to pneumococcal pneumonia with penicillin or to appendicitis with surgery.

In the field of nutrition, the linear approach also had successes, some spectacular. For instance, these included the rapid responses of beriberi and scurvy to appropriate vitamin administration, and the lower incidence of goiter and rickets following fortification of appropriate foods with iodine and vitamin D.

Typical of the hubris of the late 19th century was the introduction of complicated "formulas" for infant feeding. They were based on gross algebraic approximations, which attest to the human infant's adaptability to the metabolically inappropriate. The pseudoscientific absurdity of the formulas of the percentage schools of infant feeding earlier in the century are paralleled by the rise of conditions that are, in large measure, "cow's milk bottle-feeding syndromes," particularly infantile obesity, neonatal hypocalcemia, and hypernatremic dehydration.

In retrospect, it is obvious that Western linear-type medical practice was so successful with a segment of disease (especially infections) that a narrow superstructure was built on the assumption that its approaches were universally appropriate and likely to be successful with all other forms of ill health. In fact, it may well be that Western allopathic medicine is to some extent in a cul-de-sac, striving overexclusively for the technological "breakthroughs" so beloved by journalists, but usually misreported or ephemeral.

The need is rather to appreciate the high value of Western linear medicine *as one part of wider possibilities.* Its partial quality is readily evident. Many conditions do not respond to attempted therapy—for instance, multiple sclerosis or atheroma, and many organisms are increasingly insensitive to chemotherapy (e.g., malarial plasmodia, meningococci). There is rightly concern over iatrogenic ill consequences of some potent linear approaches, and, above all, it is slowly being recognized that most disease is not caused by one agent, but by many circumstances in combination. This is certainly the case with malnutrition.

An important consequence of the dominance of linear Westernism has been the difficulty of having preventive medicine taken seriously, apart from the dramatic linear prophylaxis of immunization. One result has been the almost incredibly hard, and as yet unachieved, task of introducing nutrition into the curricula of medical students anywhere in the world.

Innumerable instances of a preference for linear techniques permeate hospital practice. For example, there is often an unnecessary emphasis on intravenous feeding when it is no longer necessary; on highly elaborate, costly electronic monitoring systems for the birth process, even though only a small percentage of pregnant women are receiving prenatal care; and on the expensive undertaking of screening by costly laboratory examinations without specific indication, although little attention is given to the social or dietary history.

"BIOTRADITIONAL CURVED CULTURES"

All cultures in the world, including those of Western Europe and North America prior to the Industrial Revolution, are biotraditional—that is, based on biological adaptations by the species over millenia, and on practices and customs gradually evolved by the community and handed down from generation to generation.

Biotraditional cultures may be categorized as curved—with characteristics almost the opposite of linear Westernism. For example, their approaches tend to be more biologically based, slower, and not so concerned with efficiency, speed, or precise numerical proof. They are in considerable harmony with wider aspects of community life, including the family and the spirit world.

An unbiased general view indicates clearly that methods of healing and techniques for social support in such biotraditional cultures are often much more effective for some conditions and circumstances in which linear Westernism alone has been shown to be insufficient. Some of these have been termed *lessons from developing countries* (5), and include perinatal social support for the pregnant woman, the management of lactation, and the mother–infant contact, exemplified by traditional methods of baby-carrying.

Similarly, long-tested techniques of food preparation may have unappreciated virtues. Pellagra swept through the polenta-eaters of southern Europe after the introduction of corn, whereas it did not occur in the tortilla-eaters of Central America, the ancestral home. Conversely, the medical systems, dietary patterns, and agriculture in biotraditional cultures plainly also have many inadequacies and ill consequences, in part because of their imprecision and lack of emphasis on proof.

Interestingly, the effectiveness of curved approaches to the improvement of health was reported from the Western world at various stages in the Industrial Revolution. The Armstrong brothers in 18th-Century London reduced child mortality by simple curved means long prior to antibiotics or immunization (6). Another example is the emphasis by Florence Nightingale toward the end of the 19th Century on good food, cleanliness, and fresh air. The successful activities of the early lay health visitors in the United Kingdom in the 1920s were for the most part based upon nontechnological approaches feasible within the home milieu (7).

LINEAR ⋧ CURVED INTERACTION

The great successes of the Industrial Revolution in transport, communications, war potential, and industry led to the rapid spread of Westernism throughout much of the world. In colonized countries, cultural change was in part imposed, but in addition, the dramatic and efficient results of some aspects of Western culture were everywhere compellingly beguiling—for example, the rifle, the railway, and, more recently, the radio.

In the medical field, totally out-of-context Western models of service and education were eagerly adopted; hospitals became centers of higher technology, physicians were high priests, and the laboratory the acme of endeavor. Conversely, the biological and traditional tended to be almost automatically downgraded and underemphasized as old-fashioned and archaic, if not retrogressive and barbaric.

The approaches used most often in young child nutrition programs in developing countries in the decades since World War II have very frequently been linear—as suggested by the generic term often used, *intervention programs.* Examples include widespread supplementary feeding programs (particularly using dried skimmed milk), amino acid fortification programs, and the introduction of bottle feeding with cow's milk formulas as the mathematically linear way to nourish babies. All have been of partial benefit at most, and have also had considerable ill consequences. In particular, the disastrous decline in breast feeding is belatedly being recognized as an entirely Western-induced change of very great public health significance, in part "commerciogenic" and in part "iatrogenic."

Other unfortunate effects of the psychological overdominance of Westernism include the loss, or decreased status and hence use, of some important indigenous foods (e.g., *quinoa* in the Andes, many traditional dark green leafy vegetables); the neglect, or block to acceptance, of some traditional practices of nutritional consequence–for example, the nutritional, anti-infective and contraceptive value of "prolonged" breast feeding. The pattern of behavior in Westernized maternity units acts as a barrier to the successful initiation of lactation (8,9), and the hospitals are assumed to have inherent quasi-mystical healing virtues. In fact, many overcrowded, understaffed pediatric wards in developing countries instead become negative factors (10).

Apparent Needs

Neither linear Westernism nor curved biotraditional cultures has a monopoly of answers for health and nutrition; both usually show benefits and defects. In everyday terms, the fly-breeding hazards of animal manure (curved) have been succeeded by the respiratory problems of smog (linear).

The limited effectiveness of most linear nutrition programs for young children, including supplementary feeding, has become apparent. Moreover, such approaches are not feasible economically or organizationally on a wide scale. One of the least helpful characteristics of many well-intended small-scale pilot projects is that there is no practical possibility that they can be replicated. However, the possibility of using economical and effective linear approaches must always be considered.

In any consideration of the advantages and disadvantages of linear and curved cultural approaches, a significant recent development must be noted. This has been the "naturalism" movement, including the resurgence of concern with breast feeding, the widespread and spontaneous change in methods of baby-carrying (11), the natural childbirth trend, and, with all its absurdities, exaggerations, and commercial exploitation, the interest in "health foods." This represents a grass roots change–certainly without support from health professionals–and a spontaneous shift from linear to curved practices. Interestingly, the value of some of these new/old methods can only be accepted by medical orthodoxy when validated by respectable linear scientific, hard facts. For example, the obvious anti-infective and growth-promoting effects of breast feeding have been given linear legitimacy with the demonstration of secretory IgA and specific patterns of nucleotides and polyamines in human milk (12).

Fundamentally, there is need for conceptual flexibility to search for compromises–for syntheses between the best of Western medicine ("allopathy") and other healing systems, and between the direct linear technological and the improved curved biotraditional. Potential examples abound. Infant feeding programs can be based on breast feeding and village-level multimixes, derived from traditional foods, together with supplementary foods when indicated; contraception can be based on breast feeding together with newer technical methods that least interfere with lactation; nutritional surveys need to be based on statistical sampling and appropriate scientific testing together with information of a qualitative, "soft" nature, gained by observation.

Recently, some nutrition planners are beginning to think in curvilinear terms. Examples include the DEIDS programs being initiated by the APHA (13) and the programs encompassed by the Zagreb Guidelines (14). These are intended to be based on the local culture and ecology, with the village health auxiliary as the primary worker. At the same time, they include linear components when required—for example, supplementary food for specific indications and dermojet apparatus for immunizations. Difficulties with such curvilinear approaches will be considerable, but linear Western science rarely has rapid, feasible breakthrough answers. Do people, politicians, or even professionals understand this?

ACKNOWLEDGMENTS

We thank Mr. Stuart Cloete and Dr. James Moloney for much stimulus.

REFERENCES

1. Jelliffe, D. B., 1968, *Infant nutrition in the subtropics and tropics,* World Health Organization Monograph Series No. 29, WHO, Geneva, pp. 32–84.
2. Jelliffe, D. B., 1956, Cultural variation and the practical pediatrician, *J. Pediatr.* **49:** 661.
3. Jelliffe, D. B., 1967, Culture, social change and young child nutrition, *Am. J. Clin. Nutr.* **20:** 279.
4. Jelliffe, D. B., 1975, Cultural factors and nutrition, *in: Brenneman's practice of pediatrics,* Harper-Medical, Harper & Row, New York.
5. Jelliffe, D. B., and Jelliffe, E. F. P., 1976, Lessons from developing countries, *in: The cost, quantity and quality of child health services in Africa,* Dag Hammarskjöld Foundation, Addis Ababa, Ethiopia, in press.
6. Maloney, W. J., 1954, *George and John Armstrong of Castleton. Two eighteenth century pioneers,* Williams & Wilkins, Baltimore, Maryland, and Livingstone, Edinburgh.
7. Williams, C. D., and Jelliffe, D. B., 1972, *Mother and child health: Delivering the services,* Oxford University Press, London.
8. Raphael, D., 1973, Breast feeding in a bottle-feeding culture, *Ecol. Food Nutr.* **2:** 121.
9. Jelliffe, D. B., and Jelliffe, E. F. P., 1974, Doulas, confidence, and the science of lactation, *J. Pediatr.* **84**(3): 462.
10. Jelliffe, D. B., and Jelliffe, E. F. P., 1970, The children's ward as a lethal factor, *J. Pediatr.* 77: 895.

11. Jelliffe, E. F. P., 1975, Recent trends in infant carrying, *J. Trop. Pediatr. Environ. Child Health.* **21:** 93.
12. Jelliffe, D. B., and Jelliffe, E. F. P., 1976, *Human milk in the modern world,* C. V. Mosby, St. Louis, Missouri, in press.
13. American Public Health Association, 1972, *Guidelines to DEIDS (Delivery and Evaluation of Integrated Delivery Systems),* Mimeographed Document, APHA, Washington, D.C.
14. Jelliffe, D. B., and Jelliffe, E. F. P. (eds.), 1973, *Nutrition programs for pre-school children: Report of a working conference, Institute of Public Health, Zagreb, Yugoslavia,* International Maternal-Child Health Section, U.S. Department of Health, Education and Welfare, Bethesda, Maryland.

COMMENTS

Carl E. Taylor · *Department of International Health, School of Hygiene and Public Health, The Johns Hopkins University, Baltimore, Maryland.*

The Jelliffes offer a curvilinear compromise. Some of us, using a curvilinear approach, have climbed the Volcano Pacaya. We used a linear approach where the footing was good and a curving approach in the soft, sliding areas of cinder and ash. In the health field we can be linear where we have measurements and data, but where we must proceed intuitively, without measurements, we must be more circuitous and tentative. Linear methods have tended to deal with single causes that are easily measured. Now we need a whole new approach to make simultaneous measurement of multiple causes to be able to deal with the more complex problems.

Nancie L. González · *Program Director for Anthropology, National Science Foundation, Washington, D.C.*

In 1955 I first studied changing social and cultural patterns in the INCAP study village of Santa Maria Cauqué as they related to the acceptance of dietary supplements and health care by mothers and preschool children (1). For some time after, only a handful of anthropologists worked on subjects related to health and disease, and practically none on nutritional problems per se. The field has come a long way since. There is now an autonomous Society for Medical Anthropology of well over 1000 members, and a subgroup of anthropologists interested in nutrition has been formed.

George Foster, at a recent conference, (2) suggested that medical anthropology be viewed in terms of two distinct types of endeavors. The first, "anthropology *in* medicine," deals with the use of anthropological data and insight within the field of medicine in order better to accomplish the goal of preserving or restoring a state of health. The second, the "anthropology *of* medicine," takes as its subject matter the medical system itself, seeking ways to understand how that system is structured in our own or any other society.

The Jelliffes' remarks, with which I am in essential agreement, have made a contribution to the second of these domains. Indeed, the majority of medical anthropologists make their contributions here, and the fact that our science holds so little prestige within the field of medicine even today is perhaps explained by the note that our methodology is more curved than linear! In the early days, the problems with which most of us concerned ourselves lay in the area of what are often called "beliefs and practices." The work was primarily descriptive, and the "results" frequently more intuitive than scientific. Perhaps for this reason we were not held in high regard by many of our colleagues either within or outside anthropology.

In any case, after my early field work in Santa Maria Cauqué, I did not immediately continue to pursue health systems. Instead, I spent 14 months in 1956–57 in the Black Carib village of Livingston on the north coast of Guatemala. There my major observations centered on household and family forms and their relations to the economic system (3). I observed that 40% of the Carib households in Livingston included no person regularly present in the role of husband/father; the central and most stable figure was the mother. I hypothesized that this household form might be viewed as an adaptation to modern conditions of poverty in societies living on the margins of the world industrial system. Furthermore, I suggested that under such circumstances one might expect to find the kinship unit known as the nuclear family (parents and children) living dispersed in various households. I also collected data on health and nutrition, although I did not at that time relate these specifically to my primary concern with the family and household. I did observe, however, that public health officials as well as private physicians, such as those employed by the United Fruit Company for their employees, were as upset by what they saw as immoral and indecent marital arrangements as they were by the malnutrition and sickness they tried to treat. I often heard women admonished to feed their babies more *and* to get married to the father—all in one breath of Western medical advice!

Since 1955 anthropologists working in the medical field have moved considerably beyond the beliefs and practices stage. By this I mean that they have increasingly been concerned with more basic and fundamental structures by means of which societies wittingly or unwittingly affect the physical and mental well-being of their members. They are also more inclined to move beyond the purely descriptive stage to suggest interrelationships that may have deeper explanatory value. The primary characteristic of their work, which in my opinion also distinguishes medical anthropology from medical sociology, is a special concern with the interface between biology and culture. Many advances have been made by anthropologists working in the field of human genetics.

William Stini (4), for example, has suggested that selective factors may now be operating in populations similar to those with which INCAP is concerned when they are deprived of adequate calories and protein. The interaction between culture and biological factors is now generally accepted as having played an important part in the evolution of human beings (5).

The relatively new interest in what we call cultural ecology stresses the importance of the broader environment, including both social and natural factors, in influencing or even determining various cultural forms and processes, which in turn have an effect upon the body. The "new" medical anthropology, if I may be allowed such a term, attempts to expand its view beyond the earlier concentration upon beliefs and practices, which were frequently of interest to Westerners primarily so that they might better plan how to change them.

A systems analysis often shows that the customary ways of handling problems related to nutrition and health were perfectly adequate, within the context of the original sociocultural system. That is, the so-called health problems of non-Western peoples are often (a) not really problems at all, and/or (b) the product of interference with their system by the industrial world. Many of the worst problems are brought about simply by poverty, which, as Oscar Lewis (6) has reminded us, tends to take similar forms and has similar results today wherever it is found. Thus, the impingement of the outside world upon once independent and integrated societies most often works to the disadvantage of the latter in both political and economic terms, and ultimately in the deterioration of health. The Western system in its arrogance then reenters these societies in order to teach the people how to feed and care for themselves and their children. A more important endeavor is to sort out the different factors involved so as to help the people understand recent changes and their causes. Only then may restructuring of their lives and their social systems occur—it is to be hoped at higher levels than the merely therapeutic.

Susan Brown (7) compared two groups of households in the Dominican Republic, all of which were characterized by themselves and other villagers as the poorest in the rural community she studied. In one group the women had histories of what Brown termed "multiple-mating" practices. Husband/fathers were unstable household members, yet they provided varying levels of financial and moral support. Although a woman might have liaisons with several men during her lifetime (usually only one at a time), she could count on these men for some assistance to their children even after her own relationship with the men had terminated. The other group consisted of women who were legally married and remained monogamous, even though in some cases the husbands were no longer present in the household.

Brown discovered that the households headed by multiple-mating women were better off in terms of dietary adequacy (especially in terms of protein intake), and size and condition of the house. In addition, they raised more children to maturity over a three-generation period than did the women who married monogamously. This clearly tends to confirm the hypothesis I suggested after my work in Livingston; i.e., under conditions of industrial-related poverty, some family/household arrangements seem more advantageous than others in allowing people to cope. The circumstances under which these conditions arise in Latin America, the Caribbean, and perhaps elsewhere, tend to be in cities and near industrially organized modern plantations, mines, or seaports.

In most Guatemalan villages the nuclear family, sometimes extended to include three generations or an occasional lateral relative, is still the primary household unit. These may well persist so long as the villages and the peasant economy upon which they are based remain intact. However, as industrialization proceeds, it is clear that many changes are imminent. There will be more migration to towns and cities to supplement the meager incomes the overworked land provides. I suggest that multiple-mating patterns will become more prevalent in both rural and urban zones, and that we should further examine the role of the household composition in determining health, as it relates to the individual *and* to the population as a whole, through time.

With this in mind, I plan to gather further data in Livingston on contemporary patterns of marriage, household form, health, and general economic status, and I predict that those households exhibiting monogamous marriage forms and nuclear families will be viable forms for those whose men are employed in secure and reasonably well-paid occupations. For others not so fortunate, however, such social arrangements may contribute substantially to poor nutrition and higher morbidity. By maximizing the resources contributed by both males and females, the multiple-mating households may turn out to be healthier environments for all concerned. In such cases, public health practitioners will have to adopt a more relativistic attitude toward what they consider moral precepts.

I thank the Jelliffes for their long-standing and well recognized efforts to include social factors in the health equation. This volume demonstrates that they and others like them have had some effect. Nearly every chapter gives at least lip service to "culture," "relativism," "social factors," the "human factor," "beliefs and practices," and the like. However, this is not enough. We must now work together to discover the immediate and the long-range effects of these factors upon health and vice versa. Our task is complicated both by our own ethnocentrism and by the constantly changing milieu within which we work. The changes triggered by the industrial world today are often totally opposite to the changes intended by those who desire to improve the lot of those they study. I believe this is also the message of the Jelliffes' discussion.

Acknowledgments

Grateful acknowledgment is made to the Henry L. and Grace Doherty Charitable Foundation, Inc., for grants that made the original field work and the following year's study in Livingston possible. Assistance was also rendered by INCAP and by the United Fruit Company.

References

1. Solien, N., and Scrimshaw, N. S., 1957, Public health significance of child feeding practices observed in a Guatemalan village, *J. Trop. Pediatr.* **3** (3): 99–104.
2. Foster, G., 1974, Comment during the Symposium on Medical Anthropology, Meetings of the American Anthropological Association, Mexico, November (1974).
3. Gonzalez, N., 1969, *Black Carib household structure: A study of migration and modernization,* University of Washington Press, Seattle, Washington, 163 pp.
4. Stini, W., 1971, Evolutionary implications of changing nutritional patterns in human populations, *Am. Anthropol.* **73** (5): 1019–1030.
5. Washburn, S. and Moore, R., 1974, *Ape into man,* Little, Brown and Company, Boston, Massachusetts, 196 pp.
6. Lewis, O., 1970, *Anthropological essays,* Random House, New York, 523 pp.
7. Brown, S., 1973, Coping with poverty in the Dominican Republic: Women and their mates, *Current Anthropol.* **14** (5): 555–557.

Robert F. Chandler, Jr. · *The Asian Vegetable Research and Development Center, Shanhua, Taiwan.*

An example of favorable cultural patterns is the eating habits of the Chinese. Over the centuries they have worked out a highly nutritious and varied diet, with a large variety of meats and vegetables. They eat all parts of animals and relatively large quantities of green leafy vegetables. They cook all foods and boil their water, drinking mostly tea, thus minimizing food-borne infections.

When one travels from the Philippines to Taiwan, the improvement in the health of the people is notable. Much of it can be attributed to the varied and rather well-balanced diet of the Chinese.

24

Food Attitudes to Actualize Community Nutrition Education

Marina Flores

Division of Applied Nutrition
Institute of Nutrition of Central America and Panama
Guatemala City, Guatemala

Dietary patterns are culturally determined, but limited by the availability of food products. Economic and educational factors are important and largely determine the acceptance of new food products. For the success of a nutrition education program, however, it is necessary to observe the food attitudes of the people in their own environment.

Among the lowest income groups, very little can be accomplished by educational activities; only economic changes can be effective. A little higher in the social structure, families may improve their diets if they are exposed to an effective nutrition education program. Until now, most nutrition education activities have failed, not because of ignorance of the importance of sociocultural factors, but because the educators have followed a traditional educational system without investigating the practical changes they would have to promote in order to improve the food habits of the people. For many years it has been observed that teaching nutrition has largely consisted of looking for appropriate schemes, such as the "basic food groups," to facilitate popular learning of what constitutes a good diet. Instead, the real nutritive value of the indigenous staple in the local diet and the logic and wisdom in the food behavior of the people should be determined first (1). It is discouraging to see an educator trying to transfer knowledge to children or adults in rural areas about a set of foods classified in three or four groups, when the poor child or mother is accustomed to seeing only one basic food in the family dish, plus a pot of coffee. When such mothers and children see a variety of food products, it may have negative emotional results.

Our dietary study results among preschool children illustrate these basic points. For example, two Central American countries with very different cultural backgrounds–Guatemala (2), whose ancestors are predominantly Mayan, and Costa Rica (3), with Spanish antecedents–show some similarities in food attitudes. Such information has been obtained while recording food intake of children and families during three consecutive days, weighing the food, and observing how families handle and prepare the different foods.

Figures 1–6 show the food intake of children in Guatemala and Costa Rica, by age, with respect to consumption of corn tortillas, rice, beans, milk, meat, and sugar. Differences between the countries are expressed in quantity, and the differences in amounts consumed reflect availability of those products in the homes.

In Guatemala, where corn tortillas are the staple food, children consume larger quantities than Costa Rican children do; the reverse is true for rice. The consumption of beans and meat in both countries is quite similar; only small amounts are given to children up to the age of three years. There is then some increase, especially of beans in Guatemala. The greater consumption of milk in Costa Rica is impressive. Sugar consumption is also higher in Costa Rica than in Guatemala.

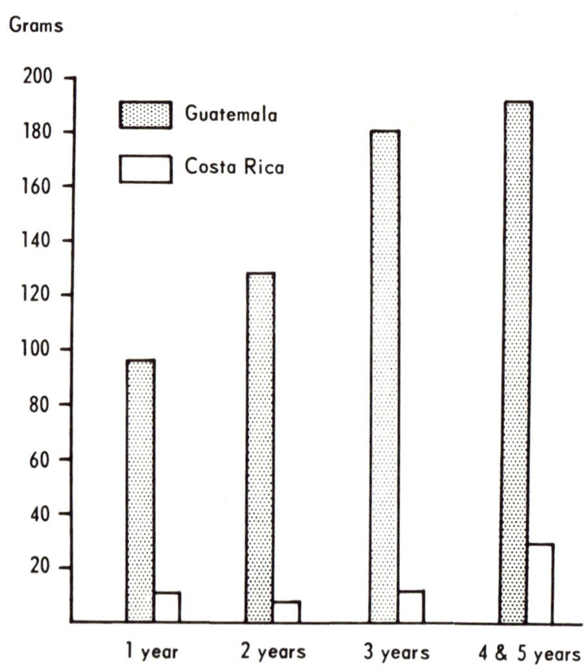

FIG. 1. Consumption of corn tortillas per child per day in Guatemala and Costa Rica.

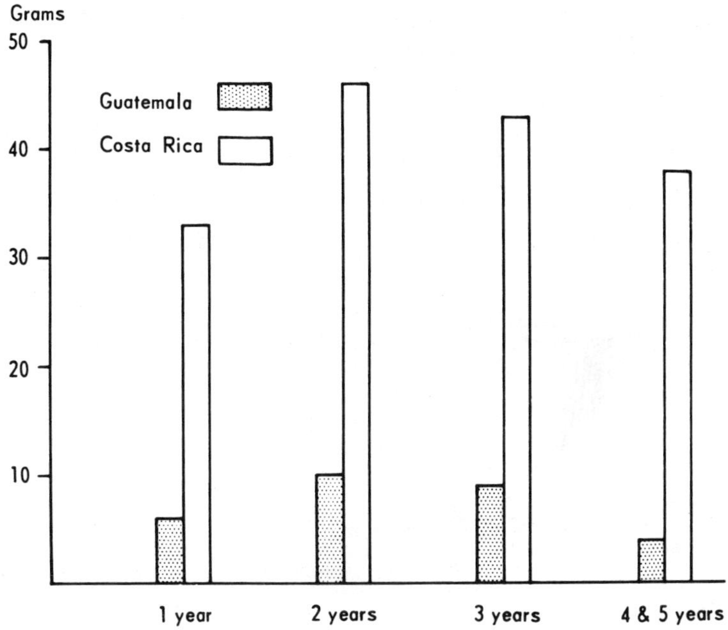

FIG. 2. Consumption of rice per child per day in Guatemala and Costa Rica.

When the effect of the socioeconomic level on the calorie and nutrient content of the children's diets is compared, there are marked differences among the socioeconomic groups (Tables I and II), although deficiencies in calories are similar in both countries, with a little improvement according to socioeconomic level. All of the populations studied had diets deficient in calories.

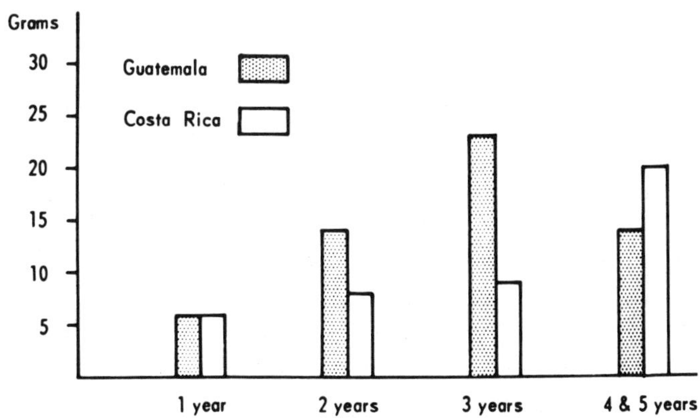

FIG. 3. Consumption of beans per child per day in Guatemala and Costa Rica.

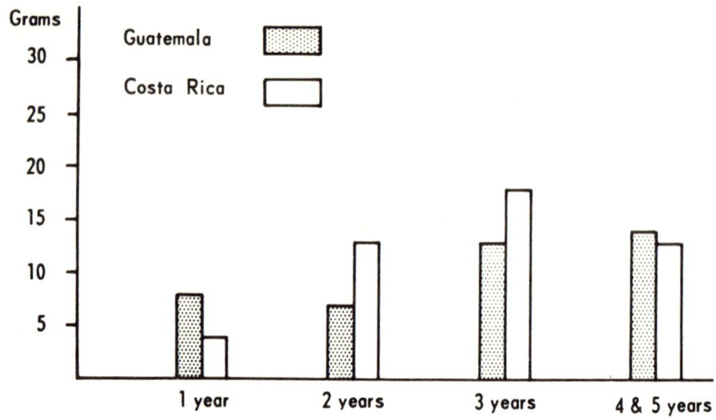

FIG. 4. Consumption of meat per child per day in Guatemala and Costa Rica.

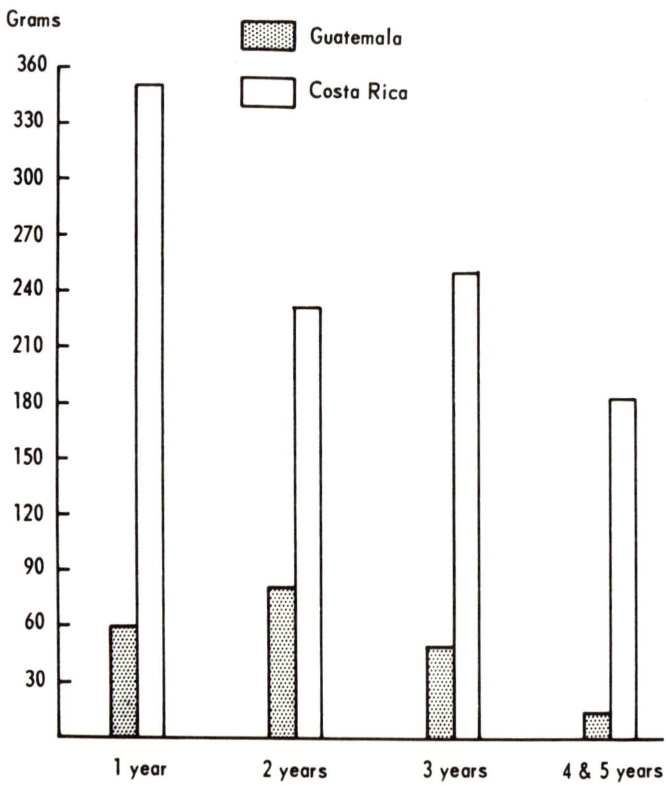

FIG. 5. Consumption of milk per child per day in Guatemala and Costa Rica.

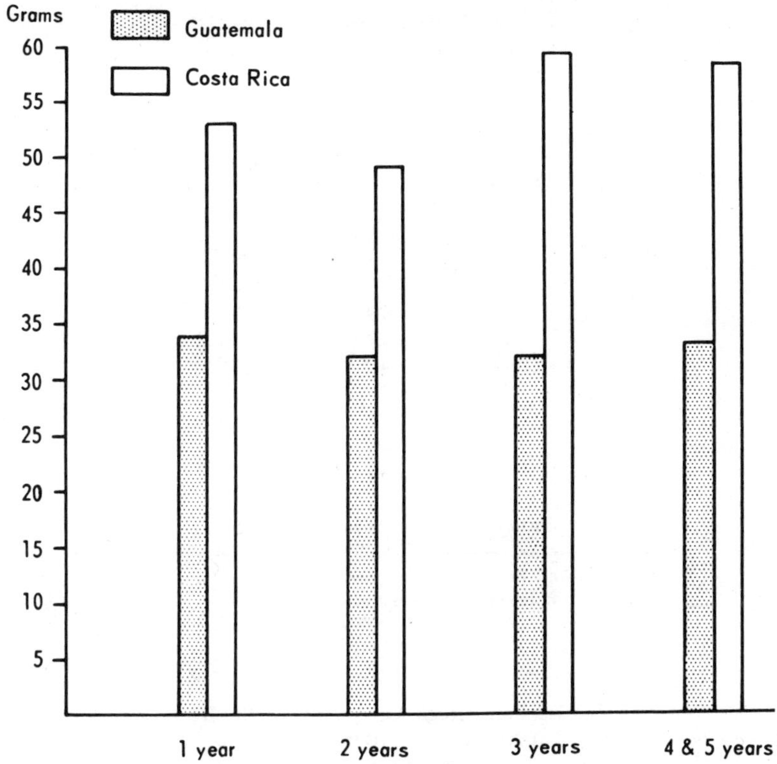

FIG. 6. Consumption of sugar per child per day in Guatemala and Costa Rica.

The relationship between family intake and child intake of calories was then investigated. To compare the percentage of adequacy of calories at the family level and at the child level by age group for the two countries, a series of graphs were constructed. Figures 7–14 illustrate the regression lines obtained for the relationship compared with a slope of 45° for a direct association. A closer association was anticipated, because the more calories available to the family, the more calories should be available to the child; this was not the case in either of the countries. Practically no relationship was found between the intakes of families and their children in any of the age groups except in Costa Rica, where for the two-year-olds the correlation coefficient reached significance at the 5% level.

Some of the reasons for such a lack of correlation are:

1. Families do not give sufficient food to children even if they have it, because they believe children have a limited capacity to consume greater amounts.

Table I. Percentage Adequacy[a] of the Dietary Intakes of the Children in a Rural Area of Guatemala

Dietary components	Socioeconomic groups		
	Low	Middle	High
	%	%	%
Calories	58	73	87
Protein	70	94	109
Calcium	79	97	120
Iron	73	89	89
Vitamin A (retinol)	40	45	94
Thiamine	86	115	130
Riboflavin	34	64	102
Niacin[b]	48	58	59
Vitamin C	53	77	105
Number of cases	28	75	24

[a]Reference 4.
[b]Niacin from Tryptophan was not considered.

Table II. Percentage Adequacy[a] of the Dietary Intakes of the Children in a Rural Area of Costa Rica

Dietary components	Socioeconomic groups		
	Low	Middle	High
	%	%	%
Calories	64	78	83
Protein	85	121	148
Calcium	93	159	240
Iron	43	52	48
Vitamin A (retinol)	43	87	118
Thiamine	72	98	106
Riboflavin	86	141	211
Niacin[b]	37	49	46
Vitamin C	38	75	110
Number of cases	22	49	7

[a]Reference 4.
[b]Niacin from Tryptophan was not considered.

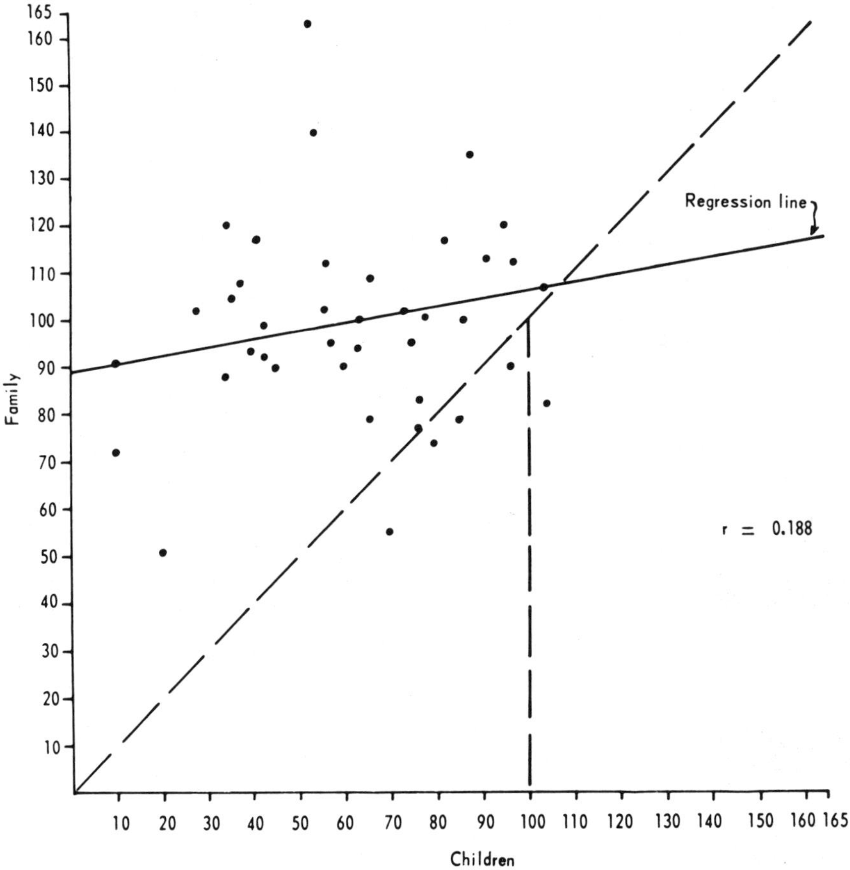

FIG. 7. Correlation of adequate calorie intake between the family and the child of one year of age, Guatemala.

2. The presence of anorexia because of frequent infections may sometimes keep children from accepting more food.
3. Some foods, like milk, eggs, or noodles, are considered specifically for children, and when they are not available the children do not receive enough of other kinds of food.

The relationship between calories and proteins in the diets also deserves special analysis, because the types of staple foods in these areas provide sufficient total protein when calories are consumed at requirement levels. When the caloric adequacy of the diets of children was compared with their protein

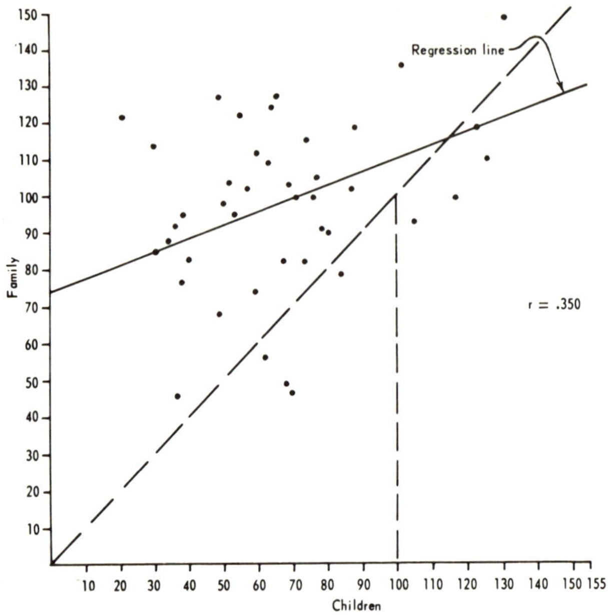

FIG. 8. Correlation of adequate calorie intake between the family and the child of two years of age, Guatemala.

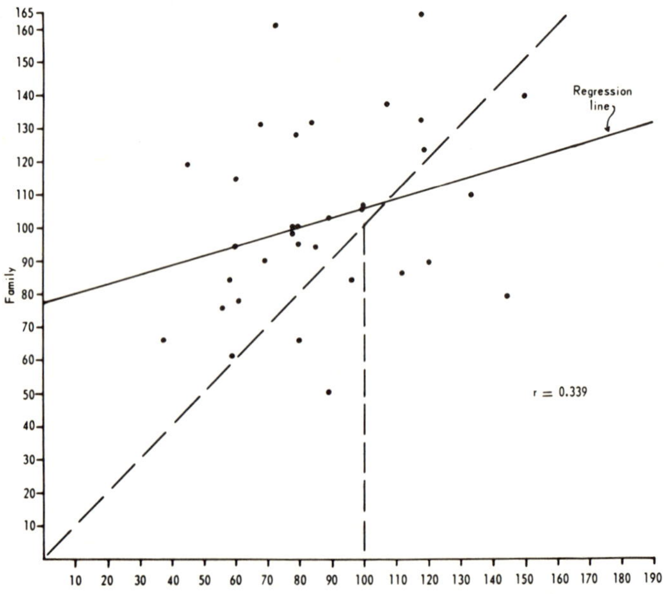

FIG. 9. Correlation of adequate calorie intake between the family and the three-year-old child, Guatemala.

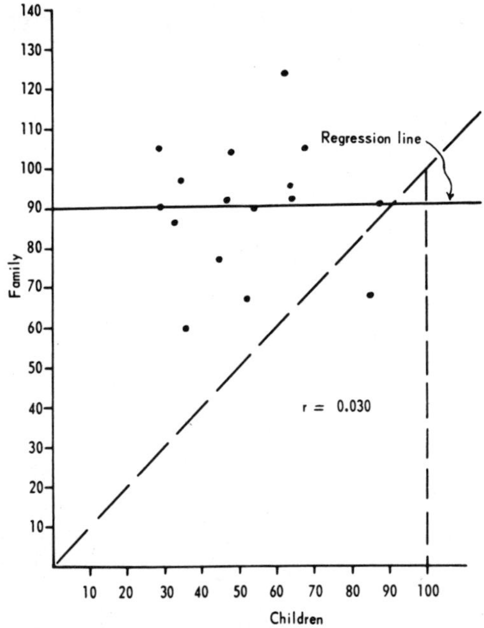

FIG. 10. Correlation of adequate calorie intake between the family and the child at age four and five years, Guatemala.

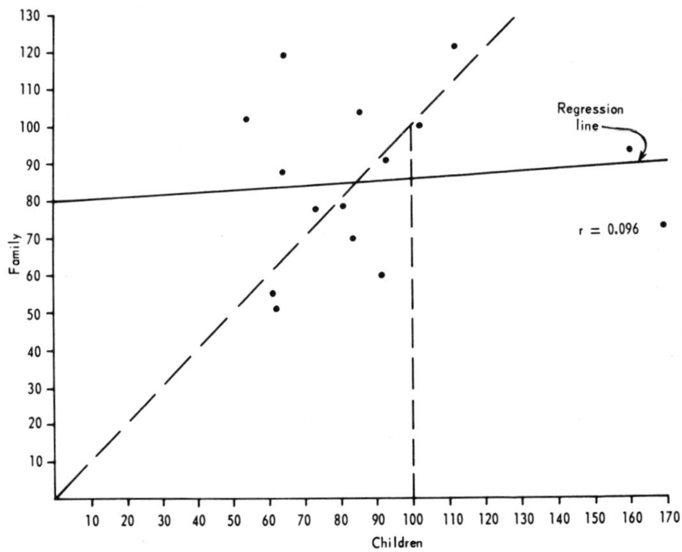

FIG. 11. Correlation of adequate calorie intake between the family and the one-year-old child, Costa Rica.

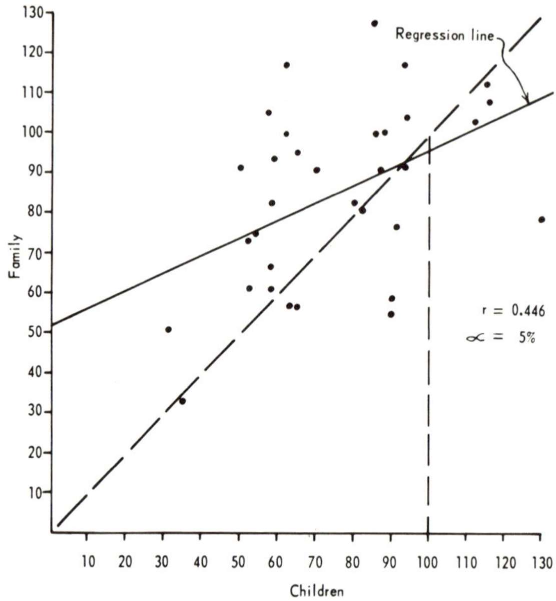

FIG. 12. Correlation of adequate calorie intake between the family and the child of two years. Costa Rica.

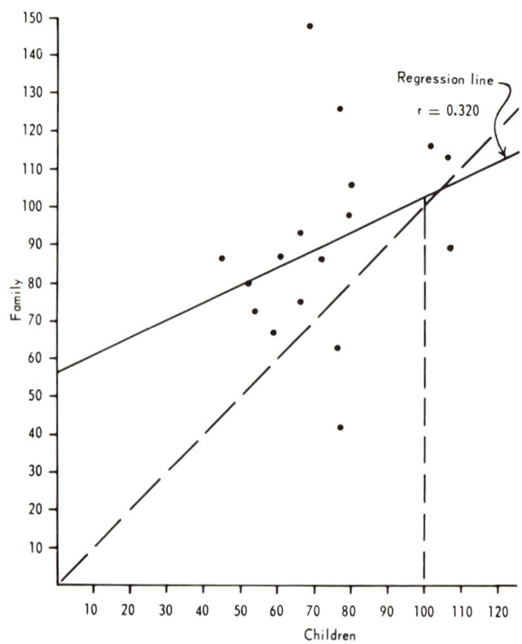

FIG. 13. Correlation of adequate calorie intake between the family and the three-year-old child, Costa Rica,

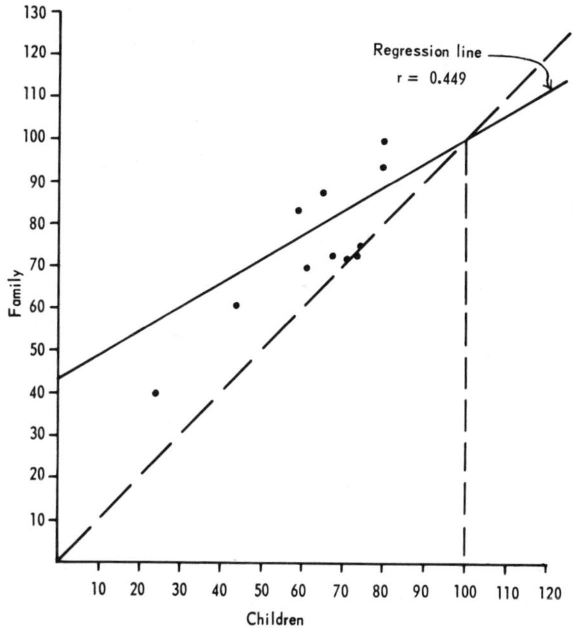

FIG. 14. Correlation of adequate calorie intake between the family and the child at age four and five years, Costa Rica.

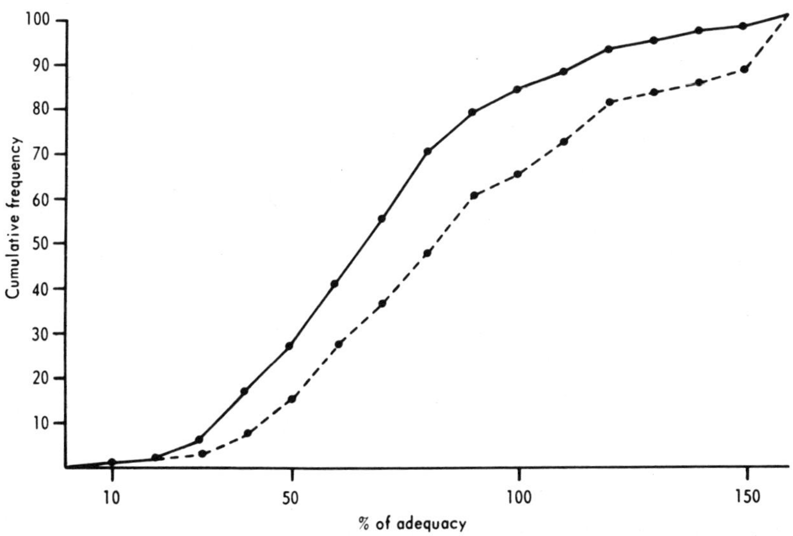

FIG. 15. Distribution of the percent adequacy of levels of calorie (——) and protein intake (- - -) in the diets of preschool children in a rural area of Guatemala.

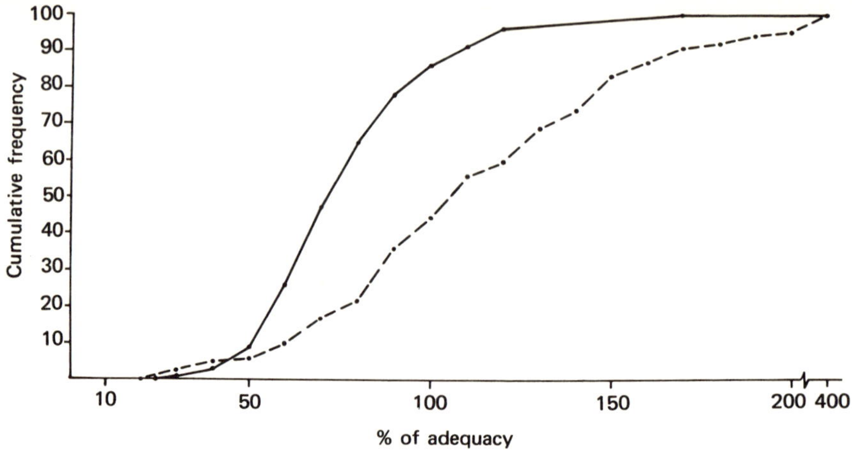

FIG. 16. Distribution of the percent adequacy of levels of calorie (—) and protein intake (- - -) in the diets of preschool children in a rural area of Costa Rica.

intakes, the situation was similar in the two countries. The data for both countries, presented in Figures 15 and 16, reveal an appreciable number of inadequate intakes for both calories and protein. The distributions show that calories are more deficient than protein, and this becomes more evident in Costa Rica. About 34% of children consume the recommended levels for protein in Guatemala, but only 15% consume adequate calories. In Costa Rica, 55% of the children have adequate intakes of protein, but only 4 or 5% have diets approaching calorie requirements.

These observations indicate that nutrition education should be reoriented to teach families, not by using fancy food charts, but by persuading the mother to give children more of the food available in the home, even when they are sick. More realistic approaches for nutrition education, especially at the community level, would be as follows:

1. Teach the families the value of the foods they have in their own homes: tortillas, beans, green leaves, and fruits.
2. Avoid changing good food habits; i.e., the replacement of green leaves with less nutritious vegetables, the change from yellow corn to white corn, and the change from good food habits because they seem to be lower in prestige.
3. Teach the proper preparation of foods available in the home so they can be given to the children as well as to adults.

In summary, with the information obtained from the families in the homes, nutrition education at the community level could be made far more effective.

REFERENCES

1. Ahlström, A., and Risanen, L., 1973, Review of food grouping systems in nutrition education, *J. Nutr. Ed.* **5** (1): 13–17.
2. Flores, M., Menchú, M. T., Lara, M. Y., and Guzmán, M. A., 1970, Relación entre la ingesta de calorías y nutrientes en preescolares y la disponibilidad de alimentos en la familia, *Arch. Latinoam. Nutr.* **20:** 41–58.
3. Menchú, M. T., Lara, M. Y., and Flores, M., 1973, Efecto del nivel socioeconómico de la familia sobre la dieta del niño preescolar, *Arch. Latinoam. Nutr.* **23:** 305–323.
4. Instituto de Nutrición de Centro America y Panama (INCAP), 1969, *Recomendaciones nutricionales diarias,* preparado por M. Flores, M. T. Menchú, G. Arroyave, y M. Béhar, INCAP Publication E-434, Guatemala, p. 9.

V

What Can Be Done to Break the Vicious Circle?

25

Prospects for Agricultural Production in Latin America

Quentin M. West

Economic Research Service
United States Department of Agriculture
Washington, D.C.

Fortunately, Latin America has plentiful land and water resources for agricultural development. In the early 1970s about 81 million hectares of land were cropped in the region. This is only about 17% of the estimated total land potentially suited for crop growing in Latin America, while in the world as a whole 42% of the potential farmland is actually cultivated. In some areas, such as Mexico, a large proportion of the suitable land is already growing crops, while in others, like Brazil, only a small portion of the arable land is planted. Much of the land available for expansion is currently in remote frontier areas or is now in pasture, much of which will be freed if more technologically advanced pasture use methods are adopted. In many countries, particularly Argentina and Uruguay, large areas that could be rich cropland are used for extensive grazing.

The most promising frontier areas—those fairly near markets—have already been brought into production. Examples are the Pacific coast lowlands in Central America, the north coast of Colombia, and western Parana State in Brazil. However, as transportation and marketing facilities are improved, more distant areas can be profitably brought into production.

Latin America has an extensive grazing industry. If pastures were upgraded and animal husbandry improved, much more beef and wool could be produced on less land, thus freeing land for crops. Also, as pastureland is expanded into more distant frontier areas, land closer to markets can be used for crops. In some places it appears that expansion of cropland has forced displacement and/or modernization of the grazing industry. The best example is the expansion, over the last six or eight years, of wheat and soybeans on pastureland in southern Brazil.

Expansion and improvement of irrigation offer great potential for increased agricultural production. In those areas dependent upon irrigated agriculture, such as Mexico, coastal Peru, Chile, and western Argentina, all of the easy expansion has already been accomplished. Scarce water supplies will tend to limit further expansion. However, in other countries, there is great potential for increased irrigation, if pressures of food demand warrant it. Up to now, it has been cheaper to enlarge the amount of acreage cultivated in the rainfed areas.

Existing irrigation systems in some countries could be used more efficiently. For example, productivity of irrigated land is much less than maximum because a large proportion of acreage, particularly in Chile, is under low productivity pastures or fodder crops. Also, some land in irrigated areas is not used because of present uncertainty of water supply. New investment is needed to improve and rehabilitate irrigation systems in some areas.

For many important commodities, crop yields in Latin America are below world average and are increasing at a slower rate. For example, wheat yields in the rest of the world increased 35% in the last 10 years; Latin America's declined by 3%. Corn yields jumped 25% in other corn-growing countries, while Latin American yields advanced just 11%. Potential exists for greatly expanding yields, especially of corn. There has been widespread adoption of hybrid varieties in recent years, but improper or limited use of fertilizers and other agricultural practices has limited the gains in yields.

An important source of increased yields will be greater fertilizer use. Highly commercialized export and industrial crops receive the bulk of the fertilizer at present. In many countries, cereal crops, particularly corn, receive very little. Corn happens to be quite responsive to fertilizer. The Food and Agriculture Organization of the United Nations estimated that in South America, each additional kilo of fertilizer nutrients would, on the average, yield an additional 10 kilos of corn. As a benchmark, Latin America in 1971–72 used only about 27 kilos of fertilizer per hectare of arable land compared to 98 kilos per hectare in the United States. The world average was 50 kilos.

Most recent production increases in Latin America have come from increased land use. Despite potential usable land still available, the easiest land has already been brought into production. Over the next 20 years, increasing yields are likely to play a more important role than in the past. This is why increased fertilizer use and work of research organizations, like the International Wheat and Corn Improvement Center in Mexico, the International Center for Tropical Agriculture in Colombia, the International Potato Center in Peru, and the Research and Training Center for Tropical Agriculture in Costa Rica are so important.

It is also clear to me that agriculture in this continent has a long way to go.

Yields are low compared to potential, and agricultural economic growth is slow compared to need. Yet agriculture has a great potential in expanding production for its rapidly growing population. Moreover, Latin America shows promise as well for becoming a major breadbasket for the world. An agricultural development effort unprecedented in Latin American annals will be required to lift the potential of plenty to solid reality.

26

Prospects for Improving the Production of Cereals

R. G. Anderson

International Maize and Wheat Improvement Center
Mexico, D.F.

Cereals form the major part of the diet of 70–80% of the people in developing countries. It is imperative to expand cereal protein and calorie supplies rapidly if millions are to be free of the effects of malnutrition or even starvation. If supplies currently available could be evenly distributed, the world could be fed for some years into the future. Yet it is those very countries most in need of food who are unable to buy it. In countries of rising affluence, more and more cereals are being siphoned off for animal feeds, and because of the low conversion rate, diverting supplies from direct human consumption.

Current varieties and technological means of production now available could unquestionably double world output of cereals. The problem is to make this a reality. Research, extension, wise pricing, and credit policies must be properly organized and interlinked. Inadequate seed production, nonavailability of fertilizers and pesticides, faltering economies, a shortage of leaders to make sound development policies, and a host of other problems all conspire to prevent the farmer, who is the ultimate practitioner of agricultural technology, from reaping the benefits of technology, and food production languishes.

STABILIZING CEREAL YIELDS

Total cereal production on a world scale is an important factor, but variations in production within countries from year to year have disastrous effects on the agriculturally oriented economies of developing countries, particularly in countries with large populations. Everyone is familiar with the effects of drought, disease epidemics, and insect depredations. On the other hand, in years of good rainfall, under light attack of diseases and insects, the widely adapted varieties now available for most of the cereals will give excellent returns. How, then, can we reduce the effects of water shortage, ensure adequate disease and insect resistance, and provide varieties with wider adaptation?

The cereals as a group are grown over a very wide range of conditions. In parts of the world, high rainfall or irrigation provides abundance; in other areas rainfall is infrequent and yields are scant.

Water shortage can occur as a result of too little rain and under conditions of poor irrigation management. Irrigation water from canals is often supplied free, but there is usually no coordination between supply and critical agricultural need. Too often canals are cleaned and water is withheld at the time it is most needed. This leads to overirrigation (once the water is released), wasted water, and crop damage because of the farmer's fear that his next chance for water may be greatly delayed. Shallow or tube well irrigation under the farmer's control is normally much more effective except where, in certain countries, shortage of both hydroelectric power and diesel fuel renders their operation unreliable.

Under rain-fed conditions, water supply varies from levels exceeding irrigation to near desert conditions. Within this range, cultural practices that enhance water entry into the soil profile, reduce evaporation, and prevent weed transpiration can more than double the crop in most developing countries. The technology to be used is somewhat location specific. It should be predicated on soil type, equipment available, access to power, economic resources, and similar factors. The principles of technology needed are, however, relatively well defined and all that is needed is modification to fit existing conditions.

Yield variations under irrigated culture are generally caused by power shortages, attacks of diseases and insects on the varieties grown, or untimely frosts. Thus, the task of breeding for irrigated locations is simplified to one of providing improved yield, wide adaptability characteristics, and pest resistance.

Breeding for suitability to rain-fed culture is much more complex. Varieties must be suitable for many levels of rainfall and possess sufficient buffering capacity to maintain relatively high yields in seasons of low rainfall. Where rainfall is high, the same varieties grown under irrigation are suitable, assuming disease problems are similar. For the intermediate and low range, disease becomes increasingly less important and the drought-resistance requirement increases.

Crop varieties should be chosen on the basis of their general adaptability to the local temperatures and the level of rainfall expected. Breeders should not attempt to produce varieties of every cereal to fit all conditions. Thus, where irrigation is cheap or rainfall is high, rice is well suited. Maize, wheat, and oats are best suited to controlled irrigation or intermediate levels of rainfall. In drier conditions, barley, triticale, rye, sorghum, and millets all produce higher yields than the other crops. Choice of variety and crop must also be based on the frost hazards generally encountered. This is obviously an oversimplification, because individual varieties of each crop may be grown outside the bounds set. The principle, however, is that total production of cereals can be enhanced when the species is fitted to the climate of the region. Within these general limits varieties can be bred to fit the varying levels of moisture expected.

Disease and insects are major sources of yield instability. Insects are more threatening in the raising of sorghum, maize, rice, and millets than in the production of the other cereals. Breeding for resistance and chemical control are now employed to offset attacks, and biological control may be important in the future. Insects are much less important for other cereals, although regional and seasonal damage can be severe. Where the condition is chronic, resistance must be bred into varieties, or chemical control can be applied where the attacks are seasonal and sporadic. Control can add appreciably to yield stability.

Diseases are important in all crops, but are particularly devastating in the self-pollinated cereals when grown under adequate moisture. In the latter crops, because they are genotypically similar from plant to plant, disease epidemics can develop explosively on susceptible varieties. In the cross-pollinated cereals, the genotypic variations from plant to plant check rapid buildup of disease once an equilibrium is established.

Almost all varieties of the small grains eventually succumb to new specialized forms of important diseases. Resistance in many is conditioned by specific genes. In those possessing horizontal or nonspecific resistance, the life of the variety is prolonged, resulting in greater stability. Unfortunately, it is difficult to select for and identify horizontal resistance in a nursery where both specific and nonspecific resistances are segregating. We have found, however, that international testing over a broad geographic range can sort out these types. Thus, varieties showing resistance to the wide array of virulent forms of diseases present at the many locations are likely to possess horizontal resistance. In wheat, CIMMYT has established, in addition, an international screening system and regional screening nurseries for this purpose.

It has also included a trap nursery of commercial varieties from various regions, to detect movement of new pathogenic forms of diseases. This nursery is grown in "disease hot spots" in the region. In this way we hope to provide a warning of the impending breakdown of varieties before the pathogen reaches the country where a particular variety is grown. If action is taken to replace the variety, yield stability is maintained. This system can operate for any cereal.

We are also attempting to mimic the cross-pollinated protection of open-pollinated crops by producing multilineal varieties in self-pollinated crops. Details of the procedure were outlined by Borlaug (1). In principle, a widely adapted variety is chosen. Into this are incorporated many resistance characteristics found in individual lines. Fifteen to 20 such lines, morphologically similar, are composited and grown as a mixed variety. As in the cross-pollinated crops, genotypic differences from plant to plant preclude epidemic buildup. As components become susceptible they are replaced in the new seed mixture with other resistant lines. Not classically, but by definition, this is horizontal resistance.

A Colombian multiline variety of wheat, Miramar, has retained its disease resistance for many years. Currently, a multiline in wheat for stripe rust resistance is being grown in the Netherlands (J. C. Zadoks, personal communication, 1974). We at CIMMYT are well along in developing lines in the cross 8156. Lines placed in the composite will vary from region to region, based on the disease-protection needs of the individual country. It is interesting that our preliminary results show the composite to be higher yielding than its individual components. Sources of resistance are supplied from data received from international testing. This system would seem to be a valuable way to provide yield stability for any of the self-pollinated cereals.

The third important consideration in stabilizing yields is wide adaptability of the variety. Varieties that yield well in many locations in a single year can be expected to buffer the effect of seasonal variation at any one location. In breeding, alternate generations can be grown under widely different environments. Where two generations per year are grown, the two nurseries should be selected for as wide a difference of conditions as possible. Where only one generation can be grown annually, for example winter wheat, simultaneous selection at locations with different environments will yield similar results when the performance in the two locations is combined. International testing of materials passed through such a screen again identifies the most widely adapted types. These, in turn, can be used as varieties or recycled through the breeding programs to pyramid genes for wide adaptation in the background germplasm.

These three factors—water management and conservation, stable resistance to diseases and insects, and widely adapted varieties—can minimize yield fluctuations that are so characteristic in many countries. We feel that stability of yield must be assured to form a defense line behind which the search can continue for ever higher yield plateaus.

NEW BREEDING AND PRODUCTION APPROACHES

To increase production, the limited remaining virgin lands can be opened, irrigation systems can be extended, and drainage systems for land reclamation can be installed. However, most increased production will have to come from increased yields per hectare per year. In the higher latitudes of temperate areas this means increasing varietal yield in a single crop. In the more semitropical and tropical countries, where multiple cropping can be practiced, varieties of different crops must be bred with different maturity periods to fit cropping sequences that maximize yearly food production. For example, in North India, later maturing rice varieties grown in summer and into fall delay wheat plantings, with consequent wheat yield reduction. Similarly, winter wheats are too late maturing to fit satisfactorily with rice in the Republic of Korea, hence winter barley must be grown even though wheat would be preferred. Also, varieties must be tailored to specific climates or to regional soil conditions, for example, Brazil's soil has toxic levels of aluminum.

We are crossing winter with spring wheats. We hope to select spring varieties that will lead to: (1) increased yield level from intercrossing these genetically divergent, seldom-crossed groups; (2) greater resistance to atmospheric drought, better root systems, and deeper placed crown (providing better stand establishment and root development); and (3) a wide range of maturing times to fit into different cropping systems.

We hope to obtain winter varieties that will have: (1) increased yield level, as in the case of spring wheats; (2) a range of winter hardiness to fit regional ecological locations; (3) greater disease resistance, characteristic of the spring wheats; and (4) a range of ripening times to fit cropping systems.

The evidence obtained from preliminary exploitation of these crosses indicates that most, or all, of these hopes are justified.

We hear much today of the advantages of indigenous varieties, implying that breeders should improve these strains rather than develop new ones. The fact is that they have a low yield potential, less disease resistance, poorer adaptability, and many other drawbacks when compared with the improved genetic base of the high-yielding varieties. To attempt to correct the faults in local varieties is an exercise in futility and results in improved *low*-yielding varieties. Breeders must take the opposite view and use specific genes from indigenous varieties to improve high-yielding varieties further.

Physiologic and genetic studies are being pursued in all of the cereal crops. In rice, for example, many characteristics are under investigation. These include research on: straw stiffness, height, tillering capacity, crown form, efficiency of photosynthesis, temperature requirements, growth duration, photoperiodic response, disease and insect resistance, leaf toughness, angle of leaf, dormancy of grain, ease of threshing, harvest indices, sink size, grain shape, grain appearance, protein content, and cooking properties, among many other features. The results of these studies are then used to design suitable high-yielding, nutritious varieties for the different seasons and growing conditions in which rice is produced.

In addition to such studies, empirical observations made at international test sites can be the basis for identifying common characteristics of successful varieties. Such qualities can then be incorporated into the germplasm and selection can be made for that constellation of characteristics most likely to promote yield under the different growing conditions. Certain of these qualities may be common for all varieties; others are variety specific.

The possibility of combining germplasm from different cereals in new combinations, or even wider crosses with legumes, is being investigated. One such cross, triticale, developed from wheat and rye, has now reached crop status and gives yields superior to those of wheat in certain locations. The crop appears to have tolerance to acid soils, waterlogged conditions, aluminum toxicity, and dry conditions, and has a good amino acid balance. It can be expected to join the other cereals as an important crop.

Somatic fusion is being attempted at several centers. Although many of the problems have been overcome, intergeneric hybrids have not been produced yet. In another approach, CIMMYT, in collaboration with Kansas State University, is injecting immunosuppressant chemicals into developing plants, with the aim of overcoming sterility barriers that isolate the species and genera. These are the same chemicals used elsewhere to prevent rejection of organs transplanted in humans. As a result of this work, there is good evidence that successful crosses have been made between genera, and in some cases the chromosome number has been doubled. However, in succeeding generations one of the parent's chromosome complements appears to be sloughed off. Studies are being continued to gain understanding of why this occurs and whether it can be overcome. Should this approach prove successful, the potential for new species could be enormous. For example, if N fixation capability could be transferred to cereals, this would greatly augment food supplies.

In recent years, plant breeders and nutritionists have been searching for genes in the cereal crops that would provide higher nutritional value through better amino acid balance. These genes have been located in maize, barley, triticale, and sorghum, and have long been known to exist in oats. Programs are well under way to develop varieties with better amino acid balance. The Canadian industry is developing a *protein concentrate* from oats with a protein value of 92–95%, which may make the crop a competitor with soybean as a protein source (V. D. Burrows, personal communication, 1974).

Because of the greater food value of such varieties, greater production will, in effect, have been achieved, because fewer hectares are required for nutrition.

Hybrids have been developed in maize, sorghum, millets, and wheat. We at CIMMYT do not consider this approach practical for most developing countries because of poor seed-production organizations and limited seed-distribution systems. High-yielding composite varieties in the cross-pollinated cereals such as maize have been developed, and we feel these are much more useful. These can be rapidly diffused to the farmer. In a similar fashion, we believe that work on hybrids in the self-pollinated crops is more applicable to the developed nations.

The results of mutation breeding have been disappointing. Too much manpower and too many resources have been, and are being, allotted to this activity in developing countries. It should be used only as a tool to create specific variation in characteristics for which natural variation is unknown and, because of a shortage of trained people, most of this work is better done in the developed countries.

The foregoing represents part of the breeding efforts and basic investigations that are being conducted. The last major advance in yield was the result of shortening the culms of wheat and rice. This is being extended to the other major cereals in order to make them more responsive to fertilizers and, hence, higher yielding. Whether or not similar major advances can be made in the light of new information will only be known in the future.

INDUCING AGRICULTURAL CHANGE

These remarks apply to all food crops, including the cereals. As a prerequisite for effective changes in food production, the government of the country concerned must designate solving the food supply as a major domestic issue. All governments are short of money, and the measure of their response to problems is the priority placed upon individual problems. A review of agricultural progress made in developing countries reinforces this view. I will not dwell on the various economic factors involved, but will deal only with methods of moving technology to the farmers of developing countries.

For successful diffusion of technology (i.e., varieties and agronomic practices), both research and extension must be properly organized and interlinked. The first need is for trained personnel. International centers concerned with crop commodities are now training young scientists of developing countries in an interdisciplinary crop-oriented team approach, to take a place in the research group of their respective countries, as appliers of known technology.

While some feel that a near-adequate training volume for research scientists can be done by these centers, the numbers of production agronomists needed to man extension programs worldwide are beyond the capabilities of their training programs. In our opinion, training in this field is more properly done "in country." The international centers, on their part, can teach the trainers who would return to head a training program in their own countries. Furthermore, these trainers could be assisted in organizing their country programs by center- or regionally-based training officers. These programs should be conducted at active centers of research. The trainer should be thoroughly familiar with the latest research results and employ these in farm demonstrations as a training tool. It has been popular to say that extension is ineffective, but the truth of the matter is that most extension personnel have no knowledge of research in progress, nor are they linked in any way to the research station. As a result they have little to extend. This revised approach would familiarize the extension worker with research capabilities and the research personnel to whom they could turn for advice.

Research in most countries must also be reoriented and reorganized. Too much money is being spent on nonapplied discipline-oriented research in a quest for knowledge for knowledge's sake, as opposed to funds designated for varietal improvement. Too often the scientist is only vaguely aware of the real needs of the farmer, his economic capabilities, the power available to him, or land size, for example, or what these mean in terms of his desire or nondesire to change his traditional practices. One cannot transfer, without modifications, the technology developed for mechanized farming to the bullock-powered society. The principles may, however, be the same. Properly modified, the technology of variety, fertilizer application, and water and crop management is readily accepted by the farmer, provided the advantages of change are demonstrated and he can reap greater profits. To change requires that he risk all; hence, he is risk-averting and only responds when the benefits of change are obvious to him.

Various methods have been employed in expatriate activities designed to assist in developing research and production capabilities in different countries. Two approaches are the pilot project and the country program. Viewed as an experiment, the pilot project gives valuable leads about which factors are most important in inducing change. In the process the limited land area can be, and is, improved markedly. However, such projects are supported and closely supervised in such a manner that the effort cannot be duplicated for all areas of the country because of the shortage of scientific manpower and economic resources.

The country program is much less spectacular and its immediate impact is not easily assessed. It has the advantage that it works on a countrywide basis, builds an organization within the government structure, and can enjoy wider governmental support because it benefits all sectors of the country growing a particular crop. Viewed in the longer term, it can leave the country with a research and production organization as a base on which further refinements can be made.

In each of these types of programs, expatriate personnel are generally assigned to assist national program leaders in developing their organizations. Unfortunately, the two-year appointment has been the rule. The appointee takes six months to one year to establish his bona fides and establish good will. In the second year he spends a part of his time arranging for his departure. This leaves little time in which to accomplish the objectives of his appointment. At the end of his tenure a new man takes his place and he has the same problems. What is even worse, his ideas are often different from those of his predecessor. The change in thrust mystifies and dismays the national counterpart, who does not know which one is right.

Some organizations offer career opportunities to personnel in international agriculture. In such cases expatriates are assigned to a bilateral program and continue on in this position until the aims are achieved. Periodic assessment of the progress is made, and the man is phased out when it appears that his services are no longer necessary, or he is not the correct person for that position. This approach has the advantage of continuity of thrust and the expatriate develops a close interest in assuring the success of the program (partly because its success is the basis for his own advancement). Furthermore, he carefully weighs the decisions he is instrumental in forming, and he expects to be responsible for the outcome of those decisions. The importance of choice of personnel and the tenure of their appointments is, too often, not given enough consideration when bilateral programs are drawn up.

In this age of the computer and the economist, there is a great desire to draw up long-term development plans with targeted advances, targeted time-phasing, and little flexibility. Most governments faced with the complexities of such a complete program, with all its innuendo, will despair and be immobilized like the rat staring at the snake. By contrast, the approach must be innovative, pragmatic, and liberally laced with intuition and common sense.

First, an "engine of change" such as the short-statured rice and wheat varieties, the composite variety in maize, and other types must be identified. These are introduced into the system; they respond to greater amounts of fertilizer; there is a need for seed, credit, and pesticides; and the farmers, being convinced of the need, raise a clamor for them. The government responds. Machinery is needed, wells are dug to provide more irrigation. Farm level surpluses are produced. Marketing facilities must be established. Storage and road and rail transport are found inadequate. Each new advance demands its successor.

I advocate a "first things first" approach. A whole series of vacuums are produced and the government services are forced to respond in a progressive fashion. Meanwhile, the increased production heightens its capability to do so. This plan of action is flexible and does not adhere to a specific timetable, but I am confident it is effective. The increased production leads to the development of agroindustries rurally based, slows down the country-to-slum drift, and provides increased wages for the landless.

The desirability of mechanization has been questioned by many. The social structure should dictate how far this should be instituted. In the highly populated countries of the tropics and subtropics, only two activities should be mechanized. Seed drills are essential to ensure good stands and high yields. Machine threshing removes the harvested crop from the weather and depredations of pests, while freeing the bullocks normally employed for land preparation to do so for the succeeding crop in the multiple rotation system. All other activities can be left to the plentiful supply of hand labor.

Every effort must be expended to develop new fertilizer plants if we are to maintain the race between food production and expanding populations. There is no alternative. Beyond this, a shortage of energy to power wells and agroindustries threatens to become ever more serious. Alternative cheap power sources must be forthcoming, or the crisis that has already overcome many of the developing and developed countries will engulf the world.

These are some of the critical issues. Let me conclude by stating that if governments are really serious about their food production problems, and are willing to put their resources behind research and diffusion of technology and the development of the agricultural infrastructure, the vicious circle can be broken for the immediate future. Some time can be purchased, but unless the looming population advance is brought to a halt, the entire exercise will have been in vain.

REFERENCE

1. Borlaug, N. E., 1958, The use of multilineal or composite varieties to control airborne epidemic diseases of self-pollinated crop plants, *in: Proceedings of the First International Wheat Genetics Symposium,* University of Manitoba, Winnipeg, Canada, 1959.

COMMENT

William L. Brown · *Pioneer Hi-Bred International, Inc., Des Moines, Iowa.*

In any consideration of cereal production in a developing country, three factors are particularly pertinent: (1) the producer, i.e., whether production is derived primarily from subsistence or commercial farming; (2) the availability of improved and more productive varieties that, in most developing countries, should provide the genetic potential at least to double yields; and (3) the existence of production technology to take full advantage of the genetic potential of the improved varieties.

In the tropics and subtropics of Latin America, much of the more productive land is used for the production of cash crops, most frequently sugarcane and cotton. Consequently, cereal production is usually relegated to the more marginal land consisting of small individual holdings, generally operated on a subsistence basis. Obviously, cereal production could be most effectively increased through utilization of the better land and the application of commercial farming practices. However, it is unrealistic to assume that this will happen except under unusual circumstances. Furthermore, as suggested by Quentin West, a reversal of this nature may not be in the best interest of some developing countries. The more reasonable assumption is that the competitive position of cereals relative to cash crops will be no better in the future than it has been in the past, and the bulk of cereal production will continue to come from the small farms.

It is too often assumed that little can be done to aid the small farmer to increase productivity. Recent experience indicates that, given access to the necessary inputs, encouragement, and economic incentives, the small farmer is just as anxious to adopt improved technology as is his commercial counterpart. One good example is the success of the Puebla project in Mexico. Over a seven-year period, maize production among small landholders of the Puebla area rose about 48% because they used better varieties, more fertilizer, and improved methods. It is frequently said that the small farmer cannot, or will not, pay the price for the purchase of improved seed or fertilizer, but recent experience in Central America, especially in Guatemala, proves this to be false.

In Central America maize is a staple cereal that occupies a major role in the human diet. Approximately 4 million acres are allocated to maize production in Central America and Panama. Until recently, the only types of maize available for use in this area were local varieties whose yields are 60% to 100% less than those of improved types. Although sporadic attempts to introduce improved maize varieties in Central America go back at least two decades, it was not until about 1970 that a serious attempt was made to produce and distribute seed of adapted, high-yielding hybrids throughout the area. At present only about 10% of the total maize acreage of Central America and Panama is planted with these hybrids, but the percentage is growing annually and the demand for seed consistently exceeds the supply.

It is interesting and particularly significant to note the extent to which the improved seeds marketed in this part of the world are used by small landholders. These range from 10% in Panama to 80% in Nicaragua. In Costa Rica 50% of the total available improved maize seed is utilized by small farmers. The comparable figure for Honduras is 30% and for Guatemala 70%. This goes a long way toward exploding the myth that the small farmer will not purchase improved seed. Such farmers may not be educated, but they certainly are not stupid. They do not need experts to show them that their lot has been improved when their crop yields are doubled on their own land at a cost representing only a fraction of their increased gross income.

This leads to the second aspect of improved cereal production, namely, that having to do with the availability of improved varieties of high yield potential. Regardless of the success of breeders in developing improved varieties and hybrids, the impact of such developments on food supply is zero unless these varieties reach the producer, not only in quantity, but in a state that maintains the original genetic potential. Among the cereals, the nature and requirements of seed production and distribution vary greatly, depending upon the species involved and its mode of reproduction.

With wheat and rice, both of which are self-pollinated species, the multiplication of seed is a rather simple process. All that is needed to reproduce a variety in large quantity is simply to grow, rogue, and harvest the crop, exercising care to maintain varietal purity by avoiding mechanical mixtures of seed. In contrast, in the case of maize, which is almost completely cross-fertilized, and sorghum, which is predominantly cross-fertilized, the situation is entirely different.

To maintain the purity of hybrids, fertilization must be controlled; consequently, the methods for large-scale production of quality hybrid seed are much more sophisticated than the production of seed of self-fertilizing species. I have little doubt that the large-scale and successful introduction of improved varieties of wheat and rice into several developing countries in recent years, resulting in the so-called green revolution, was, to a considerable extent, because the species involved are self-pollinating.

The importance and impact of the green revolution on the agricultural economy of countries such as India and Pakistan is unquestioned. Yet it should be recognized that the movement of large quantities of Mexican wheat seeds from the existing commercial supplies in Mexico to countries of similar latitude such as India and Pakistan was a relatively simple, straightforward process, because there was no necessity to produce additional quantities of "seed" to meet unanticipated requirements.

I am equally convinced that the limited success of the international maize programs is largely because of failure to develop satisfactory systems of seed production and distribution. The quality of breeding that has gone into international maize improvement programs is comparable to that characterizing the self-pollinated cereals, but the impact of the maize program on increased productivity has been minimal compared to that of wheat and rice.

As high-yielding hybrids were developed, first in Mexico and later in several countries of South and Central America and finally in India, the responsibility for production and distribution of seed was assumed by agencies of the respective governments involved. After 25 years of experience, I can state in fairness that, without exception, these activities represent at best varying degrees of failure. As a consequence, the fruits of some excellent plant breeding have failed to reach the farmer.

A secondary, but perhaps ultimately more important, aspect of the failure of government seed distribution systems is the influence it has had on international maize improvement schemes. Much of the maize breeding now being done by the international institutes emphasizes the development of improved varieties and largely ignores the use of hybrids. The reason usually given to justify this is that farmers in most developing countries are not sufficiently advanced in their agricultural technology to take advantage of hybrid seed. A more realistic reason is probably disillusionment with government seed agencies.

Whatever the reason, the unfortunate result is that limitations are imposed on genetic improvement by the breeding methods now employed. Stated very simply, much of the maize breeding now being done under the auspices of international programs involves the application of selection technics that, because of their very nature, effectively preclude the maximum exploitation of heterosis, a phenomenon that has played a dominant role in most maize improvement in the past.

Finally, I would like to consider briefly the third aspect of increased production–providing the technology necessary to capitalize on the full genetic potential of improved varieties. Heretofore, the greatest and most rapid increases in production have resulted from the direct transfer, not only of varieties but of complete production systems, from one developed country to another of similar latitude. One of the best examples is the transfer of maize germ plasm and maize culture practices from the United States to western Europe following World War II. Similar successful transfers have taken place between the United States and parts of eastern Europe, beginning in the mid-1960s. Among other cereals, examples are the movement of Mexican wheats to India and Pakistan and the transfer of Philippine rice and associated production technology to other areas of similar latitude in Southeast Asia.

Thus, we know that the successful transfer, not only of varieties but also of production technology, can be made from one area to another within similar latitudes and climates. We also know that transfer of varieties from the temperate zone to the tropics and vice versa is not usually possible, and we are now beginning to learn that the transfer of production technology from one climatic zone to another is usually not successful without some adaptation or modification. In such situations adaptive production research is required. It is in this area that the international institutes can play an important role, and it is encouraging to note that in Latin America these institutions are already making a significant contribution.

One example of the importance of nongenetic technology in increasing cereal production is found in some recent data from Iowa, where it is estimated that production technology has contributed 35 to 40% of the total increase in the maize yield that has occurred there during the period from 1922 to 1970. The remainder of the increased yield is assumed to be the result of genetic improvement. The important point is that without both inputs, maximum increases in productivity will not be realized and, unfortunately, nothing less than achievement of full production potential will meet the cereal requirements of many developing countries.

27

Improving the Production and Nutritional Quality of Food Legumes

Lewis M. Roberts

Agricultural Sciences
The Rockefeller Foundation
Guatemala City, Guatemala

Man has been using some legumes as important sources of food ever since the invention of agriculture, probably about 8000 to 10,000 years ago. For example, remains of peas, *Pisum sativum,* have been found in the Swiss lake dwellings of the Bronze Age (1), and the plant was cultivated by the Greeks and Romans. The broad bean, *Vicia faba,* probably native to northern Africa and the Near East, has been under domestication for at least 4000 years and probably longer. It was well known to the ancient Egyptians and to the Greeks. Records 5000 years old mention cultivation of the soybean, *Glycine max,* in eastern Asia, possibly its native habitat, but there is no record of its first domestication, which must have occurred long before.

About 20 species of the food legume crops are used in appreciable quantities in the human diet. They are most commonly consumed as mature, dry seeds, but they are also eaten as immature green seeds or as green pods with the seeds enclosed. The food legume crops have contributed enormously over the centuries to balancing diets high in cereals and starchy foods. Despite this fact, however, they have generally been taken for granted, and research on them has been treated with benign neglect with the limited exception of soybeans, field beans, peas, and peanuts. Fortunately, a good start has been made during the past four or five years to remedy this situation.

Interest and support from the Consultative Group on International Agricultural Research (CG) have been prime factors in expanding and accelerating research on food legumes. The CG is an international consortium of assistance agencies with about 30 members, including multinational institutions such as the World Bank, the Food and Agriculture Organization of the United Nations, the United Nations Development Program, and the Inter-American Development Bank, as well as governmental foreign assistance agencies and private foundations. The CG began in April, 1969, when about 15 heads of some of the major international assistance agencies met informally at the International Conference Center of The Rockefeller Foundation at Bellagio, Italy, to discuss how their organizations might work in closer concert to help the human race feed itself better. In 1971, this Bellagio Group expanded and evolved into the CG as it is now constituted.

At its second meeting in 1970, the Bellagio Group requested that five papers be prepared on areas or problems of special interest to the Group. One of these was food legumes, and the question of what might be done to expand and accelerate efforts to increase their production and improve their quality. I prepared a paper (2) that recommended that 6 of the 20 or so food legume crops be selected for increased attention on the basis of their present and potential importance. These were somewhat arbitrarily grouped according to their ecological regions of adaptation, as follows:

A. Low humid tropics
   1. Pigeon peas (*Cajanus cajan*)
   2. Cowpeas (*Vigna unguiculata*)
B. Semiarid or seasonal tropics
   3. Peanuts (*Arachis hypogaea*)
C. Tropical intermediate elevations to temperate zones
   4. Soybeans (*Glycine max*)
   5. Beans (*Phaseolus vulgaris*)
D. Cool-weather, high-elevation zone and Mediterranean winter–spring seasons
   6. Chickpeas (*Cicer arietinum*)

Later, peas (*Pisum sativum* and broad beans (*Vicia faba*) were added to the list in the cool-weather group.

It was recommended that worldwide networks for collaborative efforts on each crop be created to link three components:

1. All of the national institutions of the developing countries that have improvement programs on a particular crop and wish to collaborate in such an international network; these programs constitute the principal pillars of the network and have basic responsibility for improving a specific crop in their respective countries.
2. An international center that serves as a primary force to draw the

network together and act as a catalyst within the network; its principal objective is to help strengthen national programs and institutions in developing countries.

3. Institutions in the developed countries, which have very valuable scientific and technological resources that are not being utilized nearly as effectively as they might be to help improve the yields and quality of the major food legume crops in the less developed regions of the world.

Considerable progress has been made to implement these recommendations. For several of the species chosen for initial attention, global networks of collaborative work are in the process of development, as follows.

DRY BEANS

In 1972, the Board of Trustees of the Centro Internacional de Agricultura Tropical (CIAT) at Cali, Colombia, approved, as a major program effort, work on beans, to focus at the beginning on Latin America and the Caribbean. It is envisioned, however, that in a relatively short time CIAT's bean program will grow into the primary global center for this crop, with strong linkages with national and regional bean improvement programs throughout the world. Dry beans originated in Latin America and they are produced and consumed in much greater quantities than in any other region of the world (almost 28% of the world's bean acreage and 36% of the total production). Furthermore, there are more good national bean improvement programs (3) now under way in Latin America than anywhere else. It is logical, therefore, that CIAT assume the international center responsibilities for beans.

CIAT conducted an international seminar at its headquarters on February 26–March 1, 1973, on the topic, *Potentials of Field Beans and Other Food Legumes in Latin America.* The proceedings of this seminar (4) give a comprehensive view of the current status of work under way and the problems needing attention. Emphasis was placed on production problems, although nutritional questions were not ignored. A major contribution of the CIAT seminar was to develop a collaborative network of bean improvement programs—first in Latin America but eventually global, involving national institutions in the developing countries. These include: international and regional institutions such as CIAT, the Inter-American Institute of Agricultural Sciences (IICA), the Centro Agronomico Tropical de Investigación y Enseñanza (CATIE) at Turrialba, Costa Rica, the Institute of Nutrition of Central America and Panama (INCAP), and institutions in the developed countries that have the interest and capability to help improve field beans.

For several years, IICA, through its Northern Zone Office, has assigned a coordinator and provided technical support for the Central American Regional Project for Production and Improvement of Beans and Other Food Legumes, as a part of the Central American Cooperative Food Crop Improvement Program (PCCMCA). It has also recently published a comprehensive bibliography of bean literature. INCAP is making valuable contributions to these efforts, especially through its research on the nutritional aspects of the food legumes.

Among others, Cornell University and Michigan State University in the United States, and Hokkaido University in Japan are linked to these efforts. Breeders and physiologists at these three universities are working in close coordination, and in collaboration with CIAT, with support from The Rockefeller Foundation, to gain a better understanding of the physiology of the bean plant. Their aim is to enable breeders to change its structure in ways that will greatly increase its yield. CIAT's bean program has assembled the largest collection of germ plasm in the world and, in collaboration with other institutions, is surveying the collection for desirable genetic traits of all sorts. Details are available in CIAT's latest annual report (5).

COWPEAS

The International Institute of Tropical Agriculture (IITA) at Ibadan, Nigeria, has worldwide center responsibility for cowpeas. This species originated in Africa and today more than 90% of total world production is on that continent, although the crop has spread throughout the hot, humid tropics of the world. IITA also gives some attention to soybeans, pigeon peas, lima beans (*Phaseolus lunatus*), and African yam beans (*Sphenostylis stenocarpa*) to determine their potential in the humid tropics, but about two-thirds of the total effort of the food legume program goes into cowpeas. While the program emphasizes breeding of higher-yielding varieties with resistance to disease and insects, it is well rounded, with a multidisciplinary team working in close collaboration on production problems and on nutritional aspects of cowpeas and the other food legumes with which it is concerned. Collaborating in this interdisciplinary approach to the solution of the problems are scientists from universities in the United Kingdom, the United States, and Belgium.

A uniform cooperative cowpea yield trial was conducted by IITA in 1973 at 11 locations in five countries: Nigeria, Ethiopia, Liberia, Ghana, and Colombia. The highest yield in these trials averaged slightly less than 2000 kg/ha, which represents a several-fold increase over the yields usually obtained by farmers in the past. Worldwide cowpea yields average about 400 kg/ha. It is expected that this international network being fostered by IITA for collaborators working on cowpeas will rapidly spread to include improvement programs on this crop in all parts of the globe. Uniform yield trials have expanded quickly and include soybeans, pigeon peas, and mung beans.

PIGEON PEAS AND CHICKPEAS

The dissimilarities between pigeon peas and chickpeas are many and striking. For example, chickpeas are adapted only to cool climates such as those in the high-elevation zones of the tropics, or in the Mediterranean winter–spring seasons, while pigeon peas are adapted to the low, humid tropics. They can, however, tolerate dry, cool conditions, especially during a certain stage of their growth, as long as there are no frosts.

There are two main, though somewhat arbitrary, reasons for treating these two food legumes together—both crops are produced mainly in the subcontinent of India (more than 90% of the total world production of pigeon peas is in India and Pakistan; India produces roughly 75% of all of the chickpeas, followed by Pakistan with about 10%), and the new International Crops Research Institute for the Semi-Arid Tropics (ICRISAT) at Hyderabad, India, has accepted international center responsibilities for the two crops. ICRISAT's work on pigeon peas and chickpeas is just getting under way.

These two crops have received primary attention in the all-India coordinated research program on pulses that began about 10 years ago, with the participation of many research centers in different parts of the country. Other important food legumes that are being given attention in the Indian program are the Phaseolus group, lentils (*Lens esculenta*), cowpeas, and chickling vetch (*Lathyrus sativas*) (6). During the past decade, the Indian program, with the collaboration of the United States Department of Agriculture, has made extensive collections of germ plasm of these various food legume crops (more than 5000 entries of pigeon peas and approximately 6500 of chickpeas). Some 26,000 items representing about 10 species are being maintained by the U.S.D.A. and the All-India Coordinated Pulse Program. In addition, small collections including items of local interest are maintained in several national food legume programs around the globe.

While chickpeas are of greatest importance in India and Pakistan, they are also widely cultivated in the Middle East, the Mediterranean area, and Ethiopia. They have therefore been included, along with other pulses adapted to arid climates, such as the broad beans and lentils, in the Arid Lands Agricultural Development Program (ALAD) of the Ford Foundation.

SOYBEANS AND PEANUTS

These two leguminous crops have been traditionally considered oilseed crops, but this is changing. They are important sources of food protein both for direct and indirect human consumption, and their potential in this regard is tremendous. Soybeans contain about 18% oil and 35 to 40% protein, while peanuts contain 40% oil and 25% protein.

More research effort has been concentrated on soybeans than on any other food legume, for the most part in the United States and Canada. Recently, Brazil has given attention to soybeans and now ranks third in production behind the United States and mainland China. Soybean research is also being conducted in Ecuador, Chile, and Mexico, as well as in India, Indonesia, Japan, and the Philippines. The Asian Vegetable Research and Development Center (AVRDC) at Shanhua, Taiwan, has decided to include soybeans as one of the six principal crops on which it will concentrate, the others being mung beans, tomatoes, sweet potatoes, white potatoes, and Chinese cabbage.

In the late 1960s, the University of Illinois began its Program for International Research, Improvement, and Development of Soybeans (PIRIDS). Initially, this program concentrated on coordinated varietal and agronomic trials in India, Thailand, Pakistan, Indonesia, and the Philippines, but because it was highly successful right from the beginning, it soon grew into a global effort. During 1973 similar cooperative trials were conducted in 33 countries–90 locations in total–in Asia, Africa, and Latin America. Its success attracted interest and support from U.S./AID, which encouraged the University of Illinois and the University of Puerto Rico to work together on building an International Soybean Resource Base (INTSOY). INTSOY was launched in 1973 with major support from U.S./AID and additional assistance from the Rockefeller Foundation.

Considerable work has also been done on peanuts, particularly in the United States, Africa, and India. Among the major food legume crops, peanuts are especially deserving of expanded and accelerated attention. They are widely grown around the world, especially in the underdeveloped countries, which have over 80% of the world's peanut acreage. It is heartening that more research attention is being given to peanuts in such countries as Brazil, Ecuador, and some of the other Latin American nations, as well as in Africa and Asia. To help foster this movement, ICRISAT has recently added peanuts to its food legume program as a global responsibility along with pigeon peas and cowpeas. The University of Florida, with Rockefeller Foundation support, is also developing an international peanut program patterned generally on INTSOY.

BROAD BEANS

Broad beans are adapted to the temperate climate zones, particularly to the winter–spring season in the mediterranean region, and to the highlands of Asia, Africa, and Latin America. This crop needs research on all its aspects–production as well as nutritional–because it has really been neglected even in comparison with other food legumes. A few of the countries in the Near East and around the Mediterranean have dabbled at research on this crop, but in general these programs have been poorly supported and have lacked continuity. Some work on this crop is also being done in a few research centers in Europe and Great

Britain, with the University of Cambridge being particularly notable among these, and the ALAD program of the Ford Foundation in the Near East has included broad beans in its program.

Consideration is being given to the establishment of an international arid lands institute in the Near or Middle East, and if this comes to pass, food legumes adapted to the region, such as broad beans, chickpeas, peas, and lentils, will undoubtedly be given major attention.

PEAS

Peas are grown very largely in the temperate zone, not in the tropics. At least 75% of the world's total production comes from the USSR and mainland China, with the balance coming from Europe and the United States, and to a lesser extent from the high-altitude, cool-climate zones of Asia, Africa, and Latin America.

Peas have received research attention in several of the developed countries of the temperate zone where they are best adapted. This has come from both official research centers and private companies such as seed producers and canneries. Peas have been largely ignored, however, in the developing countries of the tropical belt and they perhaps should receive a low priority for the low altitudes in this area with respect to other species I have already mentioned that are better adapted to hot climates. They do offer possibilities for more widespread use in the Middle East and Mediterranean region for the cool winter–spring season and for the high-altitude regions of the tropics, and it is hoped that they will soon receive more research attention for these areas.

None of the principal food legumes are very well adapted to the hot, humid tropics at present. Greater attention should be given to some of the minor species, such as lima beans and African yam beans, that seem to be basically better adapted to the torrid, wet environment. Mung beans (*Vigna radiata*–Syn. with *Phaseolus aureus*) also offer possibilities in this regard, and it is encouraging to note that the AVRDC is giving major attention to this crop (6).

INTERNATIONAL CONFERENCES

A meeting organized by the United Nations Protein Advisory Group, with the cooperation of several governments and The Rockefeller Foundation, was held at the Food and Agriculture Organization in Rome in July, 1972. This meeting brought together a group of internationally recognized nutritionists, biochemists, food scientists, agronomists, and geneticists/plant breeders to review the current status of knowledge regarding nutrition and food-use problems in food legumes and to discuss how these crops might be improved by breeding. The proceedings of this symposium, published together with PAG Statement No.

22 (8), give an up-to-date, comprehensive picture of what a distinguished, interdisciplinary group of scientists feels should be done to increase the production and nutritional quality of food legumes.

A meeting held at Ribeirao Prêto, Brazil, in November, 1973, brought together about 50 leading scientists from 11 countries to discuss nutritional aspects of common beans and other food legumes. This meeting placed emphasis on storage and processing of these crops and their use in animal feeding, as well as their contribution to human nutrition. The proceedings will be published in a special edition of the monthly publication of the Latin American Nutrition Society.

IITA held its first international workshop on food legume improvement at its headquarters in Ibadan, Nigeria October 29 to November 2, 1973. This conference was attended by about 65 scientists; some came from tropical countries as distant as the Philippines and Colombia, but most were from the African tropics. Collaborating scientists from institutions in several of the developed countries also participated. This group considered the problems of food legumes in the hot, humid tropics, reviewed progress made to date, and recommended future avenues of research. The major disciplinary yields covered included agronomy, biochemistry and nutrition, breeding and genetics, entomology, pathology, and physiology. The published proceedings of the conference are available from IITA.

A workshop on grain legumes that focused on the problems of Southeast Asia was held under the auspices of the Government of Indonesia in January, 1974. Seventy-two participants, chiefly from the member nations of the Association of Southeast Asian Nations (ASEAN)–Indonesia, Malaysia, the Philippines, and Thailand–discussed technological and economic limitations to grain legume production, marketing, and utilization, and formulated recommendations for cooperative efforts to solve common problems. The proceedings of this workshop are available from the Department of Agriculture of Indonesia.

While such developments are heartening, they represent only a start in the right direction. As the world's population–food problem rapidly becomes more critical, the improvement in production and nutritive quality of the food legume crops offers one of the best opportunities for contributing to the solution of this problem.

REFERENCES

1. Schery, R. W., 1952, *Plants for man,* Prentice-Hall, Englewood Cliffs, New Jersey, p. 403.
2. Roberts, L. M., 1970, *The food legumes: Recommendations for expansion and acceleration of research to increase production of certain of these high-protein crops,* The Rockefeller Foundation, New York.
3. Pinchinat, A. M., 1973, Report on Survey of the Food Legume Situation in Latin

America, *in: Potentials of field beans and other food legumes in Latin America,* Centro Internacional de Agricultura Tropical, Cali, Colombia, February 26–March 1, 1973, CIAT's Series Seminars No. 2E.

4. *Potentials of field beans and other food legumes in Latin America,* Centro Internacional de Agricultura Tropical, Cali, Colombia, February 26–March 1, 1973, CIAT's Series Seminars No. 2E.
5. Annual Report, 1973, Centro Internacional de Agricultura Tropical, Cali, Colombia (1973).
6. Swaminathan, M. S., and Jain, H. K., 1973, Food legumes in Indian agriculture, *in: Nutritional improvement of food legumes by breeding,* Proceedings of a Symposium sponsored by the Protein Advisory Group, held at the Food and Agriculture Organization, Rome, Italy 3–5 July, 1972, and Protein Advisory Group Statement 22: *Upgrading human nutrition through the improvement of food legumes,* M. Milner (ed.), Protein Advisory Group of the United Nations System, United Nations, New York, New York, p. 69.
7. Annual Report for 1972–1973, Asian Vegetable Research and Development Center, Shanhua, Taiwan, Republic of China (1974).
8. *Nutritional improvement of food legumes by breeding,* Protein Advisory Group of the United Nations System, 1973, M. Milner (ed.), PAG, United Nations, New York, New York.

COMMENT

Clibas Vieira · *Departamento de Fitotecnia, Universidade Federal de Viçosa, Escola Superior de Agricultura, Viçosa, Minas Gerais, Brasil.*

About two-thirds of the world's population live in the less developed countries of the tropical belt, with their problems of low agricultural production, inadequate purchasing power, high rate of population growth, and deficient food supplies resulting in malnutrition and even hunger.

Most of the world's diets are based on the cereal grains, especially rice, maize, and wheat. The protein content of cereals ranges from 6 to 12%. A cereal diet consumed in adequate quantities can satisfy calorie needs, but it cannot furnish enough protein for young children and pregnant or nursing women. Thus, there is the need to complement cereal-based diets with a richer source of protein, a crucial problem in the less developed countries.

Food legumes could constitute one of the best protein sources in the human diet in developing countries and elsewhere. Unfortunately, these crops have not received the same attention from agricultural researchers as the cereals have. This neglect has led to many unsolved problems in production and to low yields. According to data presented by FAO, soybean yields in most of the developing countries are around 600 to 800 kg/ha, while in the United States the average yield is approximately 1900 kg/ha. In the case of dry beans the difference is equally great: 300 to 700 kg/ha against 1400 to 1500 kg/ha in the developed countries.

Increasing the Production of Food Legumes

In a majority of the tropical countries, varietal improvement programs have suffered from lack of continuity as well as limited resources. Even when favorable results are obtained, the new varieties have little impact because of problems of multiplication, distribution, and use of the improved seeds.

When new varieties are distributed, other problems arise. Many times farmers do not receive the full yield benefits of genetic potential of these varieties because of the lack of inputs and technical knowledge. The farmer does not provide adequate fertilizer, irrigation, weed control, and other requisite agricultural practices. This common situation raises the following question: Would it not be preferable, in the present agricultural stage of many developing countries, to create parasite-resistant varieties that would not require high levels of fertilizer? These varieties would not produce very high yields, but would give a guaranteed production to farmers with limited resources. In time, while these farmers are increasing their knowledge and financial resources, more productive varieties could be released.

Let me give an example of very successful food legume production—soybeans in Brazil. Until a few years ago Brazil was not a big soybean producer (Table I), but has become the world's third largest producer (Table II), with a yield of about 7,000,000 metric tons in 1974. Why? Contributing factors were: (a) adequate soil conditions and climate; (b) the incentive from industry and government; (c) support from research; (d) favorable international markets. Fortunately, the Brazilian harvest does not coincide with the American harvest.

Agricultural research was responsible in large measure for exploiting the soybean. Before the expansion of this crop, when soybeans were not even well known by the majority of Brazilian farmers, researchers were giving attention to

Table I. Soybean Production in Brazil[a]

Year	Acreage (1000 hectares)	Yield (kg/hectare)	Production (1000 metric tons)
1948–52	60	1300	78
1961–65	337	1050	353
1967	612	1170	716
1968	722	910	654
1969	906	1170	1057
1970	1319	1144	1509
1971	1589	1244	1977
1972	2274	1539	3500

[a]Source: FAO Production Yearbook, Vols. 25 and 26, 1971 and 1972.

Table II. World Production of Soybeans, 1972[a]

Country	Acreage (1000 hectares)	Yield (kg/hectare)	Production (1000 metric tons)
USA	18,516	1886	34,916
China	14,295	809	11,570
Brazil	2,274	1539	3,500
USSR	860	628	540
Indonesia	685	752	515
Korea DPR	405	580	235
World	38,489	1378	53,024

[a]Source: FAO Production Yearbook, Vol. 26, 1972.

soy, confident that it would have a place in the future of Brazilian agriculture. By the time farmers became interested in soybeans, productive, adapted varieties had been created and information had been developed on their best cultivation methods. There is now interest in expanding soybean production to the more tropical areas of the north. Because it is a day-length sensitive plant, the varieties that have been developed in the subtropical areas of the south cannot simply be transferred to the north. Appropriate varieties will have to be developed for the Brazilian tropics, a task that will take some years.

Despite increasing soybean production, the dry bean is still the traditional vegetable source of protein for most Brazilians. The annual per caput consumption of dry beans (*Vigna sinensis* and, principally, *Phaseolus vulgaris*) reaches almost 30 kilograms. It is the most important source of protein for poor people, who use beans with rice or cassava as their basic diet.

Although Brazil is the largest dry bean producer in the world (Table III), yields are quite low (approximately 650 kg/ha). Brazilian dry bean production is

Table III. Dry Bean Production in the World, 1972[a]

Country	Acreage (1000 hectares)	Yield (kg/hectare)	Production (1000 metric tons)
Brazil	3700	643	2380
India	6500	231	1500
China	2023	715	1446
Mexico	1700	524	890
USA	560	1458	817
Uganda	430	628	270
Japan	161	1565	252
World	22,279	489	10,899

[a]Source: FAO Production Yearbook, Vol. 26, 1972.

Table IV. Dry Bean Production in Brazil[a]

Year	Acreage (1000 hectares)	Yield (kg/hectare)	Production (1000 metric tons)
1957	2323	680	1582
1965	3272	700	2290
1968	3663	660	2420
1969	3633	610	2200
1970	3485	635	2211

[a]Source: Anuários Estatísticos do Brasil, Rio de Janeiro, Conselho Nacional de Estatística, 1960–1971.

increasing (Table IV), not because new and better technology is being applied, but because more and more land is being used. Improved technology for producing Brazilian beans has already been developed for the principal areas of production, but this technology is not being used by the majority of farmers.

How can we explain the situation in Brazil, where use of improved technology for soybeans resulted in good average yields (Tables I and II), while that for dry beans was not adopted? The answer lies in the types of farmers who plant soybeans and dry beans. The latter continue to be produced by the "traditional" farmer, who generally works a small plot of land, has difficulty in obtaining credit, and does not, or cannot, readily accept modern ideas of agricultural production. The soybean producers generally work medium to large land tracts, and have the means to obtain improved seeds and apply advanced technology. Because Brazil had no traditional soybean farming methods, farmers have had to learn how to cultivate the crop in recent times, when good technology was already available.

Increasing Productivity

Food legume yields in developing countries are generally low because the technology applied is not efficient. Allow me again to use Brazil as an example. The technology for growing dry beans, developed by agricultural researchers, permitting an increase of the national average yield from 600 to 1200 kg/ha, already exists for the major part of the country. The problem has been taking this technology to the farmer, a task of the extension agent, not the researcher. For the application of this technology, it is necessary not only to multiply and distribute seed of the best varieties, but also to apply inputs that are not always within reach of the small farmers, the traditional bean producers.

Agricultural researchers in developing countries, especially those trained in countries with advanced technology, tend to try to adapt the technology of these countries to their own. This is often unsuccessful because of agronomic, ecological, social, and economic differences. The great number of varieties of dry beans cultivated in Brazil and other Latin American countries constitutes an advantage for disease control because where there is genetic variability, diseases cause less damage. Planting uniform, improved varieties represents a danger, especially when these varieties come from a narrow germ plasm base, because genetic uniformity facilitates epidemic diseases (1).

In Latin America, the intercropping of beans with corn has been common practice for hundreds, perhaps thousands, of years. Some specialists believe that such an association has led to coadaptation in both species (2). Although at least 75% of the dry beans produced in Latin America are grown with maize (3), researchers generally study field beans and maize as monocultures, in systems similar to those used in developed countries. Attempts to increase field bean yields in Latin America should put to use the technology adapted to local conditions.

It appears that the maximum yield potential of common bean varieties is about 4000 kg/ha, a low efficiency compared with soybeans, rice, or wheat. To exceed this yield ceiling, it may be necessary to create a new model of bean plant. Ideotypes for high-yielding bean plants for monoculture were presented by Adams in Cali (2). As he suggests, plant types for mixed planting with maize should also be considered.

The yield potential of other food legumes is also low. Borlaug (4), however, thinks that "if we act aggressively, great progress can be achieved in raising production of protein grain during the next eight to ten years." He had in mind research programs of the type developed by CIMMYT and IRRI, which originated the so-called green revolution. If food legumes are to be included in aggressive research programs, it will be necessary to establish priorities in approximately the following order:

A. Common beans (*Phaseolus vulgaris*), a legume crop of the tropical intermediate elevations to temperate zones. They are one of the basic foods in Latin America.
B. Cowpeas (*Vigna sinensis*), a crop for the low humid tropics, and a very important food legume in Africa.
C. Pigeon peas, black gram (*Cajanus cajan*), also a crop for the low humid tropics, and the second most important food legumes in India. They are also widely grown in East Africa and in Central and South America. Yields in excess of 5000 kg/ha are reported (5).
D. Chickpeas, garbanzos, Bengal gram (*Cicer arietinum*), although grown in several countries, are important principally in India and Pakistan. They grow in cool-weather, high-elevation zones.
E. Soybeans (*Glycine max*) are high-yielding legumes, adapted principally for the tropical intermediate elevations to temperate zones. The United States, China, and Brazil are the leading world producers (Table II).

F. Peanuts *(Arachis hypogaea)*, a crop native to South America, is today widely grown in India, Pakistan, and Africa. Their ecological region of adaptation is the semidry or seasonal tropics.

For improving productivity of these and other food legumes, a series of research activities is needed (6).

Improving the Nutritional Quality of Food Legumes

One of the preoccupations of genetic improvement programs for food legumes is the quantity and quality of seed protein. There is enough variation in chemical composition to make nutritional improvement possible by hybridization and selection. The average protein content of seeds of the most important food legumes–common beans, cowpeas, pigeon peas, and chickpeas–is 20 to 23%. In soybeans the values are higher: 36 to 40%. These are appreciable protein contents. Unfortunately, these seeds have a lower content of the sulfur amino acids methionine and cystine, and also of tryptophan.

The creation of food legume varieties with a high content of better quality protein will not be an easy task, and will demand a close working relationship between breeders and chemists. Generally, however, research in this field has not proceeded beyond the screening stage, the determination of how much variability exists with respect to protein content and amino acids, and the study of genetic control of these characteristics.

The common bean (*Phaseolus vulgaris*) is an example. Screenings in Latin America gave percentages of seed protein that varied from 14.6% to 37.6%. In the United States, the variation observed was from 16% to 33%. Great variability was also found in amino acid content: 0.09% to 0.35% of methionine, and 0.10% to 0.36% of tryptophan. These and other data indicate the possibility of creating varieties of common bean with seeds having a nutritive value higher than at present. According to Hackler (7) of the New York State Agricultural Experiment Station in Geneva, it is possible to almost triple the methionine content in common beans by appropriate selection of varieties.

Undoubtedly, the nutritional improvement of food legumes by breeding deserves the full attention of agricultural researchers. However, at the present moment in most developing countries, this work should have second priority. The creation of varieties with high yielding capacity and resistance to parasites should still have first priority. Initially, it is necessary to obtain an abundance of food legumes, even if they have some imperfections in nutritive value.

References

1. Horsfall, J. G., Brandow, G. E., Brown, W. L., Day, P. R., Gabelman, W. H., Hanson, J. B., Holland, R. F., Hooker, A. L., Jennings, P. R., Johnson, V. A., Peters, D. C.,

Rhoades, M. M., Sprague, G. F., Stephens, S. G., Tammen, J., and Zaumeyer, W. J., 1972, *Genetic vulnerability of major crops,* National Academy of Sciences, Washington, D.C., p. 307.

2. Adams, M. W., 1973, Plant architecture and physiological efficiency in the field bean, *in: Potentials of field beans and other food legumes in Latin America,* International Center of Tropical Agriculture (CIAT), Cali, Colombia, pp. 266–278.
3. Hernandez-Bravo, G., 1973, Potentials and problems of production of dry beans in the lowland tropics, *in: Potentials of field beans and other food legumes in Latin America,* International Center of Tropical Agriculture (CIAT), Cali, Colombia, pp. 144–150.
4. Borlaug, N. E., 1973, Building a protein revolution on grain legumes, *in: Nutritional improvement of food legumes by breeding,* M. Milner (ed.), Protein Advisory Group of the United Nations System, United Nations, New York, pp. 7–11.
5. Roberts, L. M., 1970, *The food legumes: Recommendations for expansion and acceleration of research,* The Rockefeller Foundation, New York, p. 38.
6. Rachie, K. O., 1973, Research needed, *in: Nutritional improvement of food legumes by breeding,* M. Milner (ed.), Protein Advisory Group of the United Nations System, United Nations, New York, pp. 173–176.
7. Hackler, L. R., 1973, Nutritional qualities of dry beans and the potential for improvement, *in: Report of Bean Improvement Cooperative and National Dry Bean Research Association Conference,* Rochester, New York, pp. 67–69.

28

Improving the Production of Legumes and Oilseeds

Antonio M. Pinchinat

Centro Agronómico Tropical de Investigación y Enseñanza
Turrialba, Costa Rica

In working out strategies to improve the protein contribution of pulses to the human diet in the tropics, two phases can be identified. One is the stimulation of production and use through the application of existing technology, and the second would be the improvement of current technologies or the invention of new ones for continuously increasing the grain-yield capacity and protein quality of pulses. The first phase focuses on rapid, immediate impact. The second implies a longer term plan for sustained advances. Only the first phase will be considered here.

By and large, the major stimulus to production is increased profit. When farmers realize that they can make a real profit growing pulses, they grow pulses. Increased profit, of course, may mean increased prices of the product, making it harder for the low-income groups to satisfy their pulse requirements. To avert such consequences, national policies should facilitate consumer purchases while allowing a reasonable profit for the producer. The specific policies will depend on local circumstances. They may involve subsidies, reduction of costs of production inputs (especially agrochemicals and implements), governmental reserve buildups to stabilize prices, or similar measures. Also, essential services such as long-term, low-interest credits and facilities for transporting, storing, and marketing the product should be provided.

For example, the sharp decline in cropped areas (by about 40%) and production (by 30%) observed for the dry bean *Phaseolus vulgaris* in Costa Rica from 1963 to 1973 (1,2) reflected the unfavorable national policies that prevailed. El Salvador, on the other hand, almost doubled its dry bean production from 1967 to 1971 (3,4) in response to measures taken by the national government.

In the tropics, both the production and direct human consumption of certain pulses that hitherto have been used mainly for other purposes should be encouraged to lessen dietary protein shortages, especially in the marginal social groups. Soybean (*Glycine max*), now used mostly as an oil crop, is a prime example. Without any major technological change it could be consumed directly by humans. Soybeans have a higher grain content and greater yields than most other cultivated pulses, and are the cheapest. Before recent price increases, a kilogram of soybean protein cost, for example, less than one-third that of dry bean or one-thirtieth that of beef (5).

Pulse yields from farmers' fields in the tropics are exceedingly low (4), in some instances only one-eighth of those obtained experimentally from well-conducted field trials (6). The huge discrepancy between farm and experimental yields in the tropics can be ascribed to the limited application of existing knowledge by the small farmer. In El Salvador, for example, 95% of the area sown to dry beans is on farms measuring less than five hectares (7). At this level of operation, the economic capacity of the farmer to invest in new technology or to absorb losses from trying unfamiliar practices is low, and the risks are high and many. They range from continuous threats of insects, disease, and weeds to the difficulties in water management and handling of the harvested product, and heavy reliance on hand labor.

Socioeconomic constraints are responsible for most of the shortcomings in the agronomic practices of the small pulse producer. Among the common practices responsible for lower farm yields are poor quality seed (8), undersowing, inadequate land preparation, and failure to meet the nutrient needs of the crop and to give it proper maintenance, such as timely weed and insect control. Undersowing, for example, is practiced to reduce costs for seed and sowing time, or to facilitate mixed cropping, or both. Planting pulses in association with one or more other species ensures against total crop loss and allows for diversification of food crops. In Colombia, 85% of the dry bean production now comes from mixed cropping (7). Yields calculated from such a farming system, if not adjusted for actual harvested area, will appear lower than they really are.

Not all of the blame can be placed on the small pulse producer for not adopting modern agricultural technology. Traditional agricultural research in the tropics, in most instances, has assumed monoculture, unrestricted farm size, large amounts of working capital, massive use of agricultural inputs such as agricultural chemicals, and mechanization of farm operations. It has consciously or unconsciously advocated maximum yield at any cost. Obviously, these are not the conditions under which the small farmer operates, hence the limited impact of such research on pulse production in the tropics.

Fortunately, within this decade a few agricultural research centers have formally undertaken to study farming systems in and for the tropics. Pulses have been included as a major component of the cropping patterns and sequences for increased basic foods production. One such center, Tropical Agricultural Research and Training Center (CATIE), located in Turrialba, Costa Rica, directs its efforts primarily toward the Central American and Caribbean regions, adapting already established scientific knowledge to identify and develop appropriate farming systems for the small farmers of the area.

Yield potential has been shown to be high for many varieties or experimental lines of different pulse species. In a study of bean physiology, Malagamba (9) obtained yields as high as 112.25 grams of dry seed per plant. If it were possible to have field conditions similar to those of the experiment and 200,000 plants per hectare (10) for the erect type of dry bean variety that was grown, the expected farm yield would be more than 22 tons/ha. In another experiment García and Pinchinat (11), using commercial fertilizers and gravel in large (2.0 m × 1.8 m) asbestos-cement boxes in the greenhouse, obtained dry bean yields equivalent to over 6 tons/ha. Dry bean lines established in experimental field plots in Turrialba have yielded more than 4 tons/ha (12,13). It is noteworthy that high pulse yields have not been observed just in greenhouse or experimental field studies. A U.S.D.A. paper (14) officially reported yields greater than 4 tons/ha in dry beans and 7 tons/ha in soybeans, from U.S. commercial farms measuring more than two hectares. In the Dominican Republic, some commercial dry bean fields in monoculture have yielded 4 tons/ha or more.

It seems certain, therefore, that the application of present scientific knowledge can lead to manifold increases in pulse yields. Striving now for 5 to 8 tons/ha in some species, especially soybeans, may not be unrealistic. The immediate effort to increase the nutritional and economic importance of pulses in the tropics should concentrate on: (a) the establishment of national agricultural policies that stimulate farmers to produce, and (b) the diffusion and promotion of cropping practices based on existing scientific knowledge, but tailored to the circumstances of each class of farmer.

REFERENCES

1. Costa Rica, Ministerio de Economia y Hacienda, 1965, Censo agropecuario 1963, MEH. Dir. Gen. Estad. Censos.
2. Costa Rica, Ministerio de Economia, Industria y Comercio, 1974, Censos nacionales de 1973, Agropecuario, MEIC. Dir. Gen. Estad. Censos.
3. Food and Agriculture Organization of the United Nations, 1972, Production Yearbook 1971, Vol. 25, FAO, Rome.
4. Food and Agriculture Organization of the United Nations, 1973, Production Yearbook 1972, Vol. 26, FAO, Rome.

5. Litzenberger, S. C., 1973, The improvement of food legumes as a contribution to improved human nutrition, *in: Potentials of field beans and other legumes in Latin America,* Series Seminar 2E, Centro Int. Agr. Trop., Cali, Colombia, pp. 3–16.
6. Inter-American Institute of Agricultural Sciences of the OAS, 1971, Inter-American Tropical Pulses Program, IICA, Trop. Center Train. Res., Turrialba, Costa Rica, 8 pp.
7. Scobie, G. M., Infante, M. A., and Gutierrez, P. U., 1974, *Production and consumption of dry beans and their role in protein nutrition: A review,* Centro Int. Agr. Trop., AEP, Cali, Colombia, 53 pp.
8. Sanchez, F. R., and Pinchinat, A. M., 1974, Bean seed quality in Costa Rica, *Turrialba* **24:** 72–75.
9. Malagamba S., J. P., 1973, *Respuesta de compensación fisiológica del frijol* (Phaseolus vulgaris L.) *al desbalance de agua provocado por salinidad,* Tesis Mag. Sci. Turrialba, Costa Rica, IICA, Centro Trop. Enseñ. Invest., 95 pp.
10. Pinchinat, A. M., 1975, Rendimiento del frijol común (*Phaseolus vulgaris L.*) según la densidad y distribución espacial de siembra, *Turrialba* **24:** 173–175.
11. García B., J., y Pinchinat, A. M., 1973, Producción de frijol (*Phaseolus vulgaris* L.) bajo techo en solución nutritiva comercial, *Agron. Trop. (Venez.)* **23:** 419–422.
12. Instituto Interamericano de Ciencias Agrícolas, 1969–1970, Informe de labores, IICA. Centro Enseñ. Invest. Turrialba, Costa Rica, s.f. 122 pp.
13. Pinchinat, A. M., 1970–1971, Cultivos Alimenticios. Informe técnico anual, Centro Trop. Enseñ. Invest. IICA, Turrialba, Costa Rica, s.f. (mimeo), 13 pp.
14. U.S. Department of Agriculture, 1970, Agronomic potential of U.S. food crops for production of calories and protein, USDA/AID FEDS Staff Paper 2, 27 pp.

COMMENT

Robert F. Chandler, Jr. • *The Asian Vegetable Research and Development Center, Shanhua, Taiwan.*

Can the yield potential of the food legumes be increased to the same degree as has been achieved for wheat and rice? It is unlikely that the true yield potential will be doubled as it has been for certain of the cereal grains. However, we fully expect that the average yield on farmers' fields can be doubled or tripled, as barriers to yield are removed through plant breeding and crop management research.

For example, the yield of soybeans in Indonesia is no more than 700 kg per hectare, and often less. Under ideal conditions soybean yields on experimental fields in Asia have already exceeded 4000 kg/ha. We can plan on creating soybean varieties that, under farm conditions, should yield over 2 metric tons per hectare.

The mung bean is grown all over South and Southeast Asia, and yields on farms range between 400 and 1000 kg/ha, depending on management practices. It is expected that by breeding varieties with improved plant type, resistant to insect and disease attack, good farmers can expect yields of 1.5 to 2.0 metric tons within the next decade.

The pigeon pea varieties now available vary greatly in plant type and maturation time. Through selection and breeding the yield potential of this crop could well be doubled. However, most of the food legume crops do not exhibit that much variation in plant type, and increases in yield potential will depend largely on obtaining, through plant breeding, varieties that are resistant to insect and disease attack.

29

The Potential Impact of Research on Vegetable Production

Robert F. Chandler, Jr.

The Asian Vegetable Research and Development Center
Shanhua, Taiwan

The vegetable crops constitute man's richest source of vitamins, minerals, and plant proteins. They are, however, insufficiently utilized. As a consequence, hundreds of millions of people in the less developed countries show evidence of dietary deficiencies—particularly, they lack adequate protein and certain vitamins in their food. Some vegetable crops are, in addition, excellent sources of cash income for the small farmer.

Because of the lack of appropriate varieties for the tropics and subtropics, and poor cultivating practices, yields of such crops have generally been too low to provide farmers with the incentive to grow them. In this chapter, the Asian Vegetable Research and Development Center (AVRDC) will be used to illustrate how one international center selected its crops, developed its research program, and progressed over a two-year period in breaking down the barriers to increased crop yield.

IDENTIFYING THE PROBLEMS

Authorities classify more than 100 crops as vegetables. Most of them play only a minor role in feeding the world's low-income population. Therefore, if an international agricultural research organization is to benefit the small farmer and the urban poor, it must select crops for study that are important food items and that have severe production constraints to be overcome. Furthermore, consideration of such barriers to yield should be limited to those that, beyond reasonable doubt, can be reduced through good, intensive scientific research. Another essential in establishing a research program is that attention be restricted to only a few crops; otherwise it is unlikely that there will be a significant impact on any one crop.

Any national or regional vegetable crop research program should determine the research priorities for the particular area it serves. In August, 1968, a proposal for the establishment of AVRDC was sent to the appropriate government authorities of the Republic of China (Taiwan). Included in this report was a summary of the recommendations of the International Provisional Planning Committee that had made a survey of the vegetable industry in the less developed countries of Asia. The Committee listed 26 vegetable crops as being of high priority, but did not attempt to rate them according to individual importance. It did classify the 26 crops into those of high nutritional value, those that had good shipping and keeping qualities, and those of high economic value.

The list, from the standpoint of a crop selection guide for a vegetable research program, could be criticized first because it contained too many different kinds of crops, and second because the separation of vegetable crops into different categories was apparently made under the assumption that each crop fitted into only one category. This, of course, is not true. A crop can have, for example, both high economic and high nutritional value.

After AVRDC was organized and its director selected in 1971, a proposal was drawn up to present to the Technical Advisory Committee (TAC) of the Consultative Group on International Agricultural Research (CGIAR) at its meeting in February, 1972. The proposal mentioned 18 crops to receive major or minor attention. These were: Chinese cabbage (both heading and nonheading types), common cabbage, mung beans, tomatoes, eggplant, edible podded peas, okra, sweet corn, sweet potatoes, radishes, onions, and garlic. In addition, cooperative work with other centers was indicated for cowpeas, cassava, pigeon peas, chickpeas, and white potatoes.

The TAC review of the proposal suggested that the Center was trying to cover too many crops. In a second proposal prepared in August, 1972, the number of crops was reduced to 12. They included mung beans, tomatoes, eggplants, sweet potatoes, onions, Chinese radish, two types of Chinese cabbage, common cabbage, water convolvulus, sweet corn, and melons (mentioned in the report as "some of the cucurbits").

As staff were assembled and research organized, it became evident that too many crops were still included in the program.

At a meeting of the scientific and administrative staff in March, 1973, the above list was reduced to 5, but added one new crop, the soybean, to give a total of 6 crops for major consideration. The final list included the mung bean, *Vigna radiata* (syn. with *Phaseolus aureus*); the soybean, *Glycine max;* the tomato, *Lycopersicon esculentum;* the sweet potato, *Ipomoea batatas;* the white potato, *Solanum tuberosum;* and the Chinese cabbage, *Brassica pekinensis.* The purpose of this detail is to show how one crop research program sharpened its focus from an original total of 26 vegetable crops to only 6, as it advanced from an early planning stage to an actual research operation.

To be included, a crop had to have value both economically and nutritionally. Furthermore, it had to be among the crops suffering from serious constraints to high yield in the tropics and subtropics. As an example of the latter qualification, we eliminated water convolvulus (*Ipomoea aquatica*) and eggplant (*Solanum melongena*) from our original program, not because those crops were unimportant, but because varieties were already available that grow quite satisfactorily in hot, humid climates.

AVRDC selected the six crops for the following reasons:

The mung bean is an ancient and well-known leguminous crop in Asia. It is an excellent source of protein and is eaten in many forms, including bean sprouts, green beans, boiled dry beans, and noodles. In addition, in the Philippines it is widely used in soups. The mung bean has never received the level of research attention directed to most other important food crops. Yet, through a concerted large-scale research program, its yield potential, now only about 1.5 metric tons per hectare under farm conditions, might well be doubled. This would be achieved by breeding varieties that not only make more efficient use of solar energy and soil nutrients, but are more resistant to insect and disease attack.

The soybean is a major world crop, particularly in the United States, Brazil, and China. However, varieties suitable for the Asian tropics have never been developed. Those Asian countries (such as Japan and Taiwan) sufficiently affluent to support a large domestic animal population import huge quantities of soybeans for feed. Given varieties better adapted to tropical conditions, the soybean could well become an important export crop for the less developed countries of the tropics and subtropics, and a high-protein crop for local human consumption as well.

Many of the present varieties of soybeans are unsuitable for the tropics because of sensitivity to short days and high temperatures. It is AVRDC's objective to collect samples of the world's soybean germ plasm and develop improved varieties that have not only tolerance to humid tropical climates, but, also, greater resistance to diseases and insects.

The tomato is a popular crop almost everywhere. It is an excellent source of vitamins A and C and, in Asia, is an important cash crop for small farmers. Unfortunately, in the tropics it is beset by many handicaps, principally disease susceptibility and poor fruit set in hot weather. These problems are so severe that in the lowland tropics almost no tomatoes are grown during the rainy season. AVRDC has started the first really massive approach to tomato breeding ever to be conducted in the true tropics. We expect a major breakthrough in developing high-yielding varieties for hot climates.

The sweet potato, in our opinion, is an underrated food crop for the tropics and subtropics. More people can be fed from a hectare of sweet potatoes than from a hectare of rice. In addition to vitamin A, the crop is a better mineral source than rice, and the tops can be eaten as a source of protein, vitamins, and minerals. AVRDC has initiated a sweet potato improvement program with the objective of doubling the protein content and significantly increasing the vitamin A content of the roots of the varieties now commonly grown. While we are working toward these primary goals, efforts naturally will be made to develop, in the same varieties, early maturity, higher yields, and insect and disease resistance.

Although the white potato is a staple food crop in many parts of the world, it does not flourish at low elevations in the tropics. AVRDC, in cooperation with the International Potato Center in Peru, will make a major research effort to develop a white potato that will form tubers under tropical conditions, particularly during the hot, rainy months.

The heading type of Chinese cabbage is another extremely popular crop that has seasonal difficulties in Asia. Although well adapted to higher altitudes and cooler seasons in the tropics, in hot weather it does not form heads and is readily attacked by several serious diseases. AVRDC plant breeders hope to create, as has already been done for the common cabbage, new heat-tolerant, disease-resistant varieties of the Chinese cabbage. Also, the entomologist will attempt to develop improved and inexpensive methods of insect control.

In addition to weighing these specific reasons for selecting each crop, we naturally paid considerable attention to the crops undergoing research at the other international research centers around the world. None is giving major attention to mung beans, soybeans, tomatoes, or Chinese cabbage; our program will help round out the list of important crops that are being studied intensively, as only the international centers are equipped to do.

Although the International Institute of Tropical Agriculture (IITA) in Nigeria has a sizable sweet potato research program, that crop does not begin to have the importance in Africa that it does in Asia. Furthermore, in placing special emphasis on augmenting the nutritional value of the sweet potato, AVRDC aims to enrich a crop that is bound to play an increasingly important role in feeding the future populations of the tropics.

The white potato is being studied exhaustively by the International Potato Center in Peru because potatoes originated in this area. The program at AVRDC is almost entirely dependent on the Center in Peru for its germ plasm and has as its primary objective to determine, in the next few years, whether or not the development of a white potato for the lowland tropics is within the realm of possibility.

Another important consideration in selecting four of the six crops is their keeping and shipping qualities. The mung bean and soybean, with relatively inexpensive facilities, can be dried and stored for long periods. Hence, they are excellent crops for small farmers who live at some distance from the market. The white potato can also be transported and stored with relative ease. Although the sweet potato is difficult to store for long periods, it can be shipped to urban markets without difficulty.

The tomato-processing industry is developing rapidly in tropical Asia, particularly in Taiwan, Thailand, and the Philippines. Thus, it can add greatly to the cash income of farmers living near a canning factory.

PROGRESS IN RESEARCH AT AVRDC

For the sake of brevity, this discussion will be confined to a few significant advances that have been made with each of the six crops. AVRDC's annual reports contain more detail.

One of the constraints to the growing of mung beans by farmers is the low yield levels they usually obtain. Most farmers of Southeast Asia get mung bean yields of no more than 700 or 800 kg/ha. Even on experimental fields and among the best farmers, yields seldom exceed 1500 kg/ha and are usually lower, between 1100 and 1300 kg/ha. One of AVRDC's objectives is to increase the yield potential of the mung bean to at least 3 metric tons per hectare. In Table I, the yields are presented for the top five varieties in a yield trial conducted by the plant-breeding department. We were able to exceed 2 metric tons per hectare, which is twice the yield that many good Taiwanese farmers are getting, and three times the yield on most of the farms in other tropical Asian countries. Our plant physiologists are studying the relationships between yield components and population density in an effort to understand more fully the factors determining the yield potential of the mung bean.

Table I. Performance of the 5 Highest Yielding Mung Bean Varieties on AVRDC's Experimental Fields[a] (1974)

Variety	Yield[b] kg/ha
Tainan No. 1	2392
CES 140	2026
CES 55	1985
CES 87-17	1909
MG 50-10 A (G)	1817

[a]Planting density: 250,000 per hectare.
[b]Average of a spring planting (Mar. 1) and a summer planting (July 11). All plots were replicated 4 times.

Some average data obtained in two different growing seasons on AVRDC's experimental farm are shown in Table II. The number of pods per plant and the bean yield per plant decrease as the plant density increases. However, the number of seeds per pod and the 100-seed weight are not affected by planting density. The yield continued to increase up to a density of 400,000 plants per hectare. The yields were about the same in these experiments as in those conducted by the plant breeding department (Table I) for the same density (250,000 plants per hectare). Data from an experiment not reported here indicated that no further increase in yield could be expected by increasing the planting density to 500,000 plants per hectare.

The most serious disease of the mung bean in Southeast Asia and on Taiwan is the *Cercospora* leaf spot disease. Although there are several species of the genus *Cercospora* that attack the mung bean, the most important one in Asia is *Cercospora canescens.* The plant pathology department at AVRDC, in cooperation with the plant breeders, has screened the world collection (over 2000 accessions) for resistance to the *Cercospora* leaf spot disease. The resistant variety (ML 6) yielded 1240 kg/ha while the susceptible one (MG-59-6) produced only 625 kg/ha. Only resistant varieties are being used as parents in the crossing program. Undoubtedly, varieties will soon be developed that have *Cercospora* leaf spot resistance and high yield capacity.

The Soybean. As with the mung bean, AVRDC is attempting to identify varieties and management practices that will support high yields in the tropics and subtropics. Our soil scientist, studying the effect of fertilizers and compost on yield, has found that under the soil and climatic conditions prevailing in Shanhua, Taiwan (23 degrees and 7 mins. North latitude) there is a decided response to nitrogen (Table III). The crop was planted on July 4, 1974 and was harvested on September 24. All plots received a basal application of 80 kg/ha of

Table II. Yield Components, Population Densities, and Yield Data for Mung Beans[a]

	Population density (Number of plants per hectare)			
Yield component items	100,000	200,000	300,000	400,000
Pods per plant (no.)	22.90	17.60	14.65	13.25
Seeds per pod (no.)	12.35	11.55	12.25	11.95
Bean yield (gm/plant)	10.40	9.30	7.60	6.85
100 seed weight (gm)	4.86	4.71	4.77	4.73
Bean yield (kg/ha)	1040	1889	2265	2731

[a]The variety was Tainan No. 1. The data are averages for two crops—one planted September 20, 1973, and the other planted March 12, 1974.

Table III. The Effect of Nitrogen and Compost on the Pod Number and Yield of the Shi-Shi Variety of Soybeans

Nitrogen fertilizer applied (kg/ha)	Pod number per plant		Yield (kg/ha)	
	No compost	With compost	No compost	With compost
None	46.2	56.0	1750	2070
30, as basal application	58.9	87.4	2210	2760
30, as basal, plus 30 kg 28 days after planting	49.5	78.6	1780	3090
30 basal, plus 30 kg more at 28 and 40 days after planting (flowering stage)	58.3	94.8	2220	3480

P_2O_5 and 150 kg/ha of K_2O. When compost was applied it was at the rate of 20 metric tons per hectare. The nitrogen was applied in the form of ammonium sulfate. The final plant population was 150,000 per hectare, which other studies have shown is too low for maximum yield. However, the top yield of 3480 kg/ha is excellent for a summer crop in the tropics. The average yield of soybeans in Illinois, for example, is a little over 2 metric tons per hectare. However, in yield contests among farmers in that state, the highest yields reached 6 metric tons per hectare.

Table III reveals that there was a sizable response to the basal application of nitrogen. Furthermore, the 30 kg applied at flowering time gave an extra boost to both pod number and total seed yield. Our soil scientists and crop management specialists will continue to explore the reasons for the decided response to nitrogen. It is well established that in the United States soybeans do not respond to the addition of nitrogen except on some acid, rather infertile soils, where nodulation is poor.

Compost seems to increase yields of all crops on AVRDC's experimental farm. The soil varies from a sandy loam to a loam. It contains considerable silt and the clays are the nonexpanding type. Therefore the soil has poor structure and tends to become compact after heavy rains during the monsoon season. The benefit of the compost may be mostly due to the improvement in soil structure and aeration that result from its use.

Another effort in the AVRDC soybean improvement program is to develop varieties that are insensitive to photoperiod. In 1974, the soybean breeders, in cooperation with the plant physiologists, tested 1987 accessions for sensitivity to day length. Out of this number, 212 flowered within five days of each other when grown under 16- or 12-hour light periods. Twenty of the 212 showed no difference in flowering time under the two photoperiods and thus can be considered to be completely day-neutral. This means that there is every possibility that we can develop nonphotosensitive tropical varieties with wide geographic adaptability. Although nonsensitive varieties exist in temperate regions, they often flower too early when grown in the tropics. Apparently this is a heat response. AVRDC is developing varieties that not only are day-neutral, but that also do not flower until about 35 days after planting.

The Tomato. This crop is beset by many problems in the tropics. The most serious are a lack of tolerance to high night temperatures and susceptibility to the bacterial wilt disease, *Pseudomonas solanacearum.*

In 1973 and 1974, AVRDC tomato breeders tested 3799 accessions from the world collection for tolerance to high night temperatures. In Shanhua, Taiwan, night temperatures during the months of May through October are consistently above 22°C. As is evident in Table IV, most varieties of tomatoes do not set fruit when temperatures remain high at night. This is a serious limiting factor to tomato production through the lowland tropics. Several of the 31 varieties that did set fruit have been used as parents in the breeding program to introduce this essential quality into otherwise superior varieties (particularly disease-resistant ones).

The pathologists and tomato breeders are cooperating in identifying bacterial wilt-resistant tomato varieties that can be used in the breeding program. Excellent progress is being made. The contrast between resistant and susceptible lines is shown in Figure 1. The world's most resistant varieties and genetic lines have been collected from other programs. Three separate programs to develop bacterial wilt-resistant varieties used entirely different sources of resistance. AVRDC has all three sets of varieties from these programs and is now crossing them. Already segregating populations have resulted, with 62% of the plants showing high resistance after being inoculated with the bacteria that cause the wilt disease. Early trials in Thailand indicate that the level of resistance developed is the highest yet known in the lowland tropics. We are confident that in a

Table IV. Fruit Setting of 3799 Tomato Varieties during the Summer Months on AVRDC's Experimental Farm

Degree of fruit setting	Number of accessions	Number in each category (% of total)
Nil to light	3058	80.5
Light to medium	548	14.4
Medium	162	4.3
Medium to heavy	31	0.8
Total	3799	100.0

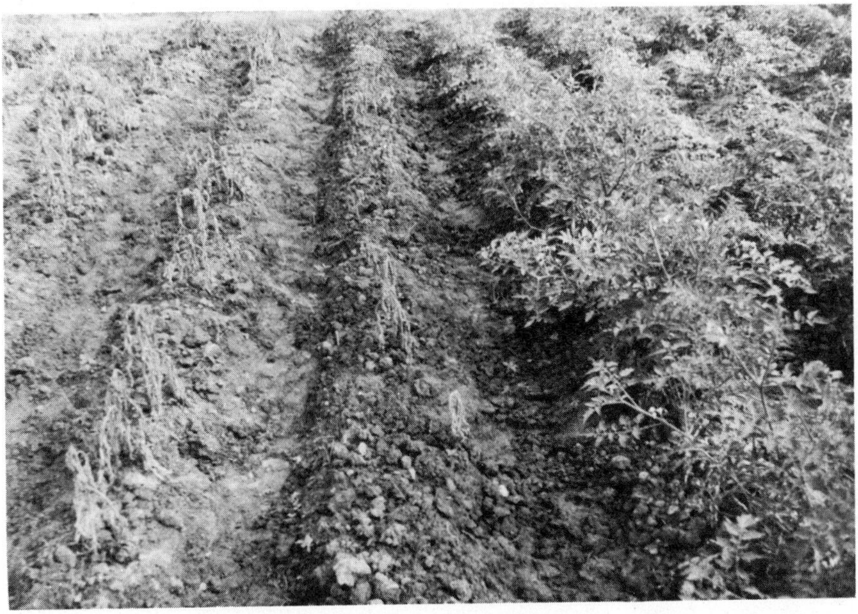

FIG. 1. Breeding for resistance to bacterial wilt in the tomato. The genetic lines on the right are resistant, while those on the left are highly susceptible.

few years AVRDC will have produced varieties that can be grown the year round in the tropics—an advantage that does not exist today.

The Sweet Potato. One of the major thrusts of AVRDC's sweet potato improvement program is to develop varieties with double the protein content, and with a much higher concentration of vitamin A than is contained in the average variety available today. Significant progress is being made. One sweet potato plant selected from among the progeny of our breeding program produced 3.5 kg of roots in 140 days. Extrapolating that per-plant yield to the yield for one hectare would be over 100 metric tons.

From their preliminary investigations, AVRDC scientists are confident that they can produce an array of sweet potato varieties that will yield 40 to 50 tons per hectare in 90 days, have a β-carotene content of at least 17 mg per 100 gm of fresh weight, and contain no less than 8% protein on a dry-weight basis.

The White Potato. AVRDC has one immediate objective of its white potato improvement program: to identify genetic lines and develop varieties that will form tubers and yield well under tropical conditions. Today, no commercial varieties exist that can be grown during summer in the lowland tropics. The International Potato Center in Peru is sending us large numbers of seeds from their segregating populations. We are testing them during the summer months in Taiwan, and the more promising ones will be tried throughout the Asian tropics. The program is new, and we do not yet know how successful it will be.

The Chinese Cabbage. Two of our research activities with the Chinese cabbage–developing varieties with resistance to bacterial soft rot and breeding for sizable heads during the summer months in the tropics and subtropics–have progressed well. As they did with the other crops, AVRDC scientists collected germ plasm from many sources and screened the accessions for resistance to diseases and for heat tolerance. They found that the best summer-heading varieties came from Taiwan, while the Korean varieties tended to have greater disease resistance. Figure 2 is a photograph of a Taiwanese parent and of the progeny of a cross between it and a Korean variety. Note how the head size and shape have been improved through breeding.

Superior heads occur infrequently in the segregating populations. Out of 2000 or so, no more than four or five plants produce heads such as the one in the photograph. However, now that we have proved this to be possible, we have high hopes of developing a Chinese cabbage for tropical summer production, which will add greatly to price stabilization and farmer income.

Bacterial soft rot resistance has been identified in the world collection, and

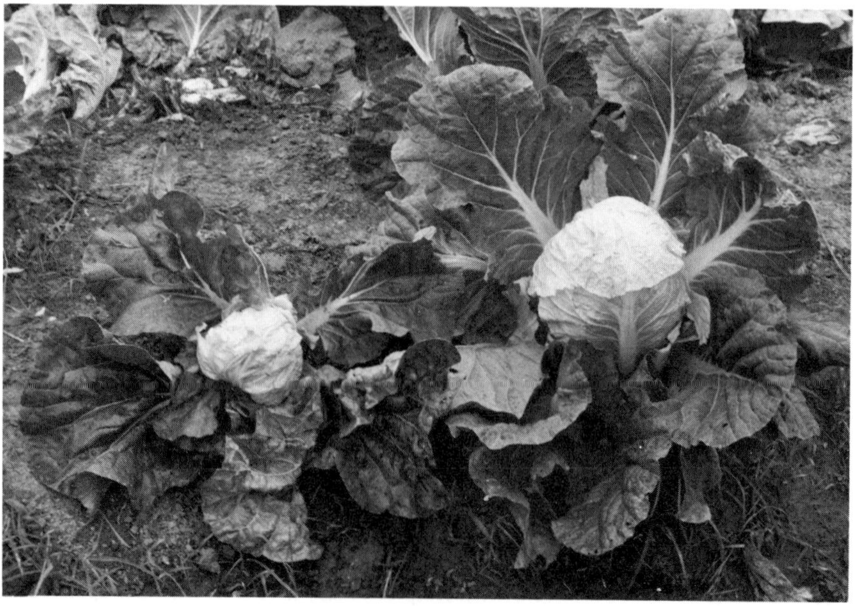

FIG. 2. Breeding Chinese cabbage for the ability to form heads in hot climates. The one on the left is the poor-heading parent; the one on the right is the improved progeny.

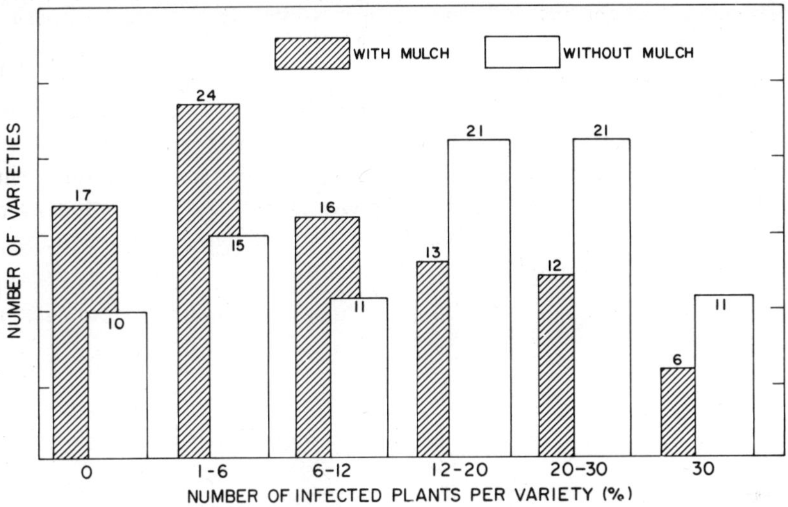

FIG. 3. The distribution of varietal resistance to the bacterial soft rot disease of Chinese cabbage in AVRDC's screening program.

the selections are being used in the crossing program. This is the most serious disease of the Chinese cabbage, and it appears that soon we can combine resistance to bacterial soft rot with heat tolerance. Figure 3 shows the distribution of the varieties in AVRDC's collection that resist disease. Note that about 17 of the accessions showed no infection and about 24% of them showed less than 7% infection. Also, in the more disease-resistant varieties, mulching with rice straw reduced the degree of infection.

CONCLUSIONS

I believe that the success of the programs of the network of international agricultural research centers is dependent, to a large degree, on the massiveness of the approach to problem-solving. An examination of their crop-improvement programs reveals that in every case an attempt has been made to assemble samples of the world's germ plasm to provide a broad genetic base for the breeding program. Furthermore, in each instance, the assembled collection has then been screened carefully for varieties that have such desirable characteristics as disease and insect resistance, plant type, and tolerance to the various climatic factors that limit yield.

After the selection of such superior varieties from the world collections, a sizable crossing program invariably has ensued. The segregating populations from these crosses have then been tested over wide areas, and the outstanding selections used where they have proved their worth. Certainly this approach is a valid one, whatever the crop being studied. Rice, sweet potatoes, and cowpeas, for example, can be improved equally well by this method of approach.

Obviously, there is no simple solution to the world's food problem. However, the massive attack on yield-limiting factors is a vital ingredient. If we can clearly identify the barriers to increased crop production and focus our research programs on them, omitting the often interesting but less important investigations, we can make increasingly significant contributions toward reducing the level of human misery in this overcrowded world.

30

Poultry and Swine Production in Latin America—Prospects for Expansion

John A. Pino

Director for Agricultural Sciences
The Rockefeller Foundation
New York, New York

National food policies will more and more be affected by factors external to the nation as the total world-food-population problem becomes influenced by a greater number of variables. How, then, do nations cope with the problem of getting an adequate quantity and quality of food products consumed by people? While political leaders must deal with national policies and strategies, agricultural experts must bring policies down to the level of the ordinary citizen. They must make things happen, often in the face of inadequate political directives and faulty administrative structures.

Unfortunately, many governments lack adequate data on which to base the formulation of sound developmental policy for poultry and livestock products, or for all agricultural development. In most cases, the result is that an enormous potential for improving people's diets, adding jobs and income, and making better use of natural resources is left unrealized. It is generally recognized by nutrition authorities that people, like certain other monogastric animals, do not *require* animal products in their diet to assure adequate nutrition. It is true, however, that the consumption of animal products—milk, meat, eggs, or fish—makes it more likely that necessary amino acid intake will be achieved, and better nutrition will result. It is also true that the consumption of animal products by people tends to rise when availability and purchasing power permit—because people *like* to eat meat. Neither of these facts means that eating animal products is indispensable.

The rationale, therefore, for promoting and accelerating expanded livestock production should be based upon the following two principles:

1. All economic strata of a society require adequate food supplies; however, those at the lower end of the economic scale are generally the ones who suffer most from qualitatively and quantitatively inadequate nutrition. Therefore, policies and efforts biased toward improving the nutrition of the economically disadvantaged are to be encouraged. In Latin America as a whole, per caput availability of pork was 2.9 kg in 1970; that of poultry was 7.8 kg. The total per caput consumption of all meat was 32.5 kg. This is equivalent to 10 grams per day (on the average) of meat products–not protein–a figure that is far too low by any standard.

Net numbers of animals have increased in all of the Latin American countries over the past decade, but per caput consumption has not risen markedly. The former parallels population growth, but lack of domestic purchasing power restrains the latter. In at least one country where swine production is only now beginning to utilize modern methods, and production and consumption is low nationally, one-third of the slaughtered animals are exported. Such an anomaly is common among developing countries and bound to continue.

2. It is incumbent upon nations to utilize their natural resources effectively and efficiently. Poultry and swine fill a niche in the agricultural complex and can convert many otherwise wasted materials into high-value food. Perhaps in no other place can this fact be more readily appreciated than in parts of Asia.

In spite of some recent clamor to discourage animal production, it should be noted that livestock has always represented for the farmer a kind of savings bank for storage of food, energy, and capital; on the national scale it serves as a buffer against high prices and inflation in times of shortage. Animals can be kept or killed, fed grain when it is cheap, and when it is not, fed something less than good feed. Because of their short reproductive cycle, lower level of investment, and more rapid turnover, smaller animals like swine and poultry are more responsive to market fluctuations than cattle or sheep. This flexibility is both an advantage and a hindrance to development of stable, productive pig and poultry enterprises in low-income countries.

The leap from subsistence livestock-raising to commercial production is wide. Labor and capital costs for the subsistence farmer are close to zero; his poultry and pigs eat refuse from the table, agricultural wastes, and whatever grain they can forage after he harvests his fields. His animals represent almost net profit when he sells or barters them–although generally they cannot compete in quality with the products of commercial farms. If he wants to become a modern poultryman or swine producer, he has to invest a fair amount of capital for equipment; he must buy quality feeds in large amounts, pharmaceutical products, and other costly inputs. He has to make deliveries, collect payments, and meet his loan or other financial obligations. The managerial skills required are not those he used for a small-scale operation in the backyard. Unless he has some expert guidance, he is likely to fail. The risks taken by the businessman are a function of his cost-benefit calculations, whether these are intuitive or made by computer. Beyond a certain level of complexity, the shrewd common sense of the most experienced farmer is likely to fail.

The result of most developmental experience in this field has been that only sophisticated operations, with a high level of capitalization, have been able to take the risks and weather the losses of commercial pig and poultry raising in Latin America. The small farmer and middle-level commercial raiser have been absorbed into larger operations that can balance a high level of investment and risk with highly efficient management and rapid turnover. If small or middle-sized operations are to survive, there must be either a governmental support mechanism to see them through periods of market fluctuation and prolonged slumps, or a sufficiently high price paid by the consumer, or both, in order to balance the cost of inputs and justify the farmer's risk.

A backyard flock of a few dozen chickens cannot be upgraded to the level of a commercial operation without cash investment above the subsistence farmer's means, which, under the rural conditions prevailing in much of Latin America, would be impractical. Raising a backyard flock improves the subsistence family's income and nutritional status, and at that level should be encouraged if resources permit, but superior poultry breeds and modern inputs are essentially wasted on a typical backyard flock. Swine-raising at the backyard level is not subject to quite as many hazards as poultry-raising, but as a general rule costly technology only pays off at higher levels of management than are usually possible on the subsistence farm. However, there is a wide gamut of operations for both species, ranging from small to medium, which can be substantially improved and can contribute to raising economic and social conditions in rural communities.

TECHNOLOGICAL CONSIDERATIONS

Technologies for poultry and swine are among the most advanced for the livestock categories; both have been the object of intensive research, and both lend themselves to improved techniques and high-level management. Furthermore, the technology is largely transferable to almost any part of the world. In the countries of Latin America, on the one extreme, one can find isolated examples of modern management methods in use for both swine and poultry; disease control services are available, and even feed formulas have been worked out reasonably well, based on locally available materials. However, there are enormous gaps between the occasional efficient, well-managed operation that can take advantage of advanced technology and the many ill-run operations. Theoretically, production technology can be applied on a large or small scale, but in practice it has not been geared for use by the small farmer. Production increases have been concentrated on commercial farms that have had access to governmental aid, credit, tax rebates on imported feeds, and other benefits.

Nevertheless, small-stock raising in most countries of Latin America remains predominantly a subsistence-level operation. As such, it is low in productivity, limited by the use of inferior types of animals, and subject to losses from diseases and parasites as well as from the effects of substandard housing, poor sanitation, and inefficient management. Production on small farms is also often wasteful of resources–feeding corn to swine or poultry without supplements, or using range for cattle without mineral supplements are examples of uneconomical uses of these inputs. In a sense, the farmers have subsidized the cost of producing livestock by assuming a zero or low cost of inputs. A realistic value placed on these inputs, however, would show that, in actuality, the cost of production is quite high. Thus we can expect that shifts toward alternative uses, changing market opportunities, taxation, or whatever places a value on the previously "free" resource, will cause the small or inefficient farmer to abandon those activities that do not return a profit in a real sense.

What are we to conclude from these observations? Two things: (1) that the livestock industries in Latin America are caught in the web of worldwide problems of population growth, market competition for grains and protein sources, food and energy shortages, domestic inflation and unemployment, the foreign currency squeeze, and a number of related pressures that are not the monopoly of any single country or region of the world; and (2) that the barriers to productive swine and poultry industries are not primarily technological (although technical improvements are still necessary); they are institutional, socioeconomic, and political.

INSTITUTIONAL CONSIDERATIONS

While many of the countries of Latin America have made important progress in development of their institutional base for agricultural research and education, most countries lack adequate mechanisms to provide technical services to farmers. Small farmers especially are largely unaware that such information exists or is applicable to their farms; it is the job of communications specialists, extension networks, farmer organizations, and similar agencies in cooperation with research stations to inform them. Because most countries lack the experienced manpower to carry out these tasks, one of the first priorities should be to train people in the necessary techniques, provide them with incentives, and coordinate their work within each region in cooperation with local producers of feeds, credit-granting agencies, suppliers of equipment, and similar enterprises.

The cost of maintaining a competent and adequate technical service structure is considerable. Very few nations, for example, have a network of diagnostic laboratories within reach of producers. Again, the cost of production is borne by the farmer, who accepts disease losses as a matter of course, because he has no alternative. However, the dilemma is how to structure the technical service in such a way that it is economical and sensible. Obviously, a veterinarian cannot make "house calls" to look at every backyard pig or flock of poultry; community services, however, can be provided. From the outpost diagnostic laboratory where preliminary, presumptive tests are conducted, specimens and materials for closer, more intensive study should be sent to a central laboratory that has the capability of making definitive diagnoses. Such referral capability is nonexistent in many places, although, fortunately, it has reached an excellent level in others.

In Africa, the veterinary and husbandry officers have auxiliary personnel called "scouts." These are subprofessional people residing in the villages who act as the district veterinary officer's eyes, ears, hands, and legs. They report on troublesome diseases, vaccinate animals, encourage marketing, and provide similar services where veterinary or husbandry officers seldom go.

Mechanisms are needed for identifying the problems and potentials of introducing swine and poultry operations in the various regions, in coordination with planning for expansion of other sectors, such as the production of feedstuffs, development of markets and distribution mechanisms, and similar requisites.

Every country needs to strengthen institutional structures to narrow the gap between technological developments in the research centers and model farms and their application on small and large farms throughout the country. The new emphasis being placed by educators on training for intermediate-level production specialists, the progress being made toward introduction of interdisciplinary training for agriculturalists–technologists as well as planners and administrators–is part of the effort toward strengthening and coordinating the national institutional network that undergirds agricultural development.

Strong national institutions are the indispensable base; these can then form strong links with regional and international organizations doing research and offering planning assistance and promoting exchange of scientific information on swine and poultry production. In view of the high cost of maintaining these institutions and the technical capability they represent, there needs to be a division of labor based upon mutually reinforcing interaction. Thus, the universities, the technical schools, the ministries of agriculture, and the local governments should be interlaced so that each function is carefully carried out. Weak links should be strengthened by mutual consent and understanding rather than divisive professional, political, or institutional policies.

ECONOMIC CONSIDERATIONS

The development of the livestock sector, and of swine and poultry in particular, is closely interwoven with overall economic development in each country. The demand for meat is a particularly sensitive indicator of economic development. In several countries of Latin America, where beef is raised primarily for export, and where purchasing power and domestic demand are low, encouragement of small-stock raising can help meet the local demand for meat, contribute to protein needs, and prevent such unpopular measures as export quotas for beef.

Peru's Ministry of Agriculture reports that the government is encouraging substitution of poultry, swine, and other meat products for beef. Targets for 1980 include raising consumption of poultry meat from 26 to 38% of all meat consumed and reducing beef from 27 to 16% (E. P. Enrique Valdez Angulo, Minister of Agriculture, Peru, personal communication, 1974). However, such encouragement needs careful scrutiny in terms of its total economic impact; market saturation can depress prices and put the small entrepreneur out of business. Mexico, Venezuela, and Chile have all experienced the effects of saturating the market for poultry by overproduction on an industrial scale, without sufficient planning. On the other hand, Argentina, traditionally a beef-eating and beef-exporting country, reports that poultry is gaining favor with consumers on its own merits; the trend is attributed to the desire for more varied diets as well as to the improved quality of poultry meat and to better processing and marketing procedures (Horacio Giberti, Secretary of the State of Agriculture and Livestock, Argentina, personal communication, 1974).

Dr. Pedro Solana, Director General for Livestock in the Mexican Department of Agriculture, sums up a situation that is common throughout Latin America: "Poultry raising is the only livestock industry that has achieved sufficient development to meet national demand, the chief limiting factor being the low level of consumption due to the people's lack of purchasing power. Compared with the development of production, systems for processing, distribution and commercialization have remained in a deplorable state of stagnation" (personal communication, 1975). To a large extent, the same can be said for swine.

Perhaps no other factor will so strongly influence the nature and size of the agricultural enterprise as basic economic considerations. Nevertheless, economic relationships do change, and what is not feasible in one set of circumstances can become workable under different conditions. The cost and availability of services, production inputs, labor, land, and the cost of marketing the product are all important factors. Furthermore, it is all too common that prices paid to farmers are determined by their limited access to markets. Market news reporting will encourage the flow of products to consumers. Soundly based economic technology is no less important than production technology.

POLITICAL CONSIDERATIONS

Finally, there are political barriers to improvement of agricultural development, including swine and poultry development. Specifically, in the case of the swine and poultry industries, little attention has been given to encouragement of small and medium-sized enterprises through appropriate policy interventions.

A study (1) prepared by the Ministry of Agriculture and Livestock and the Ministry of Economic Affairs of El Salvador reports that commercial production of eggs and poultry is concentrated in a small number of operations, whose production determines consumer price levels. The proportion of family poultry farms has been markedly reduced. Expansion of commercial farms has made it possible for these producers to dominate the market and benefit from economies of scale in such areas as imports and credit. Feed-concentrate manufacturing in the country has expanded in similar fashion—600% in 11 years—but two companies alone supply 78% of the domestic market.

Recommendations to encourage small and medium-sized commercial operations include: integration of small enterprises into economically efficient associations, which would permit them to compete with the large enterprises that dominate the market; drafting of a law for regulating the poultry industry to protect and organize small and medium producers; large-scale government imports of inputs and equipment to be sold at cost to associations of small and medium-sized poultry producers; intervention to stabilize prices when imbalances occur in supply and demand.

It is this kind of special concern with small farmers that will be significant in assuring national food supplies. Ministries of agriculture must be able to rely at the policy-making level on individuals who have training in agricultural sciences and economic development; scientists as well as politicians should have a say in decisions affecting national priorities, so that recommendations like those above can be implemented where appropriate by the passage of laws, allocation of funds, and other concrete measures.

A better knowledge of the agricultural sector is a prerequisite for adequate planning. Existing statistics are incomplete and show only general trends. For example, statistics on the number of animals mean little. What is significant is the productivity of these animals. For example, a million high-producing hens under modern management are capable of producing 250 million eggs, but if most of the 25 million chickens reported are *criollo* types, the implications for food production are completely different. The same is true for swine, cattle, and other livestock. It is of no more use to quote numbers of animals than to characterize a nation's agriculture by giving the total agricultural area or the area cultivated. One needs to know something about the yield.

There is also inadequate knowledge of the resource base in terms of availability of feed materials, price relationships, and similar factors. In too many instances government programs are not geared to stimulate or promote production. Controls are confused with supportive measures. Policies must remain the province of policy makers, but as scientists and technicians, we have a responsibility to provide the policy makers with information with which policy decisions can be made.

CONCLUSION

The Latin American countries know that time is pressing for the implementation of new agricultural policies. At present rates, their populations will double in 20 to 25 years, and a very high proportion of these people—estimates for some areas indicate up to 80%—will be in the low-income, largely rural sectors of the population. These people will demand decent housing, adequate food, a fair share of health and educational services. High-technology agriculture, which employs fewer and fewer people and has to sell its products at high prices to pay for energy use, feed-grains, and other costly inputs, cannot be grafted onto a predominantly agrarian economy with low per caput incomes. Countries struggling with massive urban problems, unemployment, poverty, malnutrition, dislocation of essential services, and the resulting explosive frustrations, must act swiftly and decisively if these problems are not to worsen. Integrated planning for agricultural development must take account of these factors; it is a job for statesmen, politicians, and lawmakers, but in the complex economic situation of today, they must rely increasingly on economists, agriculturalists, environmentalists, and other scientists, both from their own countries and from the world community.

Today, at a time when the animal industry faces unfounded criticism, when it is challenged to pioneer new approaches, the lack of response by leaders in this field is appalling. This is the time for action, not timidity. It is time for agriculture to be tuned to social, political, economic realities. Science is a vital base for agricultural development, and should be applied in the context of human values in each culture.

REFERENCE

1. República de El Salvador, Ministerio de Agricultura y Ganadería, Ministerio de Economía. Estudio de la Avicultura en El Salvador (Serie Estudios Agro-ecónomicos No. 2), October 1973, pp. 1–6.

COMMENTS

Manuel Cuca García · *Colegio de Postgraduados, Escuela Nacional de Agricultura, Chapingo, México.*

In the last decade, the rapid increase in the poultry industry in Latin America has stimulated research and the cultivation of crops such as sorghum and soybeans that were practically unknown before, or used in only a limited way. Poultry matures earlier than other animals do and can transform products of vegetable and animal origin into meat and eggs more efficiently. In Latin America, conversions of 2.4:1 can be obtained for broilers and 3:1 for eggs.

In Mexico, poultry supplies 25% of the animal protein consumed, and it is almost the only product that has dropped in price for the consumer. This year, for the first time in 20 years, because of inflation, the price of eggs was higher than U.S. .85¢ per kg. One limitation to expansion is the fact that poultry competes with man for direct grain consumption. However, it offers other advantages: relatively efficient feed conversions, short reproduction time, low land requirement, and the high nutritive value of eggs. Eggs can contribute importantly to a balanced diet.

A wide range of protein sources, i.e., microbial and yeast protein produced on vegetable wastes, algae, wild plants, and even, to a limited extent, dry poultry manure can supplement conventional feedstuffs. Poultry can use many different sources of protein for feed, and can still provide protein of good quality for human consumption. Poultry raising can be highly efficient if newer techniques are applied. In the industrialized countries, feed conversions of 2:1 are attained. By using advances in nutrition, management, and disease control, developing countries could lower the feed conversion ratio and increase egg production. Even the productivity of poor-quality hens (*criollos*) could be improved through better nutrition, although they cannot compete with modern commercial breeds.

Transport and management of poultry and eggs will need to be improved because adequate care of eggs and broiler meat during transport from farm to market is important in cost reduction. The local mixing of feeds incorporating indigenous feedstuff is also essential to reduce costs.

Jerome H. Maner · *Centro Internacional de Agricultura Tropical (CIAT), Cali, Colombia.*

The swine industry, if it is to contribute to the well-being of mankind in the tropics, must make efficient use of available resources. There are slightly more than 100 million head of swine in Latin America–15% of the world swine population–but because of low extraction rates and low slaughter weights, they produce only 5% of the world total of 35 million metric tons. This embarrassingly low level and inefficiency of production is explained by the distribution of pigs on farms and the husbandry and feeding practices employed in their production.

Only about 20% of the pigs in Latin America are produced on commercial or semicommercial swine farms, and on many of these a sow may produce only 8 to 10 pigs per year. These require 5 to 6 kg of feed per kilogram of pig produced and seven to nine months to reach market weight. Diseases, such as brucellosis and leptospirosis, which cause abortion and prenatal mortality; swine dysentery, which causes morbidity and reduced rate and efficiency of growth;

and foot-and-mouth disease, which causes morbidity, mortality, and very high economic losses, are common on many commercial farms.

Even these poor conditions are much better than for the remaining 80% of the swine produced on medium, small, and subsistence farms. These farmers use the pig as a means of marketing grain and other farm products that would not be sold because of quality, distance to market, price, or other factors, as a way of saving for periods of the year when cash is scarce, and as a source of high-quality food for their families.

Under the present system of production, native pigs are allowed to roam freely in the fields and villages and are fed farm by-products, scraps, maize, and sorghum. In the traditional system, large litters are born, but because of poor management and inadequate nutrition for the sow, only two to three of these pigs live to be weaned at 4 to 6 kg. Moreover, they take 6 to 7 months to reach a body weight of 18 to 20 kg and 18 to 20 months to achieve market weight. This traditional system of production, so widespread in Latin America, is extremely wasteful of the available feed energy and protein, and of the farmer's available resources. Almost two years and 600 kg of feed are required to produce a 60-kg, marketable pig.

For the commercial farmer, there are few biological and technological restraints, the notable exception being the control of foot-and-mouth disease, that would prevent us from increasing pork production by 40 to 50% even with little additional feed. Production efficiency can be increased through the application of available technology. Well-trained swine specialists are needed to transfer this production technology to these commercial producers, and government pricing policies must fairly reflect production inputs and reasonable profit margins. Much effort must be given to the training of technicians who can efficiently and effectively carry out these functions.

As to the improvement of the backyard production on medium, small, and subsistence farms, recent work in Colombia has shown that, with the exception of the subsistence farmer with less than 1.5 hectares, farmers will respond with technical assistance. They will accept and build simple swine housing facilities, improve their feeding systems, including the use of purchased protein supplements, and will use improved breeds of boars. By simple management, feeding, and breeding techniques it has been possible to change the farm's production from a loss of approximately $12.00 Colombian pesos per kg of pig to a net profit of $3.00 pesos per kg. This change, accepted by approximately 50% of the farmers in a test village, required: (1) continued and close supervision from well-trained technicians; (2) availability of credit; and (3) institutional cooperation to make protein supplements available for purchase in small quantities.

Although this has been possible, it is unlikely that there will be a great change in the traditional swine production system of the majority of the small farmers in Latin America because most governments and institutions of Latin America continue to follow the same stagnant policies of nonactivity. They are failing to provide the leadership, technical assistance, credit, and stimulus that could improve and increase swine production without increasing the swine population or the present level of feedstuffs being utilized.

31

Ruminant Production in Increasing Animal Foods in Latin America

Tony J. Cunha*

Department of Animal Science
University of Florida
Gainesville, Florida

There is a tremendous undeveloped potential for increasing ruminant production, both beef and dairy cattle, in Latin America. Less potential exists for augmenting the number of sheep and goats. The improved animal husbandry technology currently available could greatly expand ruminant production on the vast underutilized land areas of Latin America. Most of this land is not suitable for intense tillage for human food crops, and some of it will not be needed for this purpose for decades. Increasing ruminant production is a means of making this land more productive and helpful to the total economy of Latin America without competing for man's food sources. Because forage is of no direct use to man, ruminant production is the best method for converting it into animal products for human food and other uses, and of adding quality and palatability to the diet.

ECONOMICS OF EXPANSION

Before ruminant production can be greatly increased in Latin America, there needs to be a market and people must be able to purchase animal products. Equal in importance to solving animal production problems are economic and social programs designed to make it possible for people to have better living standards, including ability to buy the meat, milk, and other foods they need. Increased ruminant production needs to be kept in line either with market

**Present address:* School of Agriculture, California State Polytechnic University, Pomona, California.

Table I. World's Livestock and Poultry Production in 1962 in 1000 Metric Tons[a]

Area	Meats					Milk	Eggs	Total animal products	Percent of world production
	Pork	Poultry	Bovine	Other	Total				
United States	5,430	3,265	7,747	1,483	17,925	56,828	3,806	96,484	19
Developed countries	12,356	5,404	15,840	5,795	39,395	187,464	8,682	274,936	54
Less developed countries	3,021	1,241	10,420	3,816	18,498	74,275	2,496	113,758	22
Total world production	23,045	8,155	31,840	12,010	75,050	346,880	13,929	510,909	–

[a]Reference 2.

demand for it within each country, or with the demand for export of animal products.

A limiting factor in the expansion of ruminant production in Latin America is that the market price paid for live animals is low. Consequently, the returns to cattle producers make it uneconomical for them to buy better quality breeding stock and all the supplemental feeds needed in conjunction with the forage program, nor can they afford to purchase many other items necessary for high-level productivity. Thus, the demand for beef and milk, and their price levels at the farm, will be key factors in determining how much expansion can occur, and how well cattlemen raise the quality and productivity of their farms.

REASONS FOR LOW RUMINANT PRODUCTIVITY

Most of the cattle producers in Latin America are still not using much of the new technology now used routinely in the more developed countries. As a consequence, it takes four to five years or more for Latin American beef cattle to reach market weight. The number of animals slaughtered per year amounts to less than 12% of the cattle population, as opposed to 38% in the United States. In most cases, breeding selection is mostly for survival and not top productivity. The calving rate is estimated to be between 40 to 50% compared to 86% in the United States. Most evidence indicates that the cattle mortality rate is at least 12 to 15% versus 5 to 6% in the United States (1).

The 80 developing countries, including those of Latin America, have about 60% of the world's livestock and poultry, but produce only 22% of the world's supply of meat, milk, and eggs (2,3) (Table I). Table II shows how far developing countries lag behind the developed countries in pounds of animal products per year for ruminant animal production in terms of beef, veal, and milk (4). Latin America has twice as much land area and twice as many cattle as the United

Table II. Kilograms of Production per Animal,[a] Yearly

	Production in developed countries	Production in developing countries
Beef and veal	71	16
Milk	811	97
Mutton, lamb, and goat meat	6	4
Pork	83	40
Eggs	5	3

[a]Reference 4.

States has, yet produces only one-half as much beef. The ratio of productivity of 1 to 4 means that Latin America is feeding four times as many cattle as is the United States to produce a ton of beef (5,6). With this low level of animal productivity in Latin America there is tremendous potential for increasing and improving ruminant animal husbandry.

NEED FOR RESEARCH

Ruminant research programs in Latin America are on a small scale compared to the need. Very little research is being conducted in the hot, humid areas where the largest land areas are located. Results of animal husbandry studies from the United States and other countries in the world are of some value in Latin America, but are limited in application to the tropics and will not substitute for adaptive research to meet the local conditions. This research must include the breed of animal used, the forage and other feed supply available, the level of management required, the level of productivity desired, the disease and parasite problems encountered, the market price and demand, and many other factors associated with a total ruminant production and marketing program (7).

FORAGE PRODUCTION

In Latin America ruminant animals depend, to a large extent, on forage production. Even in the United States, in 1971 (8) 72% of the feed consumed by beef cattle, 66% by dairy cattle, and 90% by sheep and goats came from forages, both in the pasture and harvested. In Latin America this percentage is even higher. Latin America has the advantage of plenty of sunlight, a long growing season, and a warm climate, all important in forage production. However, in many areas the soil is infertile and long seasonal dry periods greatly restrict the continuous year-round production of quality forage. Research information is required on how to correct mineral deficiencies, extend the grazing season, preserve forage, and supply other needed nutrients if economic returns justify doing so. Proper use of fertilizer can greatly increase forage production in Latin America, but its cost is a practical limitation. Crop rotations need to be developed that will minimize the need for fertilizer when land is used for pasture. The development of legumes to use in combination with forage grasses would also lessen the need for fertilization. Adapted forage varieties, disease control, and other problems also require attention.

BEEF CATTLE

Expansion of beef cattle herds has great potential in Latin America. This is because of the very large land areas available in sparsely populated, underdeveloped locations where beef cattle grazing is the preferred method of utilizing the land and the resources available. The problems to be solved in order to increase beef production in Latin America include: better quality cattle, improved breeding programs, proper feeding and nutrition, better disease and parasite control, improved management, and many other production problems that need to be solved or ameliorated. Development of an improved marketing program is also important. This includes a simplified beef grading system to reward the rancher producing the better quality beef. Until he can obtain more money for his cattle, he does not have much incentive to improve the quality of the animal produced. Exports of beef provide some incentive for increasing beef production in Latin America, but problems associated with a fluctuating demand for beef exports should be carefully considered.

DAIRY CATTLE

It is difficult to predict how much expansion in dairy cattle production will occur in Latin America. There are some who feel that it is more economical to import dried milk powder and reconstitute it into fluid milk, and also that butter, cheese, and other milk products can be imported more cheaply than they can be produced in Latin America. A lack of proper transportation, pasteurization, processing, and marketing facilities for milk in many areas adds credence to the belief that the dairy industry in Latin America will not expand very much. Others disagree. Modest expansion will probably occur as better transportation, processing, and marketing facilities are developed. Some very good dairy operations already exist near the larger cities of Latin America. As better quality cattle and feeding practices, production, management, marketing, and other factors are improved, the level of milk production per cow will increase. This is important, because Latin America produces less than 30% as much milk as North America does (C. J. Wilcox, University of Florida, personal communication, 1974). There will, of course, be more demand for milk as the human population continues to increase in the future. To begin with, more emphasis should be placed on improving the productivity of present dairy herds, as this in itself could result in a 50 to 100% increase in milk production.

SHEEP AND GOATS

Expansion in sheep and goat husbandry in Latin America will be small. In tropical areas, severe parasite problems exist, especially for improved breeds brought in from other areas. In Florida, native sheep are relatively resistant to parasites, but high death losses from parasite infestation occur when improved sheep breeds from other states are brought to Florida (9–11). It is logical to assume that any move to increase sheep production in Latin America should make use of the native sheep as the basis for commercial flocks in each area. Interest in raising sheep in tropical Latin America is not great. Sheep would fare best in the cooler, higher altitudes of Latin America. They perform better than cattle in the mountainous country and in areas where the amount and quality of forage is low.

Goats could be used more in Latin America as a source of milk as well as meat for the small farmer and the poor people who otherwise would have little or no milk or meat for their families. They can be staked out to consume forage along roadsides, in ditches, and in other areas where the forage might otherwise be wasted. This forage, plus some mineral supplementation, would result in fairly good milk and meat production. This would be an important income supplement for the poor farmer whose earnings may average only \$100 to \$200 per year. It would also supply much-needed protein and other essential nutrients to their diet.

REFERENCES

1. McDowell, L. R., and Conrad, J. H., 1973, University of Florida Research Proposal to US/AID, pp. 1--81.
2. Caton, D. D., 1970, Growth in demand for feed grains, U.S.D.A. Foreign Agric. Service, Econ. Report No. 63, p. 205.
3. Van Horn, H. H., Cunha, T. J., and Harms, R. H., 1972, The role of livestock in meeting human food needs, *Bio Science* **22**: 710–714.
4. Phillips, R. W., 1972, Towards an intensified animal agriculture, Proceedings, 7th Symposium on International Production, Milan, Italy, April 15–17, pp. 62–72.
5. Cox, M. L., 1966, Animal agriculture in Latin America: Present status and possibilities for expansion, Proceedings, 15th Annual Meeting of Agriculture Research Institute, Washington, D.C., Oct. 10–11.
6. Cunha, T. J., 1971, The role of the livestock and meat industry in meeting human food needs, Proceedings, National Biological Congress, Miami, Florida, Oct. 25.
7. Cunha, T. J., 1967, Positive suggestions for the future, *in: Rural development in tropical Latin America,* K. L. Turk and L. V. Crowder (eds.), Cornell University Press, Ithaca, New York, pp. 413–429.
8. Hodgson, R. E., 1971, Place of animals in world agriculture, *J. Dairy Sci.* **54**: 1–6.
9. Loggins, P. E., Koger, M., Warnick, A. C., and Cunha, T. J., 1964, Spring lamb production in Florida, University of Florida Agric. Exp. Stat. Bull. 669.
10. Radhakrishnan, C. V., Bradley, R. E., and Loggins, P. E., 1972, Host responses of worm-free Florida native rambouillet lambs experimentally infected with *Haemonchus contortus, Am. J. Vet. Res.* **33**: 817–823.
11. Bradley, R. E., Radhakrishnan, C. V., Patil-Kulkarni, V. G., and Loggins, P. E., 1973, Response in Florida native and rambouillet lambs exposed to one and two oral doses of *Haemonchus contortus, Am. J. Vet. Res.* **34**: 729–735.

COMMENTS

J. K. Loosli · *University of Florida, Gainesville, Florida.*

In support of Cunha's summary of the problems and potentials for increasing protein production with ruminants in Latin America, I will cite some experiences in other countries. Whether or not the tremendous potentials for increasing animal protein production in many tropical areas will be achieved in any country depends on: (a) control of diseases and parasites; (b) upgrading of the genetic merit of the animals; and (c) improved nutrition and management to make economic production of animals a reality.

Ruminants have the advantage that they can be fed grass, weeds, and food crop wastes. They can add to the total food supply without competing with the land used to produce food. They can effectively use waste products from the breweries, sugar refineries, and fruit and vegetable processing plants. They can be integrated into small farms and add income, and improve human nutrition. Large beef cattle and dairy farms could be developed if incentives were available. Past attempts to modernize cattle production in tropical countries have often failed because of the lack of adequate inputs, especially nutrition and management, but there have been some recent successes.

Traditional livestock owners in West Africa and areas of East Africa are nomadic. They do not own land or have permanent homes, but move their families with their cattle as they search for feed. They range across national boundaries into the Sahel during the rainy season, then south again in the long dry season. The cattle are milked and the milk is used by the family or exchanged for cereals, clothing, and other necessities. Surplus bulls are sold after they reach maturity and provide the beef for the villages and cities. The cows are all kept to maintain the breeding herd. Only 30 to 50% of the cows produce a live calf each year, compared to at least 85% in the United States, and death losses are high. Carcass weights of the animals are about one-third of those in Europe and the United States.

Formerly, the tropical climate and disease problems were blamed for the low productivity of the cattle in these areas. Much progress has been made in reducing losses from diseases and parasites, but there are still some unresolved problems. Very little progress has been seen in improved management except in isolated instances. Recent experience has shown that European breeds of dairy and dual-purpose cattle are able to grow rapidly and produce two to five times more milk than do native tropical cattle, if they are protected from diseases and fed and managed to minimize stress. At elevations above 1000 meters, there is no important heat stress problem.

In the rain forests of Africa, the slash and burn bush fallow system of farming is the only method that has maintained a reasonable level of soil fertility over centuries. Domestic animals play no part in this system, except for a few native goats, pigs, and chickens as scavengers. It would seem that a grass rotation using ruminants would be more productive. There are more difficulties in producing and processing milk in the humid tropics than there are for meat. Striking success has been achieved, however, in Kenya, where grass crop rotations are stimulating milk and beef production on small farms. Government assistance with credit, land, and cattle, and training in production methods, as well as price stabilization to give needed incentives, have made this possible. This could serve as a model for other tropical countries.

In Batangas, Philippines, the small farmers keep one to three cows to graze coconut groves and consume rice straw, weeds, corn stalks, and vegetable and fruit residues. They supply some milk and significant cash income when sold for beef. In Nigeria, government-owned cattle ranches have met with only limited success. Some private ranches now being started should become more productive, but financial returns on these enterprises are lower than for industrial development or housing units. There is much unused, or poorly used, land in Africa that could be used for livestock if people were trained in husbandry and assisted in starting the operations.

A few sheep and goats live with the migratory herds of cattle in Africa and supply meat for the family. Dwarf goats are widely distributed in the villages throughout tropical Africa and Southeast Asia, where they survive as scavengers, consuming the grass, weeds, and brush on the roadsides and garbage in the streets and markets. Most of the sheep exist in the drier regions and higher altitudes of the tropics, but some dwarf types are found in lowland humid areas of Africa, along with the goats. Both sheep and goat meat are well accepted. The smaller size of these animals is an advantage in rural villages without refrigeration, where distribution and use of the meat is easily made on the day of slaughter.

No mention has been made of the water buffalo, a most important ruminant in southern Asia and India and, to some extent, in the Middle East, as a source of power for farming and transport, as well as meat and milk. Domesticated buffaloes are not found in tropical Africa, and there are only a few in the Amazon basin in Brazil in Latin America. There are vast areas of swamps and wetlands, largely unused, along coast lines, rivers and lakes where water buffaloes could thrive with limited care and without competing with other animal production or crop farming. They could greatly increase the efficiency of the labor-intensive food crop production in tropical Africa. The meat is comparable to beef, and the milk is higher in protein and fat than milk from cattle or goats.

Robert F. Chandler, Jr. • *The Asian Vegetable Research and Development Center, Shanhua, Taiwan.*

During nearly 16 years in Asia, I have been tremendously impressed with the performance of the water buffalo in the humid, lowland tropics. It converts roughage into meat much more efficiently than cattle do. It is tolerant to heat, and resists parasite and disease attack. The Murah strain from India, for example, is a good milk producer. Some individual females have produced over 4000 kg in one lactation. Also, of course, they are excellent draft animals under humid conditions. Should not the water buffalo be introduced into the humid, tropical lowlands of Latin America?

32

The Role of Ruminants in Tropical America

Hernán Fonseca

University of Costa Rica
San José, Costa Rica

The area devoted to grasslands in Latin America in 1967 consisted of 446 million hectares, accounting for 79.9% of the agricultural land available (1). However, the ratio of man to bovines, formerly 1:1, has decreased in recent years because of the growth in human population, and will continue to diminish if adequate measures are not taken to stimulate livestock production (2).

The availability of meat from cattle, sheep, and goats per person in tropical America is 17.2 kg per year, compared with 49.1 kg for the United States (3). In the past 20 years Latin America has increased meat production by 64.5% and milk by 86%. Because inefficient production methods are responsible for the low production in Latin America, a new technology has to be developed.

Until a few months ago, the high prices of beef on the U.S. market and the unlimited import quota stimulated Latin American cattlemen and government and credit agencies to increase beef production on an unlimited scale, to the point that large forest areas were being cut to increase grasslands in an attempt to speed up national incomes from beef exports. However, when North American housewives began to reject the high costs of beef, consumption and imports decreased drastically. There is an overcrowded population of fat cattle in Latin American pastures, and cattlemen are waiting for better prices to ship their steers to market. As the dry season arrives in many of these tropical areas, millions of kilograms of beef will be lost because of steers suffering weight loss due to lack of adequate forage (4).

In contrast to meat, milk is increasingly short every year and imports grow correspondingly. However, vast areas adaptable for dairy cattle are found in the tropics and should be developed in order to meet the demands of a population that will number 364 million by 1980 (5). Sheep and goat raising is not likely to increase significantly, mainly because these species require special husbandry techniques generally unknown to most Latin Americans.

A question that arises is whether to increase the area devoted to grasslands, or build up the already existing ones. If the land devoted to grass were managed properly, it should increase ruminant production manyfold without any further need to increase the area planted in grass. As an example, a 28.3% increase in beef production per hectare was obtained in Mexico by applying nitrogen to Pangolagrass pastures, and this figure extended to a 41.3% increase when the animals were fed supplements of molasses with 3% urea. The combined effect was a 92.8% increase in beef production (6).

The World Bank has assisted in developing many thousands of acres into productive pasture by allowing credit to Latin American governments. Such is the case in Chile, where the dairy industry is being developed, and it is expected that within the coming years Chilean milk will be exported to neighboring countries (7), as opposed to the $40 million worth of imported dairy products otherwise predicted for Chile by 1980 (8). In Uruguay, bank loans have made it possible to develop over 100,000 hectares of land into high-producing pastures, the majority devoted to dairy cattle (7).

In many countries, especially the smaller ones, there might be competition between humans and ruminants for use of land to produce food. This is true in those with a high proportion of mountainous areas, such as in Honduras, El Salvador, Costa Rica, and Ecuador, where tillable land is scarce and the best agricultural lands have been devoted to pastures.

With increasing scarcity of basic foods for man, grain products necessarily must bring better prices for the farmers, and obviously more land should be turned over to food crop production. Vicente-Chandler (9) recommends the use of flatlands in the tropics for machine-cultivated crops, such as soybeans, which are capable of producing about 10 times as much protein as can be obtained with grass-fed cattle.

Even though export markets for beef are doubtful at the present time, production must be increased if all Latin Americans are eventually to obtain adequate protein in their diets. The average animal protein intake for most people in Latin America is 30 to 35 grams per day compared to 95 grams per person per day in the United States (10). Moreover, not all of the countries in Latin America are able to supply their own animal protein needs. Thus, if purchasing power increases throughout the area, those countries that produce ruminant products in excess of their own demand will have regional export markets.

Total beef production increased slowly during the 1960s, providing some growth in per caput consumption, but beef exports were possible for only a few countries. In 1971 beef supplies, at present national average income levels, allowed less than 20 kg of beef per person annually in all tropical Latin American countries (11). It must be understood that with the great differences in individual incomes, there are people who had no beef at all, while others may have consumed as much as five times the average given. Only Jamaica, Panama, Peru, and Venezuela showed significant increases in average per caput beef consumption (12,13).

Milk and beef are the main animal products in Latin America. However, the annual increase in the ruminant population (2.7%) is below that for humans, while the demand for animal products increases at an estimated rate of 5% per year (14). A main reason for this slow increase in ruminant numbers and for their low productivity is poor reproductive efficiency, estimated at a 45% level, with a mortality rate of 12 to 15% (15,16). Marketing weight of beef cattle in Latin America varies from 250 to 500 kg (16), and market age for beef cattle varies from two to six years (16).

Tolerance to high temperatures of the indigenous criollas is associated with lower milk production (17). Methods for increasing milk production have been widely applied, and a large number of herds are now made up of crossbred Native-Brahman and European cattle. Success is achieved only when sound management and nutrition practices are employed. Average milk production has been reported to range from 2,187 kg of milk per lactation (18) to 1,738 (19) and 1,420 kg (20). A crossbred Native-Holstein herd studied in Honduras, comprising 45 head, averaged 3,422 kg of milk per lactation (21).

A vast portion of Latin America is located in the tropics, thus adequate sunlight, a warm climate, and abundant rain provide good conditions for a long grazing season in most areas. However, soil fertility is low in many regions, and the lack of fertilizer is the main barrier to abundant forage production of adequate nutrient content; consequently productivity is low. Most soils of tropical America do not fix enough nitrogen over a long period of time for satisfactory forage and pasture production (22). High forage yields and increased protein production are achieved only by liberal nitrogen applications. Numerous experiments conducted in the tropics indicate that no matter what amount of nitrogen is applied, favorable responses are always obtained (9). Increases in dry matter yield from 5 tons/ha to 14 tons/ha, a carrying capacity increase from 0.5 animals/ha to 5.5/ha, and animal weight increases from 100 kg/ha to 1100 kg/ha have been reported after applications of 400 kg N/ha per year (23).

Under tropical conditions where it is possible to grow grasses the year round, phosphorus losses can be extremely high, and phosphorus applications need to be considerably greater than those in temperate regions. This is because the highly weathered soils in the tropics are generally very deficient in phosphorus, and also many soils fix large quantities of added phosphorus (24). It has been demonstrated in British Honduras that even though a level of 64 ppm of added phosphorus stimulated maximum yield of forages, the phosphorus content of forage was adequate only when 220 ppm of phosphorus was added (25). Phosphorus requirements for ruminants in tropical America are met at 0.15% dry matter basis for adult animals, and at 0.20% for young growing ones (26). Based on these figures, most forages are either deficient or borderline for production purposes (27–29).

Reports from several countries throughout Latin America indicate that calcium levels in forages are normal (30–33). However, a calcium content as low as 0.04% has been reported from the La Paragua region in Venezuela (26). Trace element content of forages has not been studied sufficiently, although deficiencies of zinc, molybdenum, boron, iron, manganese, copper, and iodine have been reported (27,33,34). Selenium toxicity has been described in Mexico (26) and manganese toxicity has been found in Brazil and Costa Rica (35,36). It may be concluded that trace element deficiencies are limiting both forage and animal production in the tropics, but because of a paucity of research data, no guidelines exist for proper trace element supplementation of soil to improve productivity.

Sunlight, a warm climate, and rainfall of over 30 inches per year (sometimes as much as 150 inches) provide a grazing season nearly year round in many parts of Latin America. These conditions should be ideal for ruminant production if only some steps are taken to make the best use of the forages. Many factors affect forage utilization, but among them, intake and digestibility are the main determinants of animal production in the tropics (11).

Achievements from a wide range of production practices are minimal if one considers the statistics given for ruminant production in the tropics of Latin America as a whole. Improved practices have been imported for the most part from developed countries without adaptation to the conditions prevailing here, and in many cases, trial and error procedures have produced nothing but losses. Extension services for disseminating adequate and improved practices have been limited, and seldom of benefit to the small producer who needs assistance most urgently.

The deficiencies are many, research programs are limited and vary widely among countries, depending upon available resources and trained personnel. Lack of this type of well-trained agricultural research and extension manpower is general. Agriculture schools, in many instances, have rather poor teaching programs, limited by economic constraints. Governments are so pressed with the sociological problems brought about by massive population growth that little time and few resources are available for developing sound research and educational programs aimed at increasing animal production, although it is accepted as an urgent priority. In summary, the many conditions favorable for ruminant production in the tropical areas of Latin America are counterbalanced by many obstacles and deficiencies that have to be overcome if animal production is to be satisfactorily increased.

REFERENCES

1. Food and Agriculture Organization of the United Nations, 1967, Production Yearbook, Vol. 21, Rome, 1968.
2. Caballero, H., 1971, Produccion de carne de res en América Latina, *in: Recursos proteinicos en América Latina,* Institute of Nutrition of Central America and Panama, Guatemala City, Guatemala, pp. 145–159.
3. Chicco, C. F., and Shultz, T. A., 1974, Sistema extensivos de producción de carne y leche usando pastos tropicales con y sin suplementación, VII Reunión Interamericana a Nivel Ministerial sobre el Control de la Fiebre Aftosa y otras Zoonosis, Puerto España, Trinidad. 17–20 Abril, RICAZ 7/14, Org. Panam. de la Salud, OMS.
4. Hutchinson, K. J., 1971, Productivity and energy flow in grazing fodder conservation systems, *Herb. Abstr.* **41:** 1–10.
5. Fonseca, H., 1970, Producción de Leche y Productos Lactos en América Latina, *in: Recursos proteinicos en América Latina.* Institute of Nutrition of Central America and Panama, Guatemala City, Guatemala, pp. 160–168.
6. Reta, G., 1974, Nutrición animal y desarrollo ganadero, VII Reunión Interamericana a Nivel Ministerial sobre el Control de La Fiebre Aftosa y otras Zoonosis, Puerto España, Trinidad. 12–20 Abril, RICAZ 7/19, Org. Panam. de la Salud y OMS.
7. McMeekan, C. P., *De pasto a leche,* Editorial Hemisferio Sur, Montevideo, Uruguay.
8. Keating, P. F., 1969, El desarrollo de la industria lechera, Informe al gobierno de Chile, Food and Agriculture Organization of the United Nations, Folleto mimeografiado No. AT-2629, Roma, Italia.
9. Vicente-Chandler, J., 1974, Fertilization of humid tropical grasslands, *in: Forage fertilization,* American Society of Agronomy, Crop Science Society of America and Soil Science Society of America, Madison, Wisconsin.
10. Phillips, R. W., 1969, Animal agriculture and the world's food supply, Institute of Agriculture, University of Minnesota, International Agriculture Series 6.
11. Christiansen, W. C., 1971, Livestock feeds and feeding in Latin America, Agriculture Development Paper, Institute of Food and Agricultural Science, International Programs Division, University of Florida, Gainesville, Florida.
12. Florida Agricultural Experiment Stations, 1970, Effects of changing trade systems in Latin America on U.S. agricultural exports, U.S. Department of Agriculture, Economic Research Service, Washington, D.C.
13. U.S. Department of Agriculture, 1971, Foreign Agriculture Circular FLM 1-71, Washington, D.C.
14. Mitchell, C., and Schatan, J., 1967, La Agricultura en la América Latina: Perspectivas para su Desarrollo, *in: Desarrollo agricola de América Latina en la próxima década,* Banco Interamericano de Desarrollo, Washington, D.C., pp. 47–181.
15. Christiansen, W. C., 1964, Livestock production in Argentina, Uruguay and Southern Brazil, Iowa State University/Uruguay AID Contract.
16. Rourk, J. P., 1969, The Beef Cattle Industries of Central America and Panama, Foreign Agriculture Service, U.S. Department of Agriculture FAS M-208. Washington, D.C.
17. Koger, M., 1961, Livestock improvement in tropical America, *Ceiba* 9 (2).
18. Bodisco, V., Carnevali, A., Cevallos, E., and Gómez, J., 1968, Cuatro lactancias consecutivas en vacas criollas y Pardo Suizas en Maracay, Venezuela, *ALPA Mem.* **3:** 61–75.
19. De Alba, J., and Carrera, C., 1958, Selección del ganado lechero tropical, Comunicaciones de Turrialba, IICA, Turrialba, Costa Rica, pp. 70.
20. Maltos, J., and Cartwright, T. C., 1971, Producción de leche bajo condiciones de

trópico húmedo, Hatos fundadores de Jersey y criollo en Turrialba, Costa Rica, *ALPA Mem.* **6:** 87, Abstract.

21. Fonseca, H., 1961, Resultado de mejoramiento del ganado criollo cruzado con razas de ganado lechero europeo, *Ceiba* **8** (2).
22. Blue, W. G., 1968, Soil plant relations involved in adaptation of forage crops to tropical climates, *Soil Crop Sci. Soc. Fla. Proc.* **28:** 232–240.
23. Vicente-Chandler, J., Caro-Costas, R., Pearson, R. W., Abruña, F., Figarella, J., y Silva, S., 1967, El mancjo intensivo de forrajes tropicales en Puerto Rico, Univ. de Puerto Rico Bol. 202.
24. Kamprath, E. J., 1973, Phosphorus, *in:* A review of soils research in tropical Latin America, *N. C. Agric. Exp. Sta. Tech. Bul.* **219:** 138–161.
25. Blue, W. G., 1969, Fertilizer response with Pangola grass on Puletan loam fine sand, British Honduras, as indicated by pot experiments, *Trop. Agric.* **46** (1): 25–29.
26. De Alba, J., and Davis, G. K., 1957, Minerales en la nutrición animal en la América Latina, *Turrialba* **7:** 16.
27. Aguirre, A. A., 1941, Alimentación del ganado, contribución a su estudio, Ministerio de Agricultura y Ganadería, Uruguay, Pub. No. 58.
28. Nores, J. G., 1944, Contenido de algunos elementos trazas en praderas naturales Uruguayas, Universidad de Uruguay, Montevideo, *Rev. Fac. Agron.* **35:** 23–35.
29. Grunwald, O., Ortiz, D., Romero, R. S., y Sapenc de Pollak, 1947, Una contribución al conocimiento de las plantas forrajeras de Venezuela, Ministerio de Agricultura y Cría, Venezuela, Bol. No. 5.
30. Ortiz, D. S., 1952, Composición química de plantas y factores que la determinan, *Agri. (Venezuela)* 7 (230): 39–45.
31. Azcárate, V. E., 1954, Observaciones químicas sobre el valor del Panizzo como material forrajero, *Agro* **9** (29): 17–19.
32. Iljin, W. S., 1953, Microelementos en las plantas forrajeras, *Agron. Trop.* **2** (2): 91–112.
33. Davis, G. K., 1955, Algunos micro elementos en la nutrición animal, *Turrialba* **5** (4): 114–122.
34. Cox, F. R., 1973, Micronutrients, *in: A review of soils and research in tropical Latin America,* North Carolina State University, Tech. Bull. No. 219, pp. 182–197.
35. Souto, S. M., e Dobereiner, J., 1969, Fixaçao de nitrogenio e estabelecimento de duas variedades de soja perene (*Glycine javanica* L.) com tres níveis de fósforo e de calcio, em solo con toxidez de manganes, *Pesqui. Agropecu. Bras.* **4:** 59–66.
36. Fonseca, H., and Davis, G. K., 1968, Manganese content of some forage crops in Costa Rica and its relation to cattle fertility, *Proceedings of the Second World Conference on Animal Production,* University of Maryland, Abstract.

33

Increasing the Production of Ruminants in Tropical America

Claudio F. Chicco

Centro de Investigaciones Agropecuarias
Ministerio de Agricultura y Cria
Maracay, Venezuela

The consistently low animal productivity and the limited consumption of beef and milk in tropical America restrict most of the population to predominantly cereal diets, low in animal proteins. A major political, economic, and social effort should be made to examine the possibilities for producing and consuming more animal protein. The tropics are rich in plant resources, for the most part not edible by man (1), that can be used either for industrial purposes or for conversion into animal products via the raising of cattle, sheep, and goats that can feed on a wide variety of plant materials. From 60 to 70% of a total of 1,680 million hectares in tropical America is in pasture, or is potential pasturage area. This represents a tremendous source of feed for ruminant animals. Furthermore, tropical America has over 400 million bovines, over 140 million sheep, and nearly 38 million goats, all invaluable animal resources (2).

In spite of these resources, four times the number of cattle are required to produce the same amount of beef or milk in tropical America as are needed in temperate America (3). Research and observation suggest that it is feasible to increase present productivity levels by 300 to 400%. The most important means to achieve this will be improved utilization of present and potential plant and animal resources and attention to the socioeconomic factors related to demand, marketing, development politics, education, and research.

The higher quantitative production of vegetable dry matter in the tropics depends upon natural conditions of temperature, light, and humidity. Thus, the dry season in the dry/wet tropics is a major limiting factor in the continuity of forage supplies to animals, depending on length and intensity of droughts. Irrigation facilities, when they exist, are used primarily for intensive dairy operations. It is improbable that irrigation will be feasible in tropical savannas used for raising beef cattle. Forage conservation as silage and/or hay in storage, or as standing hay, is seldom practiced unless warranted by the objectives and economics of specific cattle operations. However, extreme shortages of forage result in animal deaths, so forage conservation should be considered, not only to contribute to feed supplies, but to reduce losses from overgrazing. Flooding during the rainy season also reduces forage availability and limits cattle production in the low savannas. In the low plains of Venezuela, for instance, a dike system that would control the water level, eliminating excess water or retaining it for future necessities, is now being evaluated (4). In addition to the traditional forages, industrial vegetable wastes and animal by-products can also contribute valuable protein and energy sources for ruminant animals in tropical America.

The nutritional value of grass forages as well as their yield can be improved by introducing better grass species, use of fertilizer, grass-legume mixed cropping, better grazing management, and improved methods of conservation, harvesting, and storage. Animal body weight gains of 1,120 kg/hectare occurred in heavily fertilized grasslands in Florida (5), Jamaica (6), and Queensland (7). The capacity of the land to support grazing has been increased from 0.35 to 0.85 animal/hectare by the introduction of *Stylosanthis humilis* in the grasslands of Queensland (8); and an animal body weight gain of 630 kg/hectare was possible in heavy and irrigated soils of the flatlands of Venezuela by using *Echinochloa polystachya* (9).

Because of the low nutritive value of tropical forages and crop residues, in terms of digestibility, intake, and specific production, it is advisable to improve agronomic and managerial practices, including technological systems, such as predigestion, enrichment, and others (10) that would improve roughage utilization efficiency under certain conditions. At present, the application of much of this technological knowledge is still limited by economic barriers. Benefits could likely be derived by a more efficient utilization of fibrous material through microbiological processes, but this will require further research.

Major limitations to productivity of cattle in tropical America are low reproductive efficiency, low weaning weight, slow postweaning growth of beef cattle, and the low productivity and fertility of dairy cows. Better selection of beef cattle, in combination with adequate managerial practices, is giving promising results. In an experimental Brahman herd in Venezuela, during the first five years of the program, reproductive efficiency was improved 41%, calf weaning by 68%, preweaning and postweaning growth by 15% and 25%, respectively (11). An example of genetic improvement by crossbreeding is shown by the weight of 18-month-old steers in the Venezuelan llanos. Native Criollos reached

210 kg, the Brahman weighed 236 kg, and crossbred Criollo and Brahman animals achieved 258 kg at this age (11). In terms of carcass weight, some data from Bolivia (12) indicate a weight increment from 210 kg for the Criollo to 240 kg for the crossbred Criollo-Brahman. Therefore, through selection, crossbreeding, and efficient managerial practices, it is possible to double production levels in the majority of tropical herds in a short time.

The transfer of technology for improving milk production in dairy cows has been less successful, largely because new breeds of milk cows had to be imported from countries with temperate environments. Nevertheless, some improvements in milk production have been obtained. Starting with 858 kg milk/cow/year (12) as the average for tropical America, numerous examples have shown that it is possible to increase the milk output. Lactation yields of 2187 kg were reached for selected Criollo cows (13), 3225 kg for Brown Swiss (14), 4506 kg for Holstein (15), and yields of about 3000 kg for different crossbred cows (16). This does not mean that European breeds will give greater milk yields than the native breeds in any region within the tropics. However, in those areas where it has been possible to maintain dairy operations with European cattle, the production level is higher. On the other hand, if production and reproductive factors are evaluated simultaneously, existing knowledge shows that European breeds are producing milk at a higher level, but their reproductive performance is extremely poor. In fact, it is almost impossible to maintain dairy operations with pure European strains of cattle in many tropical areas (16) because of low fertility rates. Under adverse environmental and economic conditions, where the existing cattle have a very low potential for milk production and European breeds cannot reproduce satisfactorily, crossbreeding will be necessary (16).

There are several fundamental factors involved in the application of the innovations required that do not depend on the cattle industry itself. Marketing systems must be improved according to local conditions of production and demand. This calls for public cattle markets and the establishment of industrial slaughterhouses where the cattle would be handled by modern hygienic techniques. A refrigerated distribution network is also essential. For dairy production, peripheral collection and cooling stations are required. Prices, particularly for beef, should be established at a level appropriate to the effective demand, to market conditions in different locations, consumer preference, and producer costs.

Exportation offers advantages where the purchasing power of the population is low. The higher prices for export meat can result in greater profits for the producer, thus allowing more acceptable prices in the local market for lower quality meat and help to break the vicious circle of low demand–low efficiency. To support technical innovations and to maintain the necessary flow of operational funds, long-term credit should be ensured at reasonable interest rates.

Credit should be associated with other means to aid cattlemen, such as technical assistance, improved infrastructure, and education in methods of animal husbandry.

An adequate educational level will be required if improved production systems are to be introduced; modern technology must be utilized and efficient management assured. In addition, nutrition education of the public should be initiated to emphasize the value of animal products in a balanced diet. Improvement of cattle resources and betterment of economic and social factors will benefit from appropriate technical assistance and an active research program directed toward short-term positive results as well as long-term goals.

This cannot be done by industry alone; good judgment and vision on the part of responsible government officials will be required, with implementation by governments of sound agricultural policies, including those for encouraging animal husbandry.

REFERENCES

1. Stewart, C. A., 1970, High potential productivity of the tropics for cereal crops, grass forage crops and beef, *J. Aust. Inst. Agric. Sci.* **36:** 85.
2. Food and Agriculture Organization, 1972, FAO Production Yearbook, Rome, 496 pp.
3. Jasiorowski, H. A., 1973, Veinte años sin progreso? *Rev. Mundial Zoot.* **5:** 1.
4. Venezuela Comision para el Desarrollo Integral de los Modulos de Apure, 1974 (MOP-MAC-SAS), Caracas, 150 pp.
5. Chapman, H. L., Peacock, P. M., Kirk, W. G., Shirley, R. L., and Cunha, T. J., 1964, Supplemental feeding of beef cattle in South Florida, *Fla. Agric. Exp. Stn. Bull.* **665.**
6. Morgan Ress, A. M., 1966, The economics of tropical grassland, *in: Tropical pastures,* W. Daves and C. L. Skidmore (eds.), Faber and Faber, London, 159 pp.
7. Evans, T. R., 1969, Beef production from nitrogen-fertilized Pangola grass (*Digitaria decumbens*) on the coastal lowlands of southern Queensland, *Aust. J. Exp. Agric. Anim. Husb.* **9:** 282.
8. Stobbs, T. H., 1971, Quality of pasture and forage crops for dairy production in the tropical regions of Australia, *Trop. Grassl.* **5:**159.
9. Chicco, C. F., y Rodriguez, S., 1973, Desarrollo ganadero del tropico humedo de Venezuela, *in: Reuniòn Tècnica de Programaciòn sobre desarrollo ganadero del tròpico humèdo americano,* (IICA), Guayaquil, Ecuador, pp. III-F-I–III-F-19.
10. Proceedings of the Symposium on the Effect of Processing on the Nutritional Value of Feeds, Gainesville, Fla., 1972, published by the National Academy of Sciences, Washington, D.C., 1973, 494 pp.
11. Plasse, D., 1974, Sistema genètico para el mejoramiento de la producciòn en el tropico, *in: Seminario sobre potencial para incrementar la producciòn de carne en Amèrica tropical,* International Center of Tropical Agriculture (CIAT), Cali, Colombia.
12. Bauer, S., Plasse, D., y Verde, O., 1974, Peso de canales de ganado criollo y sus cruces con Cebú, *ALPA Mem.* **9:** 169.
13. Bodisco, V., Carnevali, A., Cevallos, E., y Gomez, J. R., 1968, Cuatro lactancias consecutivas en vacas criollas y Pardo Suizas en Maracay, Venezuela, *ALPA Mem.* **3:** 61.

14. Bodisco, V., Verde, O., y Wilcox, C. F., 1971, Producción y reproducción de un lote de ganado Pardo Suizo, *ALPA Mem.* **6:** 81.
15. Salazar, J. J., 1970, *Genetic and environmental factors affecting performance of three Holstein herds in Colombia,* Ph.D. dissertation, University of Florida, Gainesville.
16. Verde, O., 1973, Mejoramiento genético bajo condiciones tropicales, *in: Seminario sobre la producción de leche en Venezuela,* Consejo Nacional de Investigaciones Agrícolas, Caracas, 1973, pp. 23–38.

34

Fisheries Prospects for the Future—Freshwater and Marine*

John E. Bardach

Hawaii Institute of Marine Biology
University of Hawaii
Kaneohe, Hawaii

The successful nutrition research conducted at the Institute of Nutrition of Central America and Panama for the past 25 years has, understandably, not been greatly concerned with animal protein of aquatic provenience. It is fitting, however, that a future-oriented Anniversary Symposium also deal with this facet of man's protein supply, and therefore this chapter treats the production of fish and other aquatic animals, giving special emphasis to certain aspects of aquaculture and tropical capture fisheries, including a selective discussion of post-harvest technology.

Capture fisheries are akin to hunting; they take portions of the biomass of highly complex ecosystems while, ideally, restricting the take to a sustainable yield. Aquaculture in fresh, brackish, or salt water encompasses various levels of managerial manipulations resembling, in extreme cases, pure feedlot-like operations. With the exception of the environments of the latter, there are in the aquatic realm many natural feedback loops that can stand just so much distortion, by selective harvest or other events (e.g., pollution). They compose the food webs and also delimit and frame management concepts for both aquatic animal husbandry and capture fisheries.

Figure 1 (1) illustrates in schematic fashion, in a highly simplified manner, the multiple relations among primary producers, consumers, and decomposers that bring into being the small fraction of fixed carbon and nitrogen that is available to man in the form of animals large enough to be commensurate with

*Contribution no. 479, Hawaii Institute of Marine Biology.

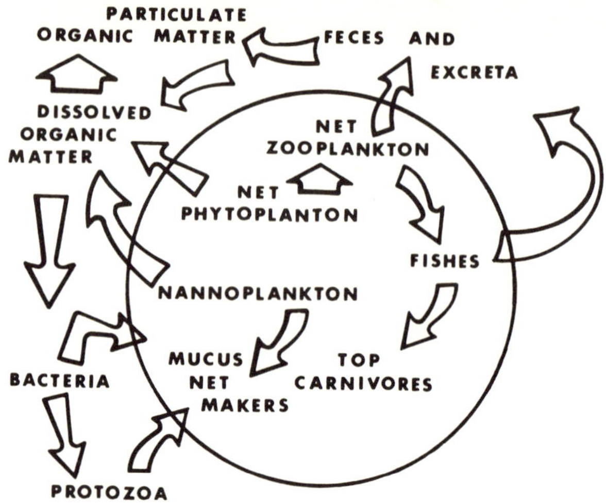

FIG. 1. The classical paradigm of the ocean's food web in simplified form is enclosed within the circle. More recently conceived pathways are outside the circle (after Pomeroy, reference 1).

his size and the nature of his gathering implements. To be noted here are the facts that—even in fertile subtropical coastal waters—between 70 and 75% of bound nitrogen is in the form of particulate and dissolved organic matter (2); nannoplanktonic photosynthesis greatly exceeds that of net planktonic algae and diatoms, which were customarily considered the base of the food chain; and respiration of microorganisms exceeds that of net plankton, often by a factor of 10. Thus, microorganisms would consume most of the energy made available by primary production (1). This need not necessarily mean that the useful harvest will be less than anticipated; in fact, under certain conditions as yet to be delineated properly, it may mean the contrary. If, for instance, assimilation efficiencies of protista and bacteria in the sea are high—as seems to be the case—and if part of their biomass finds its way into higher trophic levels, rather than representing a sink for CO_2, the channeling of energy, and therefore materials, into crustaceans and/or small fishes may indeed be more advantageous than was hitherto assumed in the rather simplistic food chain paradigm from algae to zooplankton to sardines, to larger fish—or even from zooplankton to whales.

Two prime indications for fisheries production follow from the emergence of a more complex aquatic foodchain: (a) Monospecies cropping is often wasteful, especially in bottom fisheries; (b) monospecies culture is expensive, requiring much control, environmental modification, and outside inputs; it is therefore frequently only marginally economical.

CAPTURE FISHERIES—INVENTORY

Tropical or near-tropical capture fisheries can be subsumed under three categories:

1. Truly pelagic stocks of large fish of high cash value per unit weight; that is, mainly tunas, which are taken with technologically advanced means, necessitating freezing and canning infrastructures. These fisheries are now dominated by the United States and Japan and, with the exception of one species, the skipjack tuna (*Euthynnus pelamis*) of which there probably exist unutilized stocks in the Pacific, they are either overfished or their take approaches sustained yield. Because of the high technology necessary for their utilization—in part stemming from the relatively large size and high mobility of the animals—input of medium to high technology will be necessary here, as in several other areas of promise, for an increase in aquatic protein production. Wider ranging boats will have to be developed in many regions and they will have to have ensured bait to attract and capture the fish as well as ice supplies to prevent spoilage. Such bait will often have to depend on baitfish culture of an appropriate species (e.g., *Poecilia vittata*), and with it the shaping of lures and chumming methods that tally with the bait, and perhaps also the elaboration of new bait-holding facilities (3).

2. Near- and inshore fisheries for demersal and shoaling surface stocks of intermediate unit size (jacks), gathered by small, often very small, capture units. In those tropical areas where there are better stock and yield estimates than in others, that is in the Sunda Shelf and South China Sea regions (4), additional potential catches of about three million metric tons are estimated. There are even larger, currently underused stocks in the Indian Ocean (4), and some regions of the western tropical Atlantic may also harbor unused stocks in this category, although less so than the South China Sea and the Indian Ocean.

3. Small, schooling fishes such as anchovies and sardines and other similar plankton filter feeders. Their prevalence is largely tied to areas of upwelling and not restricted to the tropics. These stocks are subject to occasional natural depressions caused by climatic and hence oceanographic events, the prediction of which still eludes near-term forecasting. Whatever the natural causes of the fluctuations of these shortlived lower trophic level stocks, they are prone to overfishing, particularly when an overcapitalized fishery is not curbed as early warnings appear of changes in fecundity and/or survival of the recruits into the fishery (5). They are, incidentally, the prime example of apparent inequities in food distribution to the protein-hungry of the world, inasmuch as they make up over 30% of the world fish catch (6), with the bulk thereof going into fish meal for animal feed in the richer nations. This is common knowledge, and unjust as one may find this state of affairs, changing it will be difficult for reasons well

beyond the biology of the fish and the means of gathering them. According to Gulland (4) and Marr (personal communication, 1974), in this realm of the small or intermediate-sized shoaling species, lies the greatest scope for expansion in the yield of capture fisheries, especially in certain areas of the tropics.

Many of these fish occur seasonally and need to be preserved in order to be usable. But even where they are more evenly distributed in time or place, more is needed than attention to increasing the catch. It was revealing to note the following consensus at the 16th Session of the Indo-Pacific Fisheries Council in Jakarta in November, 1974: "In much of the vast region served by this Council, little would be gained by a quick doubling of range and payload of traditional (small) fishing vessels, a feat certainly within technical reach. For, if the load of fish brought in by day-fishermen is often partly spoiled for lack of ice or because of slowness of vessel speed on return to port, only helping them to stay out two days instead of one would lead to twice the spoilage. Unless the management of all phases of the fishery can be changed to include preserving the harvest for local consumption, shoaling fish fisheries may be enlarged by massive extra-national efforts only to turn these surpluses once more into chicken feed for the world's rich."

After having mentioned some of the resource potentials that would permit increasing aquatic protein fare in the tropical regions, one should at least make reference to some resources that await utilization outside the tropics. Gulland (5) quotes 50 million metric tons (MMT) of krill as exploitable—this is less than whales consumed annually before they were decimated (7)—and at least 10 MMT, but probably far more, of squid; the former exist in the Antarctic and the latter mainly in the Atlantic, but squid also live in other parts of the world's seven seas. Large as these currently unused animal protein pools may be, they will require substantial research and development inputs that will most certainly be undertaken by technologically advanced nations. For krill utilization, for instance, detailed information is needed on the seasonal, diurnal, and depth distribution and density of aggregations of euphausid crustaceans (*Euphausia superba*) in the Antarctic. Upon this information, partly available now primarily from Japanese and Soviet investigations, will depend the choice of the most suitable capture methods, such as, for instance, trawling or pumping. Extraction of oils and carotenoids must be perfected, as will methods for dealing with the carapace of the crustaceans. These necessary initial steps will most likely mitigate against marketing krill as frozen shrimp, and suggest that peeling and comminution after initial boiling and/or properly integrated solvent extraction procedures may be the solution to krill preservation. Krill capture operations would, in a broad sense, require ship displacements comparable to those of Antarctic whaling, but would involve less hunting and probably cheaper catching methods than those for whales. One may therefore anticipate, once the research has been completed, that krill protein (presumably dehydrated or reconstituted and frozen) would be less costly than whale meat.

If 50 MMT of krill and some 10 MMT of squid are eventually harvestable, a rough doubling of present capture fishery yield will have been achieved. Conventional catches, the expansion potential of which was mentioned earlier, will likely add a comparable amount of, mainly, fish, but also some invertebrates, to species that may be gathered from the waters of the world. The caution applied to these projections must include mention of both increasing costs of fishing and heightened fishing efficiency resulting from more sophisticated technology that greatly increases dangers of overfishing, as well as pollution coming mainly from coastal sources, because about half of the world's fish catch comes from stocks tied to relatively nearshore marine areas (5).

AQUACULTURE

Within the clearly discernible limits of, and dangers to, the bounty of the waters, now minimally managed, but manageable, husbanding instead of capturing aquatic animals holds promise. Such husbandry is now most advanced in fresh and brackish water, but will eventually also be done in portions of the sea. The more intensive and large-scale such mariculture becomes, the more advanced will be the technology necessary to sustain it (8). It appears technically feasible to increase aquacultural yields in the world from their present level of over 5 MMT by at least a factor of six, probably by more, within several decades, if concerted efforts are made in this direction (9). Biotechnical breakthroughs are not as essential here initially as are dissemination of skills and attention to basic conceptual and economic constraints. Before discussing some aspects of these constraints, there is need for stressing similarities and differences between management and husbandry practices insofar as the aquatic realm is concerned, and to mention that animal aquaculture, although primarily producing human food, does not do so exclusively; baitfish production was already noted, and aquaculture-derived fish meal will be discussed.

First, the similarities: The properties of the aquatic food web already illustrated apply equally, in a general way, to a pond, a lagoon, a small lake, and portions of the sea. Even in a pond, which is a relatively closed ecosystem compared to the sea or a part of it, much of the bound carbon and nitrogen is present in "unusable" form. The primary difference is that, while the material and energy-flows through the ecosystems that are the bases of capture fisheries cannot yet be controlled, one attempts to control them in aquaculture. This control is directed to speed turnover and to add both nutrients and energy in the manipulation of the culture system, manipulations broadly analogous to production methods in agriculture.

Such accelerated addition of energy and nutrients, which can be further enhanced, although least so in the tropics, is achieved by raising temperatures (heated waste-water or sheltering). This should be performed in such a manner that one obtains the most output for the least additional inputs. These inputs are materials and labor for pond or enclosure construction, fertilizer, feed, fishing labor, and fuel, to name only the most obvious. It is evident, but not universally understood, probably because of the long acculturation to conceiving of fish as "free gifts" from nature, that most of the incentives for management in aquaculture lie in ownership or prolonged control (for example, by lease) over the production site and hence the harvest.

The most intensive aquaculture patterns are those employed in monoculture for single, often highly prized, species (shrimp, and to some extent, even trout and salmon). These rely—just like the U.S. maize production system so ably examined by Pimentel and co-workers (10)—on outside inputs from far and wide. An example is provided by Table I, which shows the distribution of items that enter into the cost of postlarval production on a farm of 40 ha (11) in the culture of Malaysian prawns (*Macrobrachium rosenbergii*), a promising monoculture luxury crop.

It is to be noted that Malaysian prawn farming, although a monoculture scheme, represents a level of aquaculture that relies only partially on direct feeding and is therefore semiextensive. Feed costs in intensive rainbow trout and yellowtail rearing approach or exceed 50% of the yearly running expenses of the farms (12). However, one can do aquaculture with less costly inputs for each unit of yield, even high yields per unit water surface or volume. This kind of aquaculture is well geared for, but need not be restricted to, the tropics; it can materially assist in satisfying the protein requirements of developing countries.

Some human cultures, for instance the Chinese, have achieved noteworthy success in working with nature to structure multiple feedback loops for the production of a substantial harvest per hectare. The practice, called polyculture, relies on the growing together of a number—as many as six species—of varying feeding types of fish (Figure 2) (9). One must note here that there are only two herbivores among them, not surprising if one remembers the natural aquatic bioproduction patterns described earlier. Evolution in the aquatic realm just did not lead to many bite-sized morsels that feed exclusively on plants, and fewer

Table I. Cost Distribution (in %) in Postlarval Production of *Macrobrachium rosenbergii* on a Farm of 40 Hectares

Labor	Management	Feed	Electricity and fuel	Juveniles	Miscellaneous (water, lease, repairs)
25	7.5	24	10	19.7	13.8

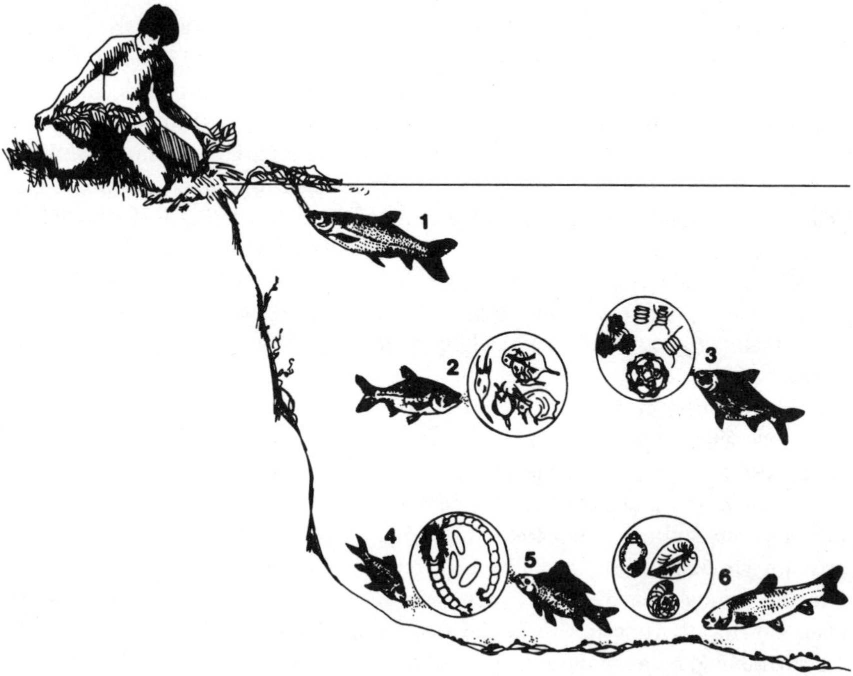

FIG. 2. Habitat and feeding niches of the principal species in classical Chinese carp culture. 1. Grass carp (*Ctenopharyngodon idellus*) feeding on vegetable tops. 2. Big head (*Aristichtys nobilis*) feeding on zooplankton in midwater. 3. Silver carp (*Hypophthalmichtys molitrix*) feeding on phytoplankton in midwater. 4. Mud carp (*Cirrhinus molitorella*) feeding on benthic animals and detritus, including grass carp feces. 5. Common carp (*Cyprinnus carpio*) feeding on benthic animals and detritus, including grass carp feces. 6. Black carp (*Mylopharyngodon piceus*) feeding on mollusks (from reference 9).

still that use large attached hydrophytes as their food. That is no obstacle, because aquatic herbivores are suitably utilized as members of a mixed feeding community; they often reingest the same food and, especially if they receive plant rations of terrestrial origin, they make nutrients available, through their metabolism, to the aquatic production chain. Welch (13) indicates that herbivores may have higher yield efficiencies than carnivores, and stresses that they may produce more flesh per unit of food available than certain carnivores do. Even then, their main virtue in the scheme lies in the fact that they are compatible in their niche occupation with several other harvestable animals that feed on various food web components (zooplankton, small mollusks, and worms, for example) not usable directly by man.

Polyculture is now practiced with a fair number of species besides those used by the Chinese. There are several compatible species of Indian carp yielding up to eight tons of fish per hectare (14), and in Israel, tilapia and carp together bring forth more fish flesh per hectare than either species reared in monoculture.

In polyculture–in contrast to monoculture–running costs have low feed and high labor components. There is, therefore, less competition for potential human foodstuffs than in the carnivore monoculture patterns (salmon, shrimp, or even catfish) of developed nations. For instance, the labor component in Chinese carp monoculture in Malaysia ranges from 36.5 to 38.2% of production costs, while in various polyculture farms in India, labor amounted to between 34 and 69% of production expenses. Feeds, in both examples described here, make up less than 5% of these costs, most often fluctuating between 1 and 3% (14). The remainder goes mostly to stocking materials and/or rental, but can include fertilizer also.

Construction costs, that is, initial expenses that have to be amortized, are highly variable, depending on size of farm unit, nature of soil, location of the farm, cost of labor and/or equipment, and the like; they have not been assessed satisfactorily in those economic appraisals that are available, but one important aspect of aquaculture ought to be stressed in connection with them: In a general way, the growing of fish can be likened to intensive, several-level chicken rearing, but the animals need neither pens nor horizontal support. Instead, special management attention has to be devoted to sanitation, inasmuch as the animals are surrounded by a medium through which disease and parasite transfer is easier than in air, where oxygen supply may be limited, and in which potentially growth-inhibiting products of metabolism surround the animals very intimately indeed.

Polyculture has developed, so far, most prominently with Asian species, but the family *Cichlidae,* to which tilapia belong, is preponderant in Africa and Latin America, and has numerous species of different feeding types that are relatively easy to breed and that tolerate brackish water conditions. Various experiments have been performed to test their suitability for culture either by using two or more species of this family, or by rearing them with other species such as common carp, mullet, or even catfish (Tables I and II in Chapter 18 of reference 9). Several viable polyculture patterns could be developed primarily with cichlids for the Central and South American tropics.

Needless to say, successful polyculture schemes eventually rely on control of breeding; such control has been achieved with Asian polyculture species and is possible with cichlids, even to achieving hybrid vigor or the production of male or sterile hybrids (9). The latter is of advantage if the species is highly prolific and breeds continuously, potentially leading to the prevalence of a very large number of runts.

Further to be noted is that ease of management, under domestication, of an aquacultural species is roughly commensurate, among other factors, with the size of the eggs (and consequently of the larvae) of the species in question. Also important are breeding habits such as nestguarding (tilapia and catfish), attachment of eggs (carp), or egg burial (trout and salmon).

It is thus not surprising that domesticated aquaculture species to date have these breeding habits. Others are barely beginning to yield to domestication and thus to selective breeding and strain selection. Most marine species and some freshwater species have very small eggs with a negative correlation between the number of eggs produced and increasing egg size. Mariculture developments have been held back by this simple fact and its implication; namely, assuring the survival of the tiny larvae in a planktonic environment that is difficult to reproduce under controlled conditions, as is shown in Table II (8).

If the eggs are very small and very numerous, however, and give rise after a relatively short planktonic life to sessile juveniles and adults, as is the case with bivalve mollusks such as mussels and oysters, they demand in their management less attention to care for larval survival than for larval capture by adequately fashioned and judiciously placed objects; mariculture with bivalves has a long tradition and can be highly successful (9).

If one were to undertake the development of indigenous polyculture schemes for Latin America and Africa, it would be advisable to perform the necessary mission-oriented research at certain key sites serving more than one country. Central America, especially, with its several relatively similar ecological patterns and small national territories, would benefit from such a regional aquaculture development scheme. As a venture of this kind would require several years of applied research, why not transfer already developed polyculture biotechnologies of Indian or Chinese carp, lock stock and barrel? Time may be saved by this procedure, but several facts favor native polyculture, especially of cichlids: breeding biotechnologies are not likely to present technical difficulties; local taste preference would presumably favor local fish; and although very occasionally overrated in the potential damage they do, new species have, more often than not, led to ecological disequilibration, including attendant problems of the inadvertent introduction of diseases and parasites potentially noxious to the native, noncultured fauna.

Whether or not indigenous polyculture systems will be developed or estab-

Table II. Relationship of Egg Size to Mass Culture of Fishes[a]

Species	Egg diameter (mm)	Larval length (mm)	Yolk usage (days)	Mass culture
Salmon	4–5.0	25.0	21–60	Achieved
Trout	4.0	20.0	21–50	Achieved
Plaice	2.0	6.5	5–7	Achieved
Dover sole	2.0	6.0	5–7	Achieved
Turbot	1.0	3.0	3–5	Difficult
Mullet	0.9	2.4	3–5	Difficult
Rabbitfish	0.5	2.0	2–4	Difficult

[a]Source: Reference 8, p. 185.

lished ones transferred, additional appurtenances of several-species animal husbandry deserve mention:

1. Ponds below a certain minimum size are inefficient because sufficient photosynthesis must occur in the enclosure to support certain food organisms and at least one of the cultured fish species.

2. In addition, most tropical regions have dry and wet seasons and water conservation may be important; therefore, water flow must balance residence time.

3. The several species, each with their peculiar feeding and spatial distribution patterns, cannot be crowded lest they suffer from nocturnal oxygen deficiencies and/or the effects of accumulating toxic wastes, not to mention disease and parasite transmittal that is facilitated by crowding. Thus, polyculture ponds of less than 1/5 ha size are inadvisable unless they are aerated by forced air or, perhaps, by wind-driven splashing recirculation devices.

Conversely, there is also an upper size limit for enclosures or ponds beyond which it becomes less and less efficient to perform the various labor-intensive management operations, including harvesting, even with machinery; fish husbandry then gives way to mere organized gathering. The size at which ponds become lakes–in this sense–is difficult to determine. Suffice it to say that ponds of 1/4 to 10 hectares have been found successful in various aquaculture systems, and that several small or medium-sized ones are more efficient than a few larger enclosures, especially under intensive polyculture.

4. Whatever the size of polyculture ponds, they have to be fertilized. Various inorganic fertilizers have been used, but the application of human and/or animal organic wastes to the ponds needs special mention because it saves a portion, and occasionally all, of a category of extraneous inputs that threaten to become both more scarce and expensive. Such waste recycling in ponds is widely used in the Orient, from simple privies placed over the ponds to more elaborate combinations of pigpens built over fishponds with the enriched water further used in market gardening. Under very special conditions of permitting sewage to enter shallow streams, annual fish production of 50 kg per square meter of stream surface has been achieved. The success, here, was due to peculiar bottom conditions promoting high growth of microbes and bloodworms in the sandy silt, facilitating cage culture that permitted the fish to engage in foraging on the bottom (9). The health caveats implied involve cooking and the discard of certain organs of the fish; often considerable inputs are needed through extension efforts from food science and community health workers.

As already mentioned, aquaculture need not be restricted to producing food directly; methods are being developed, based on the premise that livestock wastes are a biological resource that can be recycled into terrestrial or aquatic livestock feeds, again stressing a mutually advantageous relation between land and water animal husbandry.

Dried poultry waste can be incorporated into fish feeds directly (15), or the excreta can be recycled through several steps of bioconversion, as illustrated schematically in Figure 3. This process, as one of several possible such schemes, works as follows:

1. Raw wastes are collected at the site of production and transported to the location of the recycling operation.

2. Waste slurry is transferred to an aerobic digester that acts more as a nutrient storage reservoir than as a means to stabilize the waste thoroughly. The aerobic digester will be designed for less than complete digestion, which reduces the size and capital investment necessary because the retention time will rarely exceed 24 hours.

3. Mixed liquor-suspended solids are pumped continuously from the aerobic digester to a clarifier or tube settler, where the solid and liquid fractions are separated.

4. The solid fraction is fed directly to a detritus-feeding fish through a demand feeder (some species of tilapia, e.g., *T. aurea,* appear well suited).

5. Fish feces are recycled, with some wastage to prevent excessive buildup of solids in the digester.

6. By means of photosynthesis, the inorganic nutrients are stripped from the liquid supernatant of the mixed liquid-suspended solids in an algae pond.

7. Oxygen-rich algal pond water is recycled as a flushing medium for the detritus-feeding fish tank.

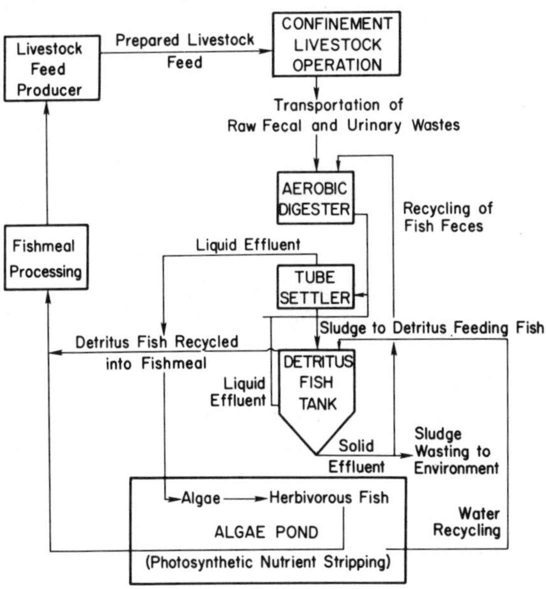

FIG. 3. Schematic representation of the animal waste recycling system. (After D. Crear, A. Cattell, R. Young, G. Dugan, and J. Bardach, 1975, Photosynthetic recycling of livestock wastes, Office of Research Admin., University of Hawaii, unpublished).

8. The fish meal feedstuffs produced are harvested, processed, and sold. Application of the scheme to sewage is possible, provided the latter is not contaminated with high technology-related chemicals (insecticides, herbicides, and the like).

While such recycling is not as simple or direct as the aforementioned techniques of direct sewage use in fish polyculture in Asia, it has some appurtenances of scale economies and may be very applicable where it is of the essence to store and/or transport the product of biological recycling. In any case, the amounts of protein-rich biomass that can be produced by organic waste recycling are impressive: Calculations from data in the literature, as well as from pilot tests at our laboratory, on nitrogen excretion by hens and pigs indicate that the annual waste of 10,000 hens, for instance, or 500 hogs (for practicality of waste handling, animals should be in one site) could optimally be turned into at least 60 tons of fish meal per year. It ought to be noted that the scheme relies on harvesting the fish at the best stage of their food conversion, that is, as small animals, thereby also easing their transformation into meal. To grow these same fishes on organic wastes to large size, consumable by man, would be possible, but it would require far larger water volumes than the fish meal scheme that utilizes small fishes and, incidentally, eliminates public health problems.

The tending and rearing of certain marine mollusks that produce a large biomass per unit input of labor will round out this treatment of aquaculture. These bivalves, most prominent among them oysters, rely on the appurtenances of open systems for their successful culture. Once the animals have settled (see the passage on larval rearing, above), food reaches them by advection, be that by tides or, in certain cases, by very special oyster-rearing practices (16): producing plankton and leading it past the sessile filter feeders. Oysters, clams, and mussels, then, require primary and secondary production, in an ecological sense, of far larger water masses than those that surround the animals at any moment in time. Yet, even though oysters occur quite copiously in the tropics, tropical oyster culture lags far behind that in the temperate zones, in part because knowledge of the biology of tropical oyster species also lags behind such knowledge in the temperate zone. Also, a not inconsiderable obstacle to culturing tropical mollusks intensively is that they are even harder to preserve than other aquatic animals. Close proximity of potential culture sites to places of consumption or fast means of transportation to them is therefore important when mollusk rearing in the tropics is being considered for the consumption of these shellfish in their fresh state.

POSTHARVEST TECHNOLOGY

While mollusks may spoil faster than many fish, all aquatic animals spoil easily and man, the fish-hunter and gatherer, has invented methods of fish saving—now called postharvest technology—for at least as long as there are records of fish preservation. It is pertinent to examine some of these from such vantage points as energy requirements and, for the most part connected thereto, levels of technology, minimal size of efficient operations, and possibilities for transfer of various methods from one region of the globe to another.

Aside from the quick and easy spoilage to which fish are prone, there are several others reasons for singling out postharvest technology in a future-oriented treatment of fisheries: (a) Fish handling is generally wasteful, especially in the tropics, shrimp fisheries being a very particular case in point. In most shrimping operations, only the shrimp are retained and the remainder of the trawl content—a volume of various fish three to four times that of the crustaceans—is dumped overboard. (b) The development of new fisheries from currently underutilized stocks is likely to be high in energy inputs, and developed fisheries produce less and less per unit of effort applied (17). Thus, fullest possible utilization of what is caught, from economic and ecological perspectives, seems to be in the interest of nations, fishermen, and consumers alike.

Fish-saving methods can be categorized from various points of view, but two principal directions are clearly apparent, both encompassing varying levels of technology and energy inputs: (a) Fish-saving processes that do not appreciably, or only partially, reduce the water content of fish, although some may transform the shape and even the taste of what was originally landed. Examples here are: Freezing (whole fish or fillets), or even as reconstituted products such as burgers or sticks made from the flesh of species of low market value for fresh consumption, fish sausages, fresh iced fish—unfortunately a vanishing retail commodity, certainly in the United States—irradiated fish, canned fish, and salted, smoked, and pickled as well as fermented and ensilaged fish. (b) Fish subjected to reduction, that is, the removal of most of their water content to enhance storage and transportation characteristics of the product. Into this category fall freeze-dehydrated fish, most prominently fish meal, and also fish protein concentrate and dried fish.

It may bear stressing that the term *fish* used here represents all aquatic animals harvested or tended, and that an attempt was made to list methods, broadly, by decreasing apparent energy inputs. Also pertinent is the trend in world fish catch utilization to more freezing and more reduction; from 1960 to 1970, freezing increased from 9 to 14% of the catch, at the expense of fresh use, and reduction from 19 to 37%, enabling commercial exploitation of small species not conveniently used for direct human consumption (18). Both freezing and keeping fish frozen, as well as their industrial reduction, require relatively large amounts of nonrenewable energy compared to some other possible methods of fish-saving, but in view of increasing quests for animal protein by the world's rich both for food and feed, the trend is likely to continue for some time.

When one discusses fish consumption and methods of saving fish, one must remember that taste for fish, and what men have made of them, are highly parochial: A French cultural attaché blanched at having to eat–for diplomatic reasons–fermented fish in floccular form at a Cambodian state dinner, yet he had recently ordered well-ripened Camembert cheese from Paris through the good offices of an Air France pilot, to be delivered on the latter's next stopover in Phnom Penh. Both are fermented proteins of animal origin, but they smell rather different. Tastes for fresh fish are culture-bound also: While mullet demand a fair price in Asia, one can hardly sell them in the U.S. Gulf states, where they abound. Raw tuna, an acknowledged Japanese delicacy, is relished by few Westerners.

Keeping foremost in mind constraints of regional tastes, and levels of technology, what can be done to save more fish, more efficiently, throughout the world? (Some bias will, inevitably, creep into the following treatment, as it must when one person deals, in a very limited space, with a field in which volumes and thousands of technical papers have been written).

Before looking at some aspects of fish meal and fish protein concentrate manufacture and utilization, one must be aware of the desirability and the already perceivable trend to use reduced fish increasingly for direct human, rather than for animal, consumption (15). Yet some instances exist where new fish meal manufacture seems possible, while making a protein additive for human fare is less feasible, at least in the near to medium term. One such example, already alluded to, is the use of trash fish from shrimping. The world catch of shrimp is over a million metric tons (19). Assuming a ratio of only three tons of trash fish to one ton of shrimp (probably an underestimate, but pertinent statistics are spotty), the fish flesh theoretically available is equivalent to about a third of the sustained yield of the Peruvian anchovy fishery when the latter is in a healthy state. Often remoteness of shrimp grounds mitigates, economically, against trash fish elaboration, but in some instances it seems possible.

Along the Pacific coasts of Mexico and Central America, shrimping operations now yield about 100,000 MT annually (H. Schafer-Escamilla, Guaymas, Mexico, personal communication, 1974), and many of these fisheries are not located very far from shore. If the crew were remunerated to perform the simple task of saving the fish, as outlined below, considering that the sorting is done as a routine operation before the shrimp are placed in the hold, the above nations may acquire 300,000 MT, at least, of a source for animal feed supplement.

The following scheme is envisaged: The fish are shoveled into inflatable rafts or tough plastic bags with an admixture of one volume percent of $Na_2S_2O_5$, commercially available as sodium bisulfite ($NaHSO_3$), which oxidizes or ferments to the sulfate, and releases gaseous SO_2. Dilute sulfuric acid would also be usable here, but in view of shipboard handling, the salt seems preferable. The gas generated would also help to float the parcels if the plastic bag method is used. Rafts or bags would be fitted with a radio signal emitter like those used for life boats or certain life vests or rafts. Bacteriostasis would be effective for two weeks at least (20) and permit a collecting vessel to gather the floats and convey them to a fish meal plant strategically located on the shore in relation to the deployment of the shrimping fleets.

Such a plant could well be operated jointly by the shrimp industries of the nations involved, or a separate factory could mount the servicing organization that buys the trash fish, pays the small remuneration to the shrimp crews to fill the floating collectors with fish, supplies them with plastic bags or inflatable rafts, and operates the collection vessel(s). If such a plant were located in Panama, SO_2-stabilized raw material for fish meal manufacture could also be derived from Atlantic tropical shrimp grounds, thus evening out, to some extent, whatever seasonal variations of supply exist because there are definite shrimping seasons along the Pacific coast of Mexico and Central America. Another possibility is the location of the rendering plant on a large barge or floating platform, as seaworthy designs for such floating bases are well worked out (21). One would place this base according to the movements of the shrimpers, thus shortening the collecting trips and achieving fuel savings. The platform would be sufficiently mobile to be towed to a safe harbor when weather conditions so indicate. Preliminary inquiries suggest that the respective shrimping seasons are sufficiently long to sustain the scheme proposed here.

The example just given intimated that there are several components for minimal economies of scale in industrial fish meal manufacture predicated on amount and steadiness of supply, season, and similar factors. Yet many instances of fish gluts exist where myriads of small fish are available for too short a time, in too small, though considerable, quantities, or in too remote a location to mount an industrial effort to transform them. Such is the case, for instance, in the postmonsoon flood periods in Southeast Asia. These fish need not be lost, because simple methods observed by the writer exist for their use. They are seined or entrapped by dikes and dams, then about 50% of their moisture is extruded by the following simple procedure: On an elevated cement slab with a gutter from which to collect the moisture pressed out of the fish (yielding a kind of stickwater to be used in pig feed), one has a cylinder fashioned out of bamboo fencing, with a post in the middle and a wooden cover through which the post protrudes, but which fits inside the circular fence. The post has a wide screw thread with a rotating horizontal shaft so that pressure can be applied on the cover for extruding the water. Next, the half-dried small fishes are spread on elevated bamboo mats permitting air circulation from below, and they are completely sun-dried in a few hours. They are then shredded into small flakes in a hand-driven shredder of simplest construction, to be turned into animal feed admixtures. Their proximate composition varies somewhat, depending on the species composition of the catch, but in Cambodia such "backyard fish meal" not only helped to reduce costs of turkey and swine production, but permitted the local upgrading of animal husbandry (R. Lafont, personal communication, 1959).

More sophisticated reduction methods that stabilize fish for human consumption hold promise on a broader scale. They require a steady supply of cheap fish and they also rely on drying after several steps of protein isolation or extraction. Therefore, research has been devoted to stockpiling; sulfur dioxide-induced stabilization has proved effective for several weeks; predrying at sea has been advocated (20), as has the use of cooked, stabilized fishmeal press cake as base material for FPC manufacture (22). For the initial reduction steps, plant-derived proteolytic enzymes proved variously effective, as did mammalian digestive enzymes (23). It appears, albeit from small-scale experiments, as if the use of stabilized bacterial enzymes, together with the fishes' native enzymes, could lead to commercially viable FPC production based on biological processes. However, the bulk of the work to date on fish protein concentrates (23) and whatever successes have been achieved are based on solvent extraction methods.

Because this book contains a contribution where technical and economic aspects of FPC are treated, and a book has been published on the subject (24), it will be given short shrift here; but certain aspects of FPC will be discussed.

Whatever the agent of reduction–solvent or enzyme–FPC is a food additive; in nations with ample protein, some of it may serve purposes other than supplying basic nutrition. It can be used as material for binding, blending, and the like (25), after further processing into so-called protein isolates. Where animal protein is scarce, it must somehow find its way into the staple foods or daily fare.

FPC advocates would like to see it mixed in bread, pasta, tortillas, soups, and crackers (26). Although such would be its ideal use, knowing the lack of centralized distribution facilities in developing countries, one foresees considerable difficulties in bringing FPC to the locations where it would count. In fact, as much or more ingenuity (although of a different kind) may well be needed to solve this latter problem as it took to make FPC tasteless and odorless. Obviously, removal of a slight remaining taint of fish after most of the extraction has been done increases the cost of the product, and probably its shelf life. It may be that a slightly fishy FPC would be more easily accepted than a completely bland product in some parts of the developing world. With the former, one may gain on the swing (in cost) what one loses on the roundabout (in perhaps not-so-essential purity). It is pertinent to note from pound by pound comparisons of costs for refining soy and fish proteins (25) that *fishmeal* contains about a third more protein than *soy flour* and yet costs less. The *bland white FPC,* still containing about 10% more protein, costs about 25% more to make than *soy concentrate.* The continuing research aim for FPC clearly ought to be to arrive at the simplest initial treatment and minimal refinement necessary that still permit preparation of a sanitary product, acceptable in a certain culture at the lowest possible cost.

Such was, in fact, the rationale underlying the development of one of the first FPC manufacturing processes. Nevertheless, FPC has so far not lived up to its theoretical promise for those most in need of protein. The reasons for this remain to be evaluated. Possible causes are: the vagaries of fish supplies; the cost of the processes–mainly the solvent materials; its Western origin; the resistance of fishermen who saw little profit in supplying the raw material; some difficult to explain reactions against it (now past) in certain U.S. Government quarters (27); perhaps some unforeseen competition with other animal products (20); or indeed the very difficult problems in its distribution. Whatever the verdict, FPC may still help in the transition from feeding fish to livestock to providing fish for people.

One can obviously learn something about the distribution of protein concentrates from the Incaparina story, and this is what some FPC researchers seem to have done by compounding a spray-dried powder from a 4% FPC, 3% fat, 10% carbohydrate, 0.2% sodium citrate, 0.3% carrageenan, and 82.5% water base. The stable powder, which lends itself to easier distribution, can be mixed in water to prepare a beverage, and further taste modifications (chocolate, fruit, or other flavors) are easily accomplished (26).

Unfortunately, no information is supplied about the economics of manufacturing such a beverage. Even if FPC prices are a somewhat unknown quantity, with one source in 1973 indicating a production cost of between 70 and 85 cents/kg, while Nabisco-Astra now wholesales its FPC product for $1.50/kg (E. Levin, personal communication, 1974), one might have bracketed the costs of the beverage by assuming a high, versus a low, cost for the raw materials. Knowing the reasonably universal acceptance of sweet foods and drinks, especially by children, the development of sweet drinks with FPC as the crucial ingredient is clearly one, albeit limited, way to circumvent the difficult problem of incorporating a food additive into staple foodstuffs in societies having no means for controlled additions.

There are also promising processes for technology transfer among the fish-saving techniques that retain the moisture in the flesh. One is the making of fish cake or sausage based on the manufacturing techniques for "Kamaboko," an elastic heat-pasteurized fish cake (28), but with flavor, texture, and appearance so modified as to simulate local foodstuffs. The making of fish sausages–or cakes–is labor-intensive and based, in the main, on separation of flesh from skin and bones of the fish by means of a simple machine (29) plus addition of various fillers. Flavor and texture can be adjusted to local culinary preferences as indicated, and small towns, if not villages, can become manufacturing sites. Inasmuch as Kamaboko was traditionally made in Japan even in the 15th century, the various manipulations in the process may be amenable to demechanization, if indicated. The fish must be fresh, and chilling is desirable for the mixing phases; steaming, broiling, or deep-fat frying accomplishes pasteurization, and the product may remain unrefrigerated, but cool, on the shelf from one to several weeks.

All fish-saving methods mentioned so far are predicated on preventing bacterial decomposition. Yet, there is a highly populous part of the tropics where methods prevail for dealing with the seasonal glut of fishes through harnessing live bacteria. These are the fish sauces and pastes of Southeast Asia, where rice is the staple, begging for a tasty condiment. In this climate, it rains frequently, firewood is scarce, and sun-drying is possible only under particular circumstances. These conditions are, most probably, related to the origin of primitive fermentation methods for preserving the bounty of the waters. The disadvantages of fish sauces and pastes are first, saltiness (in the case of sauces especially), and second, a combination of smell and taste that is highly culture-bound. Still, research into the chemistry of their manufacture might, with profit, be updated from colonial times, for it has been stated (30) that "the chemical composition of the intermediate and end products in fish pastes and sauces is for the most part *terra incognita.* Our knowledge of the beneficial influence of added carbohydrate (rice and other cereals, sugar, bran, etc.) and other materials on the properties and quality of pastes and sauces is equally deficient. Flavor problems have hardly been investigated at all. Studies in the fields of biochemistry and microbiology could do much, however, to clarify the numerous problems and underlying biochemical reactions. They might well lead to better understanding and to more standardized methods of fish preservation in this part of the world, resulting in higher quality products of better keeping capacity in the tropical climate."

A Southeast Asian regional effort for development of an improved fisheries postharvest technology, without refrigeration, is based on similar considerations. In fact, such studies could well enhance protein nitrogen yields, render taste and smell more bland, and thus become suitable for the taste preferences of other cultures, and add a set of transferable processes to the many techniques of fish saving.

FINDINGS

For the future, where numerous fisheries are threatened by pollution, and for the present, where the activities of fish catching and fish distribution are wasteful, attention to fish saving–postharvest technology–may help to augment the presence of fish proteins, or their derivatives, on the table as much as would the development of new fisheries.

Substantial expansion possibilities exist for sea fisheries production in the tropics, but the costs of such expansions are likely to be high and the developments may well benefit the richer rather than the poorer nations. Therefore, in the planning for fisheries expansion, primary attention should be devoted to the attainment of benefits for those most in need from a nutritional point of view.

Aquaculture, while not a panacea, holds substantial promise for local production of high-grade animal protein fare. However, it is not generally recognized that planning with nature (polyculture) is more sound ecologically, and cheaper, considering weight attained per input of effort, than high technology requiring attempts at greater yields through monoculture. (In that sense, aquaculture is a very peculiar "kettle of fish").

CONCLUSION

This chapter deals mainly, if selectively, with aquaculture and postharvest technology in relation to future enhancement of aquatic animal protein supplies. The two topics may seem strange bedfellows, but their juxtaposition has a purpose: In many developing countries, and even in developed ones, various processes of fisheries—from production through elaboration to distribution of fish or fish-derived commodities—are either uncoordinated or, worse still, placed under administrative management of entities that work in isolation, or are so conceived that best possible nutritional benefits are not attained.

Aquaculture, in enclosures, for instance, should be considered as a part of agriculture, while one administrative structure, although not necessarily one department, should have purview over the fate of the fish from landing to consumption by the consumer. Comparable problems beset other food production and rendering or manufacturing processes, but they are particularly pronounced in fisheries. It would transcend the framework of this chapter to discuss or speculate on various ways to remedy these dysfunctions; it must suffice here to point to them as one more example of organizational deficiencies that could be alleviated by some deviation from tradition.

Remedies are, perhaps, not as hard to come by as one might think, even in the face of bureaucratic patterns that have accentuated distances among various administrative responsibilities. Outside catalysts usually help, and one example must suffice here: In Indonesia, fisheries credits are administered by public agencies that oversee certain finance institutions and cooperatives; technical development is spearheaded by fisheries agencies and by universities; laws and ordinances are promulgated by provincial administrations; and land/water interface problems, like erosion and the silting-in of shore installations, including fishponds, are under a forestry unit, while the marketing of fish and their transportation are under different agencies still. Above it all hovers the Ministry of Planning. Rarely, if ever, have technicians and expert managers with responsible positions in these various units all talked to one another in one place until

1973. The occasion was a relatively loosely structured, but well-run, artisanal fisheries workshop that united representatives from most of the entities listed above. They discovered in a truly meaningful way that they had been chiseling away on many facets of the same stone all along. The credit for the organization of the workshop—presumably to be repeated at intervals—goes to Indonesia's energetic Director of Fisheries, to the personnel of the Agricultural Development Council in Indonesia, to the Indonesian Institute of Sciences (LIPI), and to various university participants.

True, Indonesia is one of the larger nations in need of such innovations, and it is easier to conceive of them on a national than on a regional basis, but for smaller nations adjacent to one another, e.g., the Caribbean and Central America, the regional mode is surely one to be considered. INCAP has pointed the way for regional cooperation in nutrition research. There is good rationale—small coastal strips, similarities in geography and ecology, and broadly comparable levels of technological competence—to advocate the formation of a regional fisheries research and development organization that would encompass competence in stock management and technology of coastal sea fisheries as well as postharvest technology. The organization would promote the involvement of agriculture departments with aquaculture, while interfacing the nutrition-oriented programs. At this time, the initiative for the formation of such an entity should come from one or several of the Central American nations; involvement of international organizations and foundations will follow.

Another fertile ground for national initiatives turning into regional ones lies in the political realm. The United Nations Conferences on the Law of the Sea at Caracas and at Geneva, although ending without overt agreements, have clearly shown the trend, on the part of developing nations, to claim larger portions of marine real estate than most have claimed until now. Such matters are outside the purview of direct food technology or even fisheries biology and technology, but lack of attention to them can make technologically based developments come to nought; this is why a discussion such as this should end by giving attention to them also.

Aside from managerial and operational capabilities for wide-belt ocean management, lacking in many nations, thereby inviting formation of "Neo-Hanseatic Leagues" by technologically advanced nations, it is necessary to stress the obvious disregard of man-made boundaries by marine creatures. Thus, many neighbor nations will have to manage their resources on a binational or regional basis. International technical councils currently operating under U.N. auspices, such as the Indo-Pacific Fisheries Council, seem inadequate to serve as rallying points for the resolution of joint management problems with economic and political emphasis. Single species bi- or multinational commissions, such as the International Tropical Tuna Commission and the International Salmon and Halibut Commissions, are better models, but it is easier to achieve joint management in a single-species fishery than in one comprising many species.

If coastal nation sovereignty of one kind or another is the clearly perceivable trend, worldwide, and if—as seems likely—no international regime can be developed to deal with fisheries, regional consultations should be initiated with the goal of regional resource management. It goes without saying that scientists, economists, and politicians should participate, and that the consultations should begin soon lest positions harden into stances incompatible with the conditions of the living world.

Some organizational umbrellas exist with sufficient economic and/or political orientation to serve as a forum for these consultations, at least in the beginning, until regional sea commissions can stand on their own feet. There is, for instance, ASEAN (The Association of Southeast Asian Nations), the OAS (Organization of American States), the latter with appropriate subdivisions, and there are United Nations regional fisheries commissions, possibly with their own fact-finding organizations also to be developed. It matters less which of these organizations, if any, will serve as the rallying implement for consultation than that one or another nation within a region takes the lead as it sees, out of enlightened self-interest, that the world of economics and that of ecology are one.

In this one world, largely covered by water, there exist, as has been discussed, opportunities for obtaining substantial nutritional benefits from certain parts of the hydrosphere. Their attainment is predicated on development of some new techniques and on the transfer of proven old techniques, and on more or less substantial modifications of them. Above all, it must be stressed that the days of man as a hunter of fish are coming to an end. In his place must come the sea estate manager of living resources and the fish husbandry man with new, and one hopes not necessarily complex, technologies. As technologies are applied by people who will themselves change as they apply them, the entire realm of aquatic resources development, the transfer and change of techniques, will require attention simultaneously to social, cultural, and political changes in turn, allowing those on the technical side to be effective; technology alone is not enough.

REFERENCES

1. Pomeroy, L., 1974, The ocean's food web, a changing paradigm, *BioSci.* **24:** 499
2. Caperon, J., 1975, A trophic level ecosystem model analysis of the plankton community in a shallow-water subtropical estuarine embayment, *Estuarine research, Vol. 1; chemistry, biology and the estuarine system,* Academic Press, New York, San Francisco, London, pp. 691–709.
3. Herrick, S., and Baldwin, W., 1975, The commercial production of topminnows, University of Hawaii Sea Grant Advisory Report, UNIHI-SEAGRANT-AR-7502: 18 pp.
4. Menasveta, D., Shindo, S., and Chullasorn, S., 1973, Pelagic fishery resources of the

South China Sea and prospects for their development, FAO/UNDP,SCS/DEV/73/6, 68 pp.

Aoyama, T., 1973, The demersal fish stocks and fisheries of the South China Sea, FAO/UNDP, SCS/DEV/73/3, 80 pp.

Gulland, J. (ed), 1970, *The fish resources of the ocean,* FAO Fisheries Technical Paper No. 97, 425 pp.

5. Murphy, G., 1974, Clupeoids, Chap. 3 *in: Fish population dynamics,* J. Gulland (ed.), Wiley Interscience, London, New York, p. 49.
6. Food and Agriculture Organization Yearbook of Fisheries Statistics for 1971, 33 (1973).
7. Moiseev, P., 1970, Some aspects of the commercial use of krill resources of the Antarctic seas, *in: Antarctic ecology,* M. W. Holdgate (ed.), Academic Press, London, p. 197.
8. Hanson, J. (ed.), 1974, *Open sea mariculture,* Dowden, Hutchinson & Ross, Stroudsburg, Pennsylvania, Chaps. 1 and 8.
9. Bardach, J., Ryther, J., and McLarney, W., 1972, *Aquaculture,* Wiley Interscience, John Wiley & Sons, New York, Chaps. 3 and 36.
10. Pimentel, D., Hurd, L., Bellotti, A., Forster, M., Oka, I., Sholes, O., and Whitman, R., 1973, Food production and the energy crisis, *Science* **182:** 443.
11. Shang, Y., 1974, Economic Feasibility of Fresh Water Prawn Farming in Hawaii, UNIHI-SEAGRANT-AR-74-05, 49 pp.
12. MacCrimmon, H., Stewart, J., and Brett, J., 1974, *Bull. Fish. Res. Board. Can.,* Vol. 188, 84 pp.
13. Welch, H., 1968, Relationships between assimilation efficiencies and growth efficiencies for aquatic consumers, *Ecology* **49:** 755.
14. Shang, Y., 1973, Comparison of the economic potential of aquaculture, land animal husbandry and ocean fisheries: The case of Taiwan, *Aquaculture* **2:** 187.

    Report of the Working Party on Aquaculture and Environment, G. D. Waugh, Chmn., Indo-Pacific Fish. Council, 1974, IPFC Doc. 74/5.
15. Fowler, J., and Lock, J., 1974, Inclusion of dried poultry waste as a feed ingredient in catfish rations, *Feedstuffs* **46:** 36.
16. Ryther, J., Dunstan, W., Tenore, K., and Huguenin, J., 1972, Controlled eutrophication–increasing food production from the sea by recycling human wastes, *BioSci.* **22:** 144.
17. Slesser, M., 1974, Energy analysis in technology assessment, *Technol. Assessment* **2:** 201, Gordon and Breach, London.
18. Food and Agriculture Organization Dept. of Fisheries, Fishery Development for the Future, PI/F2865/E/10.74/1/5000, Rome.
19. Peckham, C., and Patterson, P., 1974, International trade–tuna, shrimp, crab, fish meal, groundfish, IOFC/DEV/74/40, 199 pp.
20. Levin, E., 1973, *Fish protein concentrate (FPC),* Stipes Publishing, Champaign, Illinois, 38 pp.
21. Seidl, L., 1975, Limits of achievable motionlessness of large floating platforms, *in: Symposium for Seaward Advancement of Industrial Society, Dec. 2, 1974, Mar. Technol. Soc. J.* **9** (3): 12/13.
22. Pelroy, G., Spinelli, J., Miller, R., Wieg, D., and Lehman, L., 1974, Stabilized presscake for FPC manufacture, *Food Technol.* **28:** 64.
23. Knobl, G., Jr., Stillings, B., Fox, W., and Hale, M., 1971, Fish protein concentrate, *Commer. Fish. Rev.* **33:** 54.
24. Tannenbaum, S., 1975, Production and use of protein concentrates, *in: Nutrition and*

agricultural development–significance and potential for the tropics, N. S. Scrimshaw and M. Béhar (eds.), Plenum, New York, pp. 473–484.

Crutchfield, J. A., and Deacon, R., 1974, The economics of fish protein concentrate, *in: The economics, marketing, and technology of fish protein concentrate,* S. R. Tannenbaum, B. R. Stillings, and N. S. Scrimshaw (eds.), M.I.T. Press, Cambridge, Massachusetts, p. 355.

25. Spinelli, J., Groninger, H., Jr., and Koury, B., 1973, Preparation and properties of chemically and enzymatically modified protein isolates for use as food ingredients, FAO Technical Conference on Fishery Products, FII:FP/73/E-28.
26. Sidell, V., Stillings, B., and Knobl, G., Jr., 1970, The fish protein concentrate story, *Food Technol.* **24:** 40.
27. Bardach, J., 1968, *Harvest of the sea,* Harper & Row, New York, Evanston, and London, Chap. 3, pp. 159–161.
28. Okada, M., Miyauchi, M., and Kuda, G., 1973, Kamaboko, *Mar. Fish. Rev.* **35:** 1.
29. Patashnik, M., Kudo, G., and Miyauchi, D., 1973, Smooth, white spread from separated fish flesh forms a base for flavored dips, snack items, *Food Prod. Dev.* **7:** 82.
30. van Veen, A., 1965, Fermented and dried seafood products in Southeast Asia, *in: Fish as food,* G. Borgstrom (ed.), Academic Press, New York, III, p. 247.

35

Improving Patterns of Consumption

Philip R. Payne

Department of Human Nutrition
London School of Hygiene and Tropical Medicine
London, England

Up to this point, the majority of the chapters in this volume have concentrated upon the technical aspects of the problem of increasing food supplies. While it is evident that there is some connection between overall food supplies and the level of consumption, the nature and operation of this connection is by no means simple, and during the past few years there has been increasing criticism of nutrition interventions and of food and nutrition policies that have failed to take account of the need to ensure that the extra food made available could be purchased by that sector of the population most in need. In fact, while some increase in food production would almost certainly be needed in any country setting out to overcome malnutrition, it must be said that, although a necessary condition, it is by no means sufficient: Decisions about policies must also be based upon a concern for their effect upon the distribution of effective demand. In relation to improving patterns of consumption, this means that it is impossible, in practice, to separate the problems of improving the pattern of foods eaten by individuals from those of improving the pattern of distribution of food among individuals.

Levinson and Field (1) described the process of welfare planning as being about "who gets what, when, and from whom." For the nutritionist, concerned with the reduction of deprivation in the community, this means that his intention must be to improve the levels and patterns of consumption of some people *preferentially*. Broadly, there are three ways in which the distribution of effective demand might be modified:

1. *By income distribution.* This might be directly, by means of taxation

policies that effectively transfer income from the richer sections of the community, or from the more profitable enterprises, to the poor. The money collected might either be distributed directly as income supplements, or used in the form of subsidies to reduce the price of such basic commodities as staple foods. It is with food policies of these kinds that the nutritionist has traditionally been involved, and the problems of operating "two price systems" for agricultural commodities have been well reviewed in the chapter by Abbott (2). However, it must be admitted that, even given the will to do so, the capacity of many poor countries to raise money by taxation is limited.

2. *By distribution of the means of production.* Obviously, this is the method of choice followed principally, although not exclusively, by the Socialist countries, and there is little doubt that a combination of both income and resource distribution is the most immediately effective way of rapidly reducing disparities in income distribution (3). However, it is plain that many governments see it as one of their primary concerns to prevent, or at least to slow down, any such transfer of resources.

3. *Distribution of technology.* The benefits of technology and of new methods of production can be directed toward those who are most in need; i.e., to use technology explicitly and selectively to increase the capacity of the poor to generate income for themselves. In order to do this, however, the technologist must be aware of the nature of the problems poor people face, and he must become much more concerned to distinguish those kinds of projects and processes that extend the potential for productive capacity of the poorest groups in the community. Thus, it should be a matter of concern, when assessing the relevance of schemes to promote the production of new or improved varieties, that the schemes themselves are so designed that they benefit that sector of the population whose intake is believed to be critically low, and equally, that they do not result in a serious reduction of intakes of some other people.

Even the simplest schemes for changing cropping or production patterns need to be examined by the nutritionist in the light of an adequate definition of the nutrition situation, and must start, as in all aspects of nutrition planning, by asking the questions: Who is malnourished? What are they short of? When? (4).

Past history offers some sad examples of schemes whose intention was good, and whose effect was undoubtedly to increase production, but whose design was such that the pattern of consumption of needy people was not improved. One example was the introduction of dairying schemes that, by concentrating on the larger, "more efficient" farmer, led to the buying out of smaller farmers and a reduction of employment opportunities. The milk produced was shipped to the towns to be consumed by people whose needs generally were not so great. This might be contrasted with a scheme that gives cattle to landless families, utilizes marginal land for grazing, and establishes a cooperative for marketing surpluses.

There are many other such examples, and it has become almost a cliché among development planners to describe the green revolution as a technical success, but a social failure. Where this has been so, the fault lies, not with the agricultural scientists, but in the fact that the design of schemes has failed to take account of the nutritional problems of the community, has concentrated on efficiency and productivity, and has frequently failed to understand the constraints that limit the actions of the smaller farmers.

As an aside here, a feature of the present world situation that has not been mentioned is the extent to which "efficiency"-oriented agricultural development policies over the past two decades have led to the growth of the numbers of the landless in many countries. It is these people, excluded to a great extent from the benefits of development up to date, excluded also from the politicizing and participation processes of which John Field spoke, who, in the present crisis, literally find that they cannot afford to exist.

Clearly, if landlessness or the lack of effective land reform are factors that lead to the generation of poverty and malnutrition, then schemes that have as their objective merely the increased production of food will have little impact on malnutrition. Those designed to reduce the *causes* of poverty as well as augment production may. There is much to be done by the various disciplines to improve criteria for assessing the relevance of new technologies of production, in the design of effective schemes for intervention, and in discovering areas in which more research is needed. The following is an example of the kind of multidisciplinary approach that is needed in relation to assessing the potential impact of a new crop, or a new variety.

This would have as a prerequisite an adequate description of the character and situation of malnourished groups. By this is meant, not simply a physiological or age group in the population such as preschool children and expectant mothers, but rather a description in fundamental terms of the types of family in which malnourished children are most often found. These might, for example, turn out to be those families existing on less than 5 ha, in a particular ecological zone, perhaps exposed intermittently to some particular kind of environmental hazard, or to the operation of some particular kind of land tenancy. The need for such a functional classification is a challenge in itself for the nutritionists, for in many countries surveys are carried out, but the malnourished groups are not adequately characterized in these terms.

The analysis would then proceed by establishing what we might call the existing diet potential (5) of typical families in the group. I mean by this an estimate of the levels of production of various crops in both good years and bad, estimates of the present and likely future costs of inputs, of the extent and nature of marketable surpluses, and the range of market prices encountered, and also of the probable nature of existing resource constraints: land area, water, labor, and the work capacity of the adults in the family; defects in storage and marketing systems; constraints also imposed by the social structure of the community, dependency, reciprocal obligations, indebtedness. It is against this background that the dietary pattern, nutrient intakes, and the health status of the family and of its vulnerable members should be viewed, and it is this that constitutes the basis of a causal analysis of malnutrition.

It is then possible to ask the following questions. What are the most important constraints that limit the diet potential, and hence the diet patterns, of this class of family? What will be the likely effect of a particular new crop or variety; i.e., will the diet potential be extended? If so, what effect will this have upon the diet pattern?

It is very obvious that this is a multidisciplinary exercise, and has the advantage of bringing together technologists from various fields—nutritionists, agronomists, economists, and others. Frequently it also induces humility to discover that an ignorant, ill-educated peasant, who has never heard of linear programming, and is without benefit of computers, has managed to establish a pattern of behavior that is closely optimal for the long-term survival of his family unit. We are only justified in disturbing this complex and often delicate equilibrium if we can say that we fully understand its nature, and in particular, if our understanding of the risks involved in intervening is at least as good as the farmer's.

Many of the mistakes and problems in the past have arisen because at this point, each kind of technologist has seen as his function the offering of a diagnosis of the problem in terms narrowly relevant to his own discipline, in order to propose an equally narrow remedy. The nutrionist, in particular, has sought to identify the proximal causes of malnutrition with inadequate intakes of nutrients, notably, of course, protein. In doing so, he has not only run the risk of oversimplifying the problem, he has unduly narrowed the range of concerns of other disciplines, in particular that of the plant breeders. It may well be that a particular nutrient is in short supply in relation to the needs of the vulnerable family members. However, the constraints that limit the diet potential of the family may make the offer of richer vegetable sources of that nutrient a totally inadequate solution to the problem.

If we believe that in the interests of increased protein production the farmer should be urged to grow more beans, how do we decide upon the optimum proportion of maize and beans for him to grow? Traditionally, the nutritionist has fed rats with varying proportions of maize and beans in order to find a mixture that gives the maximum protein efficiency ratio; i.e., the best for feeding rats. Traditionally, also, he has failed to observe that from a fixed area of land, the yield of energy and of some other nutrients will decline as the proportion of beans rises. The small farmer needs to know what ratio will maximize his diet potential, and, if it differs from his present practice, what extra costs will be involved.

It should be evident that the need is not so much for the discovery of new criteria or new properties by which schemes and plant varieties should be examined, but rather a broader and more comprehensive approach to the process of appraisal. A list of properties for a new variety might include: (a) *yield per acre; yield of nutrients and energy per acre; yield response to moderate levels of inputs; food and general organoleptic properties,* e.g., taste, appearance, texture, bulk, and consistency when cooked. (It may well be that the capacity of the infant stomach is the factor that most frequently limits intake and, hence, nutritional status. In this case, selection of varieties on the basis of their water content and absorbing power and the jelling properties of their starches during cooking might be of much greater importance than their content of lysine, for example); (b) *labor requirements,* in particular planting and harvesting dates in relation to the pattern of labor requirements for other crops, and of seasonal availability of paid employment; (c) *resistance to drought and insect attack,* and the probable range of yields in good and bad years; (d) *variability of yield from area to area*—how representative of actual performance are the yields obtained on demonstration plots and in pilot trials?

The plant breeder knows the importance of all of these influences, but it is only in the context of the actual situation of families at risk of malnutrition that the potential value of some new variety or new species can be assessed. The nutritionist in particular, who is in a unique position by virtue of his cross-disciplinary interests, should see it as one of his major concerns to improve and refine the process of establishing the relevance of particular technologies, and thereby help to improve the direction of applied research. He is also in a position to assess the design of agricultural extension schemes in relation to their impact upon those sections of the population whose needs are greatest.

This is, in effect, to ask for a much more explicit inclusion of social considerations in planning and research activities. What it also implies is that if nutrition planning has to do with improving the pattern of consumption, which I believe to be the case, then it must be seen as an activity that begins and has its dynamic at the grass roots level rather than at the level of central government. It should, in fact, engage the attention of people of the highest professional caliber at the lowest level of disaggregation of the population.

If aiming for improved patterns of food consumption is to be seen as an important aspect of the broader activity of planning for the reduction of poverty and deprivation, then it is clear that it is also concerned with helping to expedite social change. The nutrition planner will thus find himself in one of two situations: either as a leader or an advocate of changes that are in advance of the existing set of social values of his particular community, or, alternatively, as one who is charged by his own government with the task of giving practical expression to an explicit desire for change. In either case the challenge to his professional skill requires an analysis of the nature and causes of poverty and an ability to identify, to illuminate, and, wherever possible, to extend the range of choices open to the administrators.

REFERENCES

1. Field, J. O., and Levinson, F. J., 1975, Nutrition and development: The dynamics of commitment, *in: Nutrition and agricultural development: significance and potential for the tropics,* N. S. Scrimshaw and M. Béhar (eds.), Plenum, New York, pp. 99–411.
2. Abbott, J. C., 1975, Food distribution–limitations on supplies and consumption, *in: Nutrition and agricultural development: significance and potential for the tropics,* N. S. Scrimshaw and M. Béhar, (eds.), Plenum, New York, pp. 237–245.
3. Channery, H., Ahluwalia, M. S., Bell, C. L. G., Duloy, J. H., and Jolly, R., 1974, Redistribution with growth. A joint study of the World Bank's Development Research Centre and the Institute of Development Studies at the University of Sussex, Oxford University Press, London.
4. Joy, L. J., 1973, Food and nutrition planning, *J. Agric. Econ.* **XXIV:** 165.
5. Joy, L. J., 1966, The economics of food production, *Afr. Affairs* **65:** 317.

COMMENT

Aaron Lechtig · *Human Development Division, Institute of Nutrition of Central America and Panama, Guatemala City, Guatemala.*

We are currently studying the effects of nutritional improvement on physical growth and mental development in four rural villages of Guatemala (1). In this study we have observed the apparently surprising result that, during pregnancy, caloric supplementation alone produces the same effect on fetal growth as protein-calorie supplementation does. This observation indicates that in this population, calories and not protein are the main limiting factors in the diet of these pregnant women. Similar observations have been reported recently in the literature (2), and it appears that this is a consistent finding in many regions.

With regard to alternatives available to nutritionists and planners to improve food consumption in less developed societies, technological improvement alone simply cannot accomplish this unless it is associated with appropriate social change. Furthermore, social change alone may not be enough to produce a significant and rapid improvement in the nutritional status of the population. However, social change *plus* technological innovation may exert a positive, synergistic effect on the nutrition of the poor in these societies.

References

1. Klein, R. E., Habicht, J. P., and Yarbrough, C., 1973, Some methodological problems in field studies of nutrition and intelligence, *in: Nutrition, development and social*

behavior, D. J. Kallen (ed.), U.S. Government Printing Office, DHEW Publication No. (NIH) 73-242, Washington, D.C., pp. 61–75.

2. Beaton, G. H., and Swiss, L. D., 1974, Evaluation of the nutritional quality of food supplies: Prediction of "desirable" or "safe" protein:calorie ratios, *Am. J. Clin. Nutr.* **27**: 485–504.

36

Fortification of Foods with Nutrients

Robert S. Harris

Department of Nutrition and Food Science
Massachusetts Institute of Technology
Cambridge, Massachusetts

Of all the foods consumed by man, none except human milk will give him complete nourishment, and then only during the first few months of life. In common with other animals, man is nourished by a variety of foods selected from the plants and animals present in his environment. While each of these foods usually contains small to large amounts of the 50 or more nutrients required for human nutrition, none can supply all these nutrients in correct proportions to meet the daily needs of human beings. The term *fortification* is used to describe the process by which nutrients are added to foods to maintain and improve the nutritional quality of diets (Table I). These nutrients may be added as concentrates, as extracts, or as synthetic compounds. The fortification of foods has often been described (1–4).

The trend toward urbanization, which removes the people from primary sources of food supply, has stimulated the development of foods and food products that can be shipped long distances and stored many months. The milling of cereals, and the storage, refrigeration, freezing, canning, and dehydration of fruits, vegetables, meats, dairy products, and other foodstuffs cause decreases in the nutritional values of diets consumed by urban populations (5). Such diets can be improved by: (a) blending several individual foods into food products with a better nutrient balance; (b) restoring, enriching, and fortifying individual foods and food products with selected vitamins, minerals, protein concentrates, and amino acids to produce highly nutritious foods at relatively low cost; and (c) compounding single food mixtures that will supply the entire

Table I. Some Types of Food Used in Fortification Programs[a,b]

Nutrient	Type of food	Comments
Ascorbic acid	Canned, frozen, and dried fruit drinks; canned and dried milk products; dry cereal products	Must be protected from air if in neutral solution
Thiamine, riboflavin, niacin	Dry cereals, flour, bread, pasta, milk products	With materials like rice, may be impregnated into or coated on the kernel; riboflavin may color the food; nicotinamide is usually preferred to nicotinic acid
Vitamin A (or β-carotene)	Dry cereal products, flour, bread, pasta, milk products, margarine, vegetable oils	Must be protected from air and must be added in water-miscible form to nonfat products; carotene may color product; heat losses in cooking oils may be great
Vitamin D	Milk products, margarines, dry cereal products, vegetable oils, fruit drinks	See comments for vitamin A; multiple sources may be undesirable (see section 4.2, p. 27)
Calcium	Cereal products, bread	The quantity to be added usually limits the scope of vehicles
Iron	Cereal products, bread, canned and dried milks	Availability varies with form used (see section 4.1, p. 25); may cause color or flavor changes
Iodine	Salt	Iodine usually used; iodate more stable in crude salt
Proteins	Cereal products, bread, cassava flour	Protein concentrates of various types used; the amount to be added usually limits the scope of vehicles
Amino acids	Cereals, bread, meat substitutes	Other vehicles have been proposed but not yet used; lysine or methionine now authorized in some areas

[a]In addition, a wide range of nutrients have been added to infant foods and prepared formulas.
[b]Taken from reference 4, p. 14.

nutritional requirements of infants, the aged, surgical and medical patients, and other consumers.

COMMONLY USED TERMS

The three terms most commonly used in reference to improving the nutritional value of foods are:

1. *Enrichment,* which refers to the addition of one or more nutrients to conventional foods in order to increase the consumption of these

nutrients by population groups. These nutrients are added at levels higher than those already present in ordinary food.

2. *Restoration,* which refers to the addition of one or more nutrients to conventional foods in order to restore selected nutrients that have been lost during handling and processing. The restoration is generally at the same nutrient level as that in the food before treatment.
3. *Fortification,* which refers to the addition of one or more nutrients to conventional foods, whether or not those nutrients are naturally present in that food. The amount of each nutrient added to each food is based on calculated need.

CRITERIA FOR FORTIFICATION

When foods are enriched or fortified with nutrients, it is reasonable to require that the added nutrients make a significant contribution to the diet of the consumers. To this end, in 1968 the Council on Food and Nutrition of the American Medical Association and the Food and Nutrition Board of the National Research Council issued a joint statement (6) endorsing the addition of nutrients to foods when in keeping with *all* of the following circumstances:

1. The intake of the nutrient is below the desirable level in the diets of a significant number of people.
2. The food used to supply the nutrient is likely to be consumed in quantities that will make a significant contribution to the diet of the population in need.
3. The addition of the nutrient is not likely to create an imbalance of essential nutrients.
4. The nutrient added is stable under proper conditions of storage and use.
5. The nutrient is physiologically available from the food.
6. There is reasonable assurance against excessive intake to a level of toxicity.

RESTORATION OF NUTRIENTS TO SELECTED FOODS

The Food and Nutrition Board of the U.S. National Research Council and the Council on Foods and Nutrition of the American Medical Association have discussed the need for restoring vitamins and minerals to replace those lost during the processing of foods. The August 1973 statement (7,8). stated, in part:

> The appropriate selection of a wide variety of conventional foods is important in assuring adequate intake of all essential nutrients. It is, of course, desirable that foods having undergone some form of post-harvest processing contain the variety and amounts of essential nutrients that were present at significant levels in the raw, pre-processed food. A significant level of a nutrient is considered to be 5% or more of

> the Recommended Dietary Allowance (RDA) of that nutrient in average serving. Restoration of nutrients lost in the processing of foods has been recognized for many years as an appropriate method for improving their nutritional value. Under circumstances where restoration is undertaken through the addition of nutrients as specific chemicals, it is important that all essential nutrients present at significant levels in the original pre-processed food be restored to the extent that is technically feasible. *The nutrient level achieved through restoration should be 1.0 to 1.5 times processed levels.* The principle of extensive restoration is of special importance when a label claim for the content of an added nutrient is made (Italics mine).

The basic concept adopted by both organizations is to restore significant levels of processed foods to the levels present in fresh, unprocessed food. Uncontrolled restoration could result in the addition of trivial amounts of nutrients, which might give rise to misleading promotional claims but provide no significant beneft to consumers.

The U.S. Food and Drug Administration (FDA) has proposed a concept that

Table II. Composition of U.S. RDA Diet

		Adults and children over 4 years	
Nutrient	Unit measurement	U.S. RDA	Per 100 kcal
Protein	g	65.0[a]	2.32
Protein	g	45.0	1.61
Vitamin A	IU	5000.0	178.00
Vitamin C	mg	60.0	2.14
Thiamine	mg	1.5	0.054
Riboflavin	mg	1.7	0.061
Niacin	mg	20.0	0.72
Calcium	g	1.0	0.036
Iron	mg	18.0	0.64
Vitamin D	IU	400.0	14.3
Vitamin E	IU	20.0	1.07
Vitamin B_6	mg	2.0	0.071
Folic acid	mg	0.4	0.014
Vitamin B_{12}	μg	6.0	0.21
Phosphorus	g	1.0	0.036
Iodine	μg	150.0	5.36
Magnesium	mg	400.0	14.3
Zinc	mg	15.0	0.54
Copper	mg	2.0	0.071
Biotin	mg	0.3	0.011
Pantothenate	mg	10.0	0.357

[a]If the protein efficiency ratio of protein is equal to or better than that of casein, U.S. RDA is 4.5 g.

relates vitamin, mineral, and protein content to caloric contribution (Table II), either for the addition of nutrients to foods or for establishing nutritional quality, and recommends that it be included in the general regulation regarding the addition of nutrients to foods (9). This procedure can be used, not only in controlling the addition of nutrients to foods, but also as a means for establishing a basic concept of nutritional quality for fabricated foods.

CEREAL-GRAIN FORTIFICATION

The U.S. National Academy of Sciences and the National Research Council have recommended (7) the addition of vitamin A, thiamine, niacin, vitamin B_6, folic acid, iron, calcium and zinc to food made from wheat, corn, or rice. These cereal grain products are good vehicles for nutritional additives, because they account for a significant proportion of the daily caloric intake even in the United States, with little variation by reasons of geography or income. The National Research Council is seeking cooperative studies with industry and government agencies to determine such things as stability of nutrients added, their availability, uniformity of dispersion, freedom from separation in commercial handling, and effects of possible changes in color, flavor, and odor on consumer acceptance.

Although breakfast foods in the U.S. are not subject to identity standards, the FDA has already proposed standards (9) for a number of ready-to-eat foods, including breakfast cereals. The FDA has proposed levels for the same 10 nutrients for breakfast cereals at two to eight times those recommended by the Food and Nutrition Board (Table III).

Table III. Proposed Nutrient Levels for Cereal-Grain Products

Nutrient	mg/100 gm
Vitamin A	0.48
Thiamine	0.64
Riboflavin	0.40
Niacin	5.29
Vitamin B_6	0.44
Folic acid	0.07
Iron	8.81
Calcium	198.20
Magnesium	44.10
Zinc	2.20

NUTRIENT DENSITY

The A.M.A. Council on Foods and Nutrition, in its August 27, 1973 statement, outlined its position as follows (7):

> Nutrient density is an expression of nutrient content in terms of caloric value of a serving of food as related to a standard such as the RDA . . . for nutrients and calories. For example, a serving containing 230 kilocalories might be referred to a caloric standard of 2,300 kilocalories/day. In this instance the food represents 10% of the calorie value of the standard and should be expected to contain this percentage of each of the nutrients in the standard. If a given nutrient is naturally present in an amount equal to three quarters or more of that percentage, no further adjustment is needed.

The Canadian Food and Drug Directorate reported approval (10) of a procedure that would allow controlled restoration of nutrients (vitamins, minerals, amino acids) lost during the course of food product manufacture. This proposal was similar to that proposed by the U.S. National Academy of Sciences and the A.M.A. It stated that when added to traditional foods, nutrients should be present in amounts related to the purpose of the addition, e.g., to replace those nutrients lost in the course of good manufacturing practice; if the amount originally present provided at least 10% of the daily requirement of these nutrients in a reasonable daily intake of food, the amount added should compensate for that lost in processing. The Canadian government has been applying this guideline since 1971. The concept of adding nutrients to foods when such nutrients are lost in processing, and only when the foods are recognized as significant sources of the nutrients, appears to be one acceptable approach. The Commissioner proposed 2% of the U.S. RDA as the minimum loss of a nutrient during processing if restoration is to be permitted.

The U.S. White House Conference on Food, Nutrition and Health (11) recommended that vitamin and mineral fortification be based upon caloric content. The NAS/NRC Committee, which developed the initial guidelines reports, also suggested that the nutrient levels in some foods should be related to the caloric contribution of the food. Following such a pattern, nutrient additions would be controlled by restricting the level of any added nutrients to the percentage of the U.S. RDA equal to the caloric contribution of the food to the daily caloric standard. The U.S. FDA Commissioner proposed to set the daily caloric standard at 2800 kilocalories. Thus, a food which contributes 280 kilocalories per serving (10% of the daily calorie standard) could have vitamins, minerals, and protein added per serving to a level equal to 10% of the U.S. RDA. This approach will prevent either excessive or insignificant fortification.

REFERENCES

1. Harris R. S., 1959, Supplementation of foods with vitamins, *J. Agric. Food Chem.* 7: 88.

2. Harris, R. S., 1968, Attitudes and approaches to supplementation of foods with nutrients. *J. Agric. Food Chem.* **16:** 149.
3. Filer, L. J., Jr., 1968, Enrichment of special dietary food products, *J. Agric. Food Chem.* **16:** 184.
4. Aylward, F., 1971, Food fortification, Part I., *in:* World Health Organization Technical Report Series No. 477, WHO, Geneva, p. 8.
5. Harris, R. S., and von Loesecke, H., 1971, *Nutritional evaluation of food processing,* Reprinting of 1960 edition, Avi Press, Westport, Connecticut.
6. Council on Food and Nutrition, American Medical Association, 1968, Improvement of Nutritive Quality of Foods, *J. Am. Med. Assoc.* **205:** 868–869.
7. American Medical Association Council on Foods and Nutrition, and the Food and Nutrition Board of the National Research Council, 1973, Improvement of the Nutritive Quality of Foods–General Policies, *J. Am. Med. Assoc.* **225:** 1116–1118.
8. Anon. 1973, General Policies in Regard to Improvement of Nutritive Quality of Foods, A policy statement of the Food and Nutrition Board of the National Academy of Sciences–National Research Council, *Nutr. Rev.* **31** (10): 324–326.
9. *Federal Register* 39, No. 116, 1974, pp. 20898–2100.
10. Canadian Food and Drug Directorate, 1971, Trade Information Letter No. 351 (April).
11. White House Conference on Food, Nutrition and Health, 1970, Superintendent of Documents, U.S. Government Printing Office, Washington, D.C. 20402.

COMMENTS

Guillermo Arroyave • *Division of Physiological Chemistry, Institute of Nutrition of Central America and Panama, Guatemala City, Guatemala.*

Harris has described the logistics and legal aspects of food fortification in the United States and other industrialized countries. This comment refers to the situation in underdeveloped areas.

The specific nutrients required by humans, and the daily amounts of these that should be ingested, are sufficiently well known to serve as the basis for the design of well-balanced, complete diets. A simple definition is: diets that have an adequate nutrient density; i.e., per unit of calorie in the diet, they should contain at least the amount of each essential nutrient per unit of calorie recommended for the individuals consuming them. If an appropriate variety and proportion of foods are available, consumed, and utilized in amounts to satisfy caloric requirements (the most fundamental nutritional requirement), there will be no nutrition problem. Therefore, the analysis of the food and nutrition situation of a population group should be addressed to the caloric adequacy of the diet, followed by a qualitative and quantitative analysis of specific nutrient deficits.

The diets of most underdeveloped populations are characterized by two predominant features: (1) insufficiency, which results in a deficiency of calories for the vast majority; and (2) inadequate variety of available foods to make up easily a diet with appropriate nutrient density.

Table I illustrates, in simplified form, the situation for the area of Central America and Panama, as revealed by the extensive nutrition surveys carried out in 1965–67 (1). The factor responsible for this unfavorable situation is an inadequate pattern of food production and consumption. Waiting for socioeconomic, agricultural, and educational development to improve this pattern could take many years, and the problems are so severe that short-term measures are justified. In columns 2 and 3 of Table I, a brief outline of approaches thought feasible for immediate application is given.

Data analyzed by Flores and co-workers in Central America (2,3) are examples of the number of studies that have revealed that a fundamental problem in the vast majority of low socioeconomic groups is insufficient food consumption. It has been documented that proteins per se should not constitute a primary nutrition problem where cereals and a leguminous seed are consumed together in appropriate proportions as staple foods and in sufficient amount to meet calorie needs (4). A cereal and a legume seed could thus be the simplest answer to the energy-protein deficit if their ample availability, effective demand, and consumption in adequate absolute and relative amounts could be ensured. This proposal seems the most feasible and realistic way to break the vicious cycle of undernutrition: "Populations are underdeveloped because they are malnourished and they are malnourished because they are underdeveloped."

It is inappropriate, therefore, to promote, as a first priority, costly imports or production of high-protein foods. Particularly unjustified is the importation

Table I. Analysis of the Nutrition Problem and Immediate Plan of Attack in Central America and Panama

Nutrient deficits	Source	Action
Calories Proteins	Basic foods, e.g., Corn–beans, rice–beans, wheat, sugar, etc.	The production availability and effective demand of basic foods, as defined by the National Food and Nutrition Policy, is a government responsibility, as part of the National Development Plan (by direct means: government producer; or by indirect means: subsidies, other incentives).
Other nutrients Iodine Vitamin A Iron etc.	Addition of the needed nutrients to appropriate food vehicles	Food fortification processes implemented at national or regional level.

by underdeveloped countries of protein concentrates produced commercially by industrialized countries. Enrichment and fortification are also of little use in this context; this condemns amino acid supplementation, or even efforts to incorporate protein concentrates or "protein-rich" foods into diets that already have an adequate protein-calorie ratio. Such approaches represent a waste of both effort and resources and are generally unsuccessful. The solution lies in the more adequate production, availability, effective demand, and rational utilization of basic local foods, a concept fundamental for the design of a National Food and Nutrition Policy.

In the situation described for a typical underdeveloped area, where is fortification or enrichment useful and perhaps even necessary at present? The Central American nutrition surveys revealed dietary, biochemical, and clinical evidence of deficiencies of some specific micronutrients. These were iodine, vitamin A, iron, and riboflavin. How can these particular nutrient deficits be overcome? The problem of iodine deficiency has been attacked successfully through salt iodization. In Guatemala, the overall 38% prevalence of goiter was reduced in six years to less than 5% by this means.

Table II suggests a scientific basis for designing a fortification plan with vitamins and minerals. Detailed analysis based on food composition explains that, of the nutrients listed, four are deficient in a basic corn–bean diet: vitamin A, iron, riboflavin, and ascorbic acid.

Vitamin A is a problem because food sources of retinol, the most effective form of the vitamin, are scarce and expensive, and consequently not consumed by the majority of the population in sufficient amounts. Green leaves and yellow vegetables and fruits, the carotene sources, are more available, but their consumption is very low, mainly for cultural and economic reasons. They are sold by the rural people to urban populations for cash to buy calorie-rich foods. Furthermore, carotenes are much lower than retinol in vitamin A activity. The incorporation of an appropriate amount of vitamin A in the diet of these populations, using a convenient dietary vehicle, is indicated. Based on these considerations, INCAP initiated a project in 1969 to develop such a process.

After careful studies, white table sugar was selected because it fulfilled the following four basic requirements: (a) It is "universally" consumed by the population; (b) the consumption per caput varies little from person to person and from day to day; (c) supplementation results in unappreciable changes in organoleptic characteristics; and (d) the cost and nature of the vehicle make the process of supplementation feasible on an industrial scale.

The vitamin A preparation to be used needed to: (a) be water-miscible or water-dispersible; (b) be capable of incorporation in the form of a physically stable premix with sugar; (c) be undectable by flavor, odor, color, or any other organoleptic characteristic, once mixed with the sugar at the proposed levels; (d) have a potency sufficiently stable to ensure an intake of vitamin A by the

Table II. Adequacy of a 72:28 Combination of Corn and Beans[a] to Satisfy Daily Dietary Recommended Intakes

	Calories	Protein (g) (score "70")	Calcium (mg)	Iron (mg)	Vitamin A (retinol equiv.) (μg)	Thiamine (mg)	Riboflavin (mg)	Niacin (mg)	Ascorbic acid (mg)
		Nutrient composition							
Corn–beans (72:28)	1000	33.5	244	10.8	4.7	1.16	0.33	5.4	2.2
		Recommended intakes per 1000 calories and percent adequacy							
Child 3–4 years		16.6	290	13.0[b]	161	0.40	0.55	6.6	13
Adequacy		*202%*	*84%*	*83%*	*2.9%*	*290%*	*60%*	*82%*	*17%*
Boys 16–18 years		18.0	177	5.8[b]	242	0.40	0.55	6.6	10
Adequacy		*186%*	*138%*	*186%*	*1.9%*	*290%*	*60%*	*82%*	*22%*
Girls 16–18 years		19.4	239	24.3[b]	326	0.40	0.55	6.6	13
Adequacy		*173%*	*102%*	*44%*	*1.4%*	*290%*	*60%*	*82%*	*17%*
Lactating women		22.5	423	21.6[b]	423	0.40	0.55	6.6	19
Adequacy		*149%*	*58%*	*50%*	*1.1%*	*290%*	*60%*	*82%*	*12%*

[a]50% corn protein–50% bean protein.
[b]Estimated absorption for corn–bean iron = 5%.

population in need that would contribute significantly to prevent deficiency; (e) have a cost that would not significantly affect the price of the final product for the consumer.

A process meeting these criteria has been developed (5). Tests were carried out on the fortified sugar to determine its industrial feasibility, acceptability, and physical and chemical stability as well as its biological effectiveness. These indicate that the process fully satisfies the requirements for application at national or regional levels, resulting in an entirely acceptable fortified sugar. Two Central American countries, Costa Rica and Guatemala, have already passed laws that will become effective this year, requiring the fortification of sugar with retinol palmitate.

Regarding iron, several considerations apply. The 10.8 mg contained in 1000 calories of the corn–bean combination to which I referred (Table II) would seem sufficient to prevent iron deficiency, if compared directly with the INCAP recommended intakes (6). In spite of this, microcytic, hypochromic anemia responsive to iron is very prevalent in these populations. I believe that the explanation rests in the fact that the INCAP recommendations (6), based on the guidelines of FAO/WHO, estimate iron absorption at 10%. However, iron absorption from corn and beans has been shown to be significantly poorer. Data of Layrisse and co-workers (7) indicate that iron absorption from these foods averages about 5%. For this reason the recommended iron intakes are doubled in Table II, and the corn–bean diet thus seems to be inadequate to meet the iron needs of several important groups. INCAP is engaged in intensive research to determine the best vehicle to carry iron, and the form in which this mineral should be used in fortification.

The corn–bean diet is essentially devoid of ascorbic acid. Nevertheless, all the dietary, biochemical, and clinical evidence obtained by INCAP has shown a sufficient intake of vitamin C. The reason is the availability, at practically no cost, of excellent sources of this vitamin. For example, the 20 mg per day needed by a three to four-year-old child would be provided by one-third of an orange, one-fourth of a green mango, one-third of a pineapple slice, or one-third of a guava. There are numerous other fruit sources of ascorbic acid that can be easily obtained by any rural population in Central America.

Finally, there is the dietary deficit of riboflavin. The technological problem of adding this vitamin to a vehicle like sugar has not been solved because of the yellow-green fluorescence in even microamounts of the vitamin. This vitamin is best supplied by milk. Riboflavin adequacy, even for a diet of corn and beans, would be provided by 100 ml of cow's milk per 1000 calories, which amounts to 155 ml of milk for a two to four-year-old child per day. This should be feasible as part of a National Food and Nutrition Policy. However, even if no programs could be implemented to ensure this minimum supply of milk to children, a simple technology, similar to those described for other nutrients, could be developed.

Some limitations are encountered, under certain circumstances, in the use of some staple foods as vehicles for fortification in underdeveloped countries. Corn and wheat in Guatemala are good examples. These types of food vehicles are limited by the following two factors: (a) Corn (as a model) is grown and acquired as grain; it is home-processed, rather than centrally processed, into *masa* and *tortilla.* (b) Wheat is industrially processed into flour, but is consumed principally by the more sophisticated stratum of the population—those who are most likely already consuming enough of the nutrients in question. These two limitations have to be carefully considered at the national or regional level.

A food fortification policy in an underdeveloped country must encompass economic factors. In industrialized countries, enrichment or fortification is often carried out at the discretion of the food industrialist who, independently, adds a long list of nutrients to his product and puts the list on the label. Recognizing exceptions, the instances are too many in which nutrients are added to foods without any evidence that they may be in short supply to the population. Although this may not be harmful from the nutritional viewpoint, it is economically wasteful, and an undesirable practice in countries where this would only add to the cost for the consumer.

References

1. Institute of Nutrition of Central America and Panama, and Nutrition Program, Center for Disease Control (formerly Interdepartmental Committee on Nutrition for National Development), 1972, *Nutritional evaluation of the population of Central America and Panama. Regional summary,* Department of Health, Education and Welfare, DHEW Publication No. (HSM) 72-8120, Washington, D.C., 165 pp.
2. Flores, M., Menchú, M. T., Lara, M. Y., and Guzmán, M. A., 1970, Relación entre la ingesta de calorías y nutrientes en preescolares y la disponibilidad de alimentos en la familia, *Arch. Latinoam. Nutr.* **20:** 41.
3. Flores, M., Menchú, M. T., Lara, M. Y., and Béhar, M., 1972, Dieta del pre-escolar en el área rural de El Salvador, *Arch. Latinoam. Nutr.* **22:** 205.
4. Valverde, V., Arroyave, G., and Flores, M., 1975, Revisión del aporte calórica y proteínico de las dietas de poblaciones de bajo nivel socioeconómico en Centroamérica. ¿Existe un problema de proteínas? *Arch. Latinoam. Nutr.* **25**(4): 327.
5. Institute of Nutrition of Central America and Panama, 1974, *Fortificación de azúcar con vitamina A en Centro América y Panamá*, INCAP Publication V-36, Mayo 1974, Guatemala, C.A., 18 pp. plus 6 appendices.
6. Institute of Nutrition of Central America and Panama, 1973, *Recomendaciones dietéticas diarias para Centro América y Panamá*, INCAP, Guatemala, C.A., 33 pp.
7. Layrisse, M., Cook, J. D., Martínez, M., Roche, M., Kuhn, I. N., Walker, R. V., and Finch, C. A., 1969, Food iron absorption: A comparison of vegetable and animal foods, *Blood:* **33,** 430.

George H. Beaton · *Department of Nutrition, School of Hygiene, University of Toronto, Toronto, Canada.*

I find myself in agreement that there has been an overemphasis on "protein" and that we should direct our attention to *food* rather than individual nutrients (1). However, I think it is essential that a perspective be retained; I would not wish us to be distracted by battles over protein versus energy and nutrients versus food.

Much epidemiological experience has suggested that in cases of *severe* protein-calorie malnutrition the nature of the weaning food offered to infants is an important etiologic factor. Payne has pointed out an important aspect of this: the caloric density and bulk of the diet offered. Within the framework of traditional feeding practices, can the young child eat enough of the food to satisfy energy or nutrient needs? Where this presents a problem there may be many approaches. However, *if* we choose to follow the route of formulating processed weaning foods, "protein concentrates" have an important role along with other "nutrient concentrates."

In general, it is clear that foods must be the primary focus of nutritional concern. However, we should not forget the specific situations in which nutrient intervention is warranted, feasible, and needed. Let me cite but three examples: (1) iodine and goiter; (2) Vitamin A and xerophthalmia (and blindness); (3) iron and anemia. While the ultimate control of these problems must relate to nutritionally adequate diets, the changes required will be slow in coming; there is no real prospect for short-term solutions through diet change. Specific nutrient intervention is warranted.

To return to the protein question, the need for protein concentrates and novel protein sources in the present world would seem to have been overstated. However, if the food situation and future prospects are really as discouraging as portrayed in this volume, then the technology that has been developed for unorthodox sources of protein may find broad application. We may be forced to turn to "foods" that today do not exist—we may have to couple unorthodox protein sources with unorthodox energy sources to produce unorthodox foods. The technology developed for protein may be modifiable to a much broader role.

In conclusion, while we may have overemphasized a single nutrient, protein, and perhaps distracted attention from the greater problem, food, we must be careful not to overreact and let the pendulum swing too far back. We need more food—higher energy intakes in the majority of the world's population—but we must also ensure that these foods provide not only energy but also the requisite nutrients. Moreover, there remain situations in which specific nutrient supplementation is indicated and needed.

Reference

1. Beaton, G. H., and Swiss, L., 1974, Evaluation of the nutritional quality of food supplies: Prediction of "desirable" or "safe" protein:calorie ratios, *Am. J. Clin. Nutr.* 27: 485–504.

Antonio Bacigalupo · *Universidad Nacional Agraria, Lima, Peru.*

Nutrition educators have been quite effective in popularizing important general concepts; for example, that eggs, milk, and fish are good foods. While this is not enough to solve the nutritional problems of our times, at least many more persons are aware of them and have some elementary knowledge of food values. Nutrition educators should give precise information on food selection and nutritious combinations of food at lowest cost, according to the foods available locally. The applied nutrition education trials carried out by us in Lima's slums, taking economic factors into account, are having encouraging results.

VI

Application of Science and Technology to Long-Range Solutions

37

The Application of Science and Technology to Long-Range Solutions: Multiple Cropping Potentials

Richard R. Harwood

Cropping Systems Program
International Rice Research Institute
Los Baños, Philippines

PRESENT IMPACT OF MODERN CROP TECHNOLOGY

The focus of this book is not so much on national production goals as on the welfare of people. In most Asian countries rural inhabitants constitute from 50 to 80% of the national population. A great portion of these people have been touched only marginally, if at all, by recent advances under the green revolution, even though their countries may be approaching self-sufficiency in food. In most cases these bypassed farmers either lack the capability to adopt the new technology, or do not have the physical resources to justify high investment in a technology that, for them, has only moderate production potential. Multiple cropping, or the growing of more than one crop per year, is readily adapted to areas where resources are not limiting. Special techniques may be required to achieve extra high year-round productivity in labor-intensive systems, but the approach is for the most part straightforward, using a high-input, high-return technology. Our concern with rural welfare, however, directs our attention to the bypassed majority whose production resources are limited. It is for this group that multiple cropping technology can have the greatest impact in the future. It is toward this limited-resource sector that our attention as cropping systems specialists is more closely directed.

THE ROLE OF CROPPING SYSTEMS TECHNOLOGY

In designing a technology for tropical farmers with limited resources, the key seems to lie in adapting it to meet their needs, using resources that are, or could be, made available to them. The Philippines' direct seeding program for rain-fed rice is an example of adjusting cropping practice to intensify crop production and make better use of land and water resources. In rain-fed areas having less than 9 or 10 months of good rainfall but a heavy soil that is waterlogged for part of the year, a single crop of rice is usual. After sufficient water has accumulated, normally 2 or 3 months after the beginning of the rains, the soil is puddled and rice seedlings are transplanted, using long-duration varieties that give a single crop a year. Richard Bradfield, while working with multiple cropping systems at IRRI, advocated the replacement of this method in appropriate areas with direct seeding on nonpuddled soil at the beginning of the rains, following the traditional *gogo ranca* system of Indonesia. This method has been tested in the IRRI-Philippine applied research program and extended in the Philippines. In 1974, the first year of production, it covered 50,000 hectares. An early-maturing rice variety is used for the first crop, and for the second crop the soil is puddled and transplanted if low-lying, or seeded to an upland crop if lighter and well drained (Figure 1). By this method two crops are grown per year, each producing more than the single crop that was replaced.

Several characteristics of tropical farming that influence the nature of this "suitable" technology are shared by the great majority of farmers. These are: (a) small farm size (Table I); this limits the on-farm capital investment; (b) limited

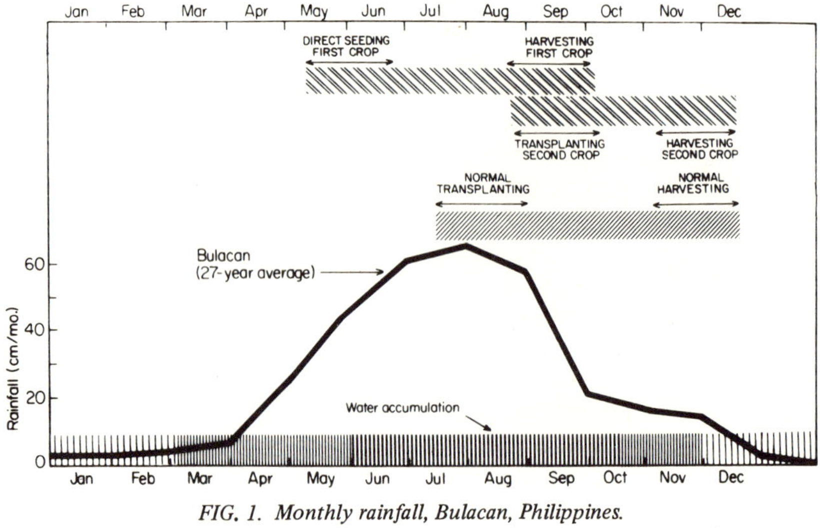

FIG. 1. Monthly rainfall, Bulacan, Philippines.

Table I. Agricultural Holdings by Farm Size in Southeast Asia[a]

Farm size (ha)	Number of farms[b] (1000)	Cumulative percent of farms	Cumulative number of farms (1000)
Less than 0.5	8,374	33	8,374
0.5–1	5,329	54	13,703
1.1–2	5,075	74	18,778
2.1–3	2,284	83	21,062
3.1–4	1,269	88	22,331
4.1–5	761	91	23,092
5.1 and above	2,284	100	25,376
Total	25,376		

[a]Based on distribution in Philippines, Thailand, and Indonesia, accounting for 70% of farms in the region.
[b]Compiled from: Food and Agriculture Organization, Production Yearbook, 1971, Vol. 25, Rome, 1972; American University, Area Handbook for Laos, Washington, D.C., 1967; American University, Area Handbook for Burma, Washington, D.C., 1968; American University, Area Handbook for Cambodia, Washington, D.C., 1963; Far Eastern Economic Review, 1972 Yearbook, Hongkong.

power for tillage, the demand being for small units as cropping is intensified; (c) high labor density; (d) uneven water availability, with seasonal variability of too much or too little; (e) heavy soils, making tillage difficult and compounding the problem of critical timing in intensive cropping systems; (f) high weathering and low fertility of many tropical soils, making the maintenance of an available nutrient source in them costly.

The corresponding needs of the small tropical farmer are: (a) an assured source of staple food; (b) a regular source of fresh food (meat, vegetables, fruits); (c) fuel for cooking; (d) fiber for building materials and other uses; (e) a steady source of cash income to purchase goods and services not available from his farm.

These needs could conceivably be met in several ways. An example is given by the opposite extremes of a grain farmer in a highly developed agricultural setting compared with one in a subsistence condition (Table II). The former produces little of what he consumes, while the latter provides for most of his own needs. We must agree that the resources and organization are not available to transform developing economies into the U.S. model of a service-oriented status overnight. Indeed, we may question whether a farm of less than 2 hectares, having limited physical resources (soil and water), will ever be of sufficient value to society to support a service-oriented economy. Neither can the rural need for services and security be met by a subsistence condition. Our goal for those having limited and nonimprovable production resources is an intermediate position where "moderate-income" farmers produce much of what

Table II. Conceptual Model of Origin of Goods and Services Used by Farmers from Countries in Different Stages of Development (Percent)

	Type					
	U.S. grain farmer		Asian subsistence farmer		"Moderate" income farmer in tropics (< 2 ha of land)	
Origin	Goods	Services	Goods	Services	Goods	Services
Own farm	< 1	–	90	–	60	–
Own town or village	10	40	–	95	20	80
Outside own town	89	60	5	5	20	20

they consume while participating in a cash economy to meet the remainder of their needs.

The key to achieving this goal lies in diversity of farm enterprises, whereby farmers make efficient use of their existing resources to meet their needs. The methodology and inputs for integrating crops into other farm enterprises (livestock, home industry, off-farm pursuits) is called cropping systems technology, and the method used is normally multiple cropping.

THE PLACE AND ROLE OF DIVERSITY OF FARMING ENTERPRISES

Labor-intensive farming systems must, of necessity, be diversified if they are to be productive. The midwestern U.S. farms of a few years ago combined two or three kinds of animal enterprises with a mixture of crop enterprises. As farm power became more plentiful and labor more scarce, specialization became more common. This shift came about because of the difficulty and high cost of mechanizing many different enterprises, and the increased ability to handle large acreages of a single crop with power. Previously used hand methods were inadequate to cope with seasonal demands at planting and harvesting time where crop specialization was attempted on large acreages.

We find the same tendency in the tropics, but with small farm sizes and adverse physical conditions, mechanization has come more slowly. We can see evidence of the interactions of power, farm size, and diversity of enterprises in the tropics today (1). The kinds of cropping patterns used and their resource characteristics are shown in Table III. A look at their power and labor requirements gives insight into their relative popularity. Intensive multicrop sequences, wherein one crop follows another in rapid succession, are high input systems, in

Table III. Types of Cropping Systems Used in Southeast Asia and Their Usual Energy and Cash Characteristics[a]

Cropping system	Energy input			Productivity	
	Human	Power	Chemical	Cash	Usable energy
1. Slash and burn (intercrop with native trees, complex crop mixtures)	H	O	O	VL	L
2. Tree monoculture	L	L	L	M	M
3. Tree monoculture intercrop with annnuals	M–H	M	L	M–H	M–H
4. Intensive tree interplanting	L	L	L	L–M	L–M
5. Homestead crops	L	O	O	L	L
6. Single crop monoculture (upland)	M	H	L	L–M	M
(lowland)	H	M	M	H	H
7. Multicrop sequences	M	VH	H	H	VH
8. Intensive vegetable (may be intercropped)	VH	L–O	VH	VH	M–H
9. Improved complex intercropping (field crops)	H	O–L	L	M	M

[a]O = none; VL = very low; L = low; M = moderate; H = high; VH = very high.

terms of both power and chemical energy. If this system is attempted without power, either animal or mechanical, the frequent soil tillage operations would make labor requirements excessive. The type of labor required, furthermore, would be largely of the heavy manual type that can only be done by a man (Figure 2). Improved complex intercrops using field crops, on the other hand, are usually of 10 months' or so duration and require only one major tillage operation a year. The bulk of labor in such a system is the light kind that can be done by women and children. This system is thus better adapted to the family's labor resource.

A diversified farming system composed of different types of enterprises, in addition to making more efficient use of labor, is better suited to meeting the needs of the farm family. Income is more regular. There is a steadier supply of a variety of foods, and the system tends to be more stable.

Biological stability (stability of production) is achieved by combining more stable but less productive enterprises with those that are more highly productive. Tree crops such as coconut, fruit, or fiber crops tend to be stable over the short-range fluctuations in weather in the humid tropics. Animal enterprises likewise add stability under such conditions. Intensive cropping patterns with annual crops, on the other hand, are more productive but have less biological stability. Their management stability is also lower. Most farmers, then, will reach

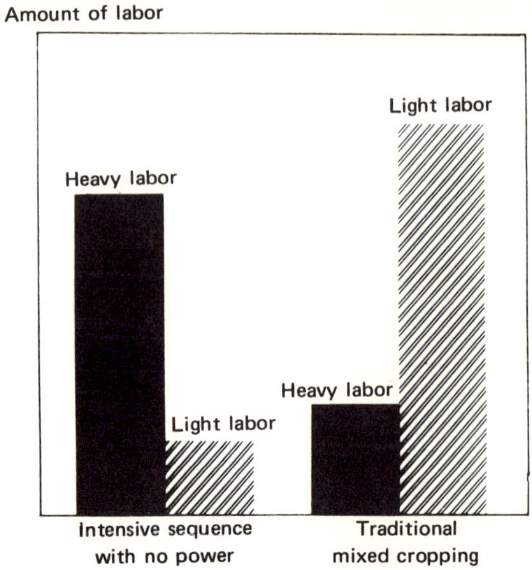

FIG. 2. Types of labor required by different cropping systems.

a balance between stability and productivity of their farm enterprises. Diversity of enterprises contributes in many ways to this balance.

Factors that shift the balance away from diversity and the need for stability are: better social organization and structure, which provides alternative forms of stability to the farmer; improved technology for a given crop, making it far more productive than other alternatives; more and larger power sources that shift the farm operation toward a power base rather than a labor base; and particular crop-suited environments such as for lowland rice, sugarcane, or rubber. Management problems often become more difficult with diversity of enterprises, as the farmer is required to master a much broader range of skills in both production and marketing.

MODEL FOR A TYPICAL SOUTHEAST ASIAN UPLAND FARM

The typical upland farm is around 1.5 ha in size and is composed of several parcels that are usually not contiguous. The study of separate enterprises is difficult because of the close interaction between them. The animal systems interact closely with crop systems in terms of both power, feed, cash flow, and recycling of nutrients. In multiple cropping programs, however, we are primarily concerned with improvement of the crop enterprises. Cropping systems studies, then, focus on this aspect, carefully considering, at the same time, interactions with other farm enterprises.

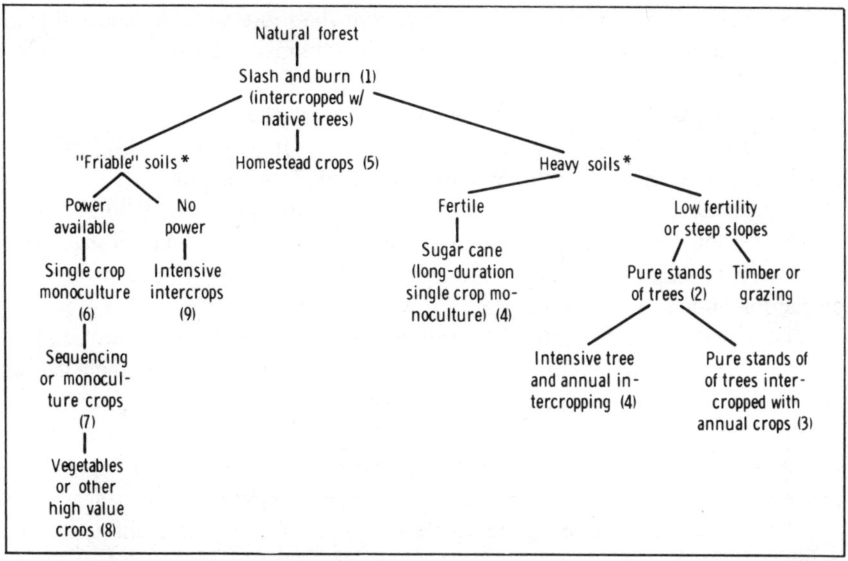

FIG. 3. Sequence of types of cropping systems on upland soil with progressive agricultural development and decreasing farm size in Southeast Asia. Asterisk (*) indicates that puddling of soil for rice is determined by water availability and drainage characteristics.

CROPPING SYSTEMS COMMON TO SOUTHEAST ASIA

The resource utilization approach is the most readily used in the understanding of the diverse tropical cropping systems. Most, if not all, farming systems have evolved as farmers learned to utilize their available physical, social, and economic resources within the influences of their environment. This was done through use of whatever technology happened to be available to them. Our data show that most of these "traditional" farming systems are a skillful blend of resources and technology to meet the farmer's needs within his environment. We will look briefly at the major types of cropping systems and their resource requirements, and then in some detail at a single system. The different systems are outlined in Table III and Figure 3.

Slash and Burn (1)*

Today we find this system confined, in Southeast Asia, to the remaining areas of natural forest or shrub regrowth that were bypassed by earlier development, usually because of poor soils or steep slopes. Farmers fell trees, often

*Numbers in parentheses refer to the ordering of the system in Figure 3.

making charcoal for sale as cooking fuel from the more suitable, and burn the rest in place after cutting. Small-scale mechanization or animal power is useless in this system because of the roughness of terrain or the residual roots and stumps of trees. Initial fertility is high because of the release of nutrients in elemental form from burning of the forest growth. In most areas this fertility is rapidly depleted through leaching under high rainfall, or the nutrients are rapidly absorbed into the soil complex in the low-fertility soils. These soils rapidly return to their low available nutrient status. At this point the natural vegetation is allowed to regrow, beginning once again the long, slow process of nutrient extraction and accumulation in the regrowing biomass.

The system is characterized by rather high labor inputs, no power, and no chemical inputs. Productivity is extremely low and usually little produce is sold. Most of the labor input goes into land clearing, with its resulting temporary fertility increase. The complex mixtures of crops are grown, not so much for their biological stability characteristics (the commonly mentioned "insurance" factor), as for their relatively high productivity with extremely low management.

The complex patterns are mixtures of crops of different plant types and growth durations. As one crop is harvested the next comes into dominance, creating a long-term period of productivity, usually covering the entire growing season. This type of pattern is essential in a hand system where tillage during the rainy season between crops would be impossible, ruling out sequential planting. We find the same principles governing "advanced" intercropping patterns where power is not available. An additional factor may be that the relatively low populations of each species, often having different root patterns and growth periods, do not place a sudden, high demand on available nutrients such as would a high-population monoculture planting of a single crop. The nutrient demand is lower and spreads over a longer period, facilitating uptake in a low-fertility situation.

Because this system is almost always unstable over time, improvement nearly always means a change of system. The steeper slopes should invariably go to trees. The more level areas should go to paddy rice. The choice of improved intercropping or monoculture with animal power depends on farm size and power availability. The farmer would probably not be in a financial position to use mechanical power for some years.

Tree Monoculture (2)

On the heavier soils, especially those on steep slopes, or in soils that are quite thin and fragile, tree cropping appears most suitable. It also seems to be adapted to areas with short periods of high rainfall, but where, during most of the year, rainfall is uncertain, or extremely variable. Tree monoculture, such as rubber or coconut, is well suited to large tenanted holdings, because the problems of management and the labor requirements are minimal. Tree monoculture has low human energy input, low labor requirements, very low power requirements, and also low chemical needs. Productivity in terms of cash or energy output is moderate. In the case of the small landowner or the tenant farmer who farms a small area, monoculture tree crops, if grown alone with no other source of either food or cash income, usually lead to a rural slum and a minimal standard of living. The reason seems to be that, although cash income is moderate, the entire food needs of the family have to be purchased, taking a large share of this cash income. This is seen to be especially true in areas of Malaysia where resettlement projects have been planted entirely in monoculture tree crops. It seems to be generally true that unless the farmer has a high cash income he must meet most of his own food needs from his own production if he is to have a satisfactory living standard. For the most part, therefore, it is only when monoculture tree crops can be combined with food-producing farm enterprises that the farmer has an acceptable standard of living.

Pure Stands of Trees Intercropped with Annual Crops (3)

One way of accomplishing this food production in farming systems where tree crops are the predominant farm enterprise is to intercrop the trees with annual crops. We often see mixtures of coconuts or rubber with bananas, upland rice, cassava, or other short-term crops that seem to tolerate some amount of shade. These intercropped products may be sold for additional cash income, but usually they are grown to meet the food needs of the farm family. In this way, the modest cash income of the farm family can be used for purposes other than meeting their food needs. This permits the family a considerably better standard of living. This system, in comparison with tree monoculture, has a moderate human labor requirement, a moderate power demand, and usually a low chemical input. Productivity in terms of both cash and usable energy is moderately high. This pattern is adapted to somewhat more marginal areas than is monoculture with annual crops, but still not adapted to the very steep slopes or poor soils.

Intensive Tree Interplanting (4)

This system is characterized by complex mixtures, often not in row arrangement, of various species of perennial, and sometimes annual, crops. We may find, for instance, that coconut is the dominant species, intercropped with a wide range of tree-fruit, or crops such as papaya, bananas, pineapples, cassava, rice, corn, or sorghum. This system has low-to-moderate labor requirements, usually low power input, and very low chemical input. Productivity is low to moderate in terms of both cash and usable energy. The system is adapted to very marginal areas with poor soils or to steep slopes where farm size is quite small. It is suited to the more densely populated areas with small farms where the land is suited primarily for forest use. It is an example of how a farmer can make use of the most marginal physical resources and still survive.

Homestead Crops (5)

Homestead crops seem very closely related, as a system, to the intensive tree interplanting, but unlike most other types of farming enterprises, a major objective of the homestead crops may be other than crop production. The homestead crops are those that are grown in the immediate vicinity of the farm homestead and are characterized primarily by mixtures of various economic tree crops. The homestead cropping system is started early in the farm development process, when the first fruit trees are planted around a temporary house. This haphazard mixture of 40 to 50 annual and perennial crop species may have as a major purpose the provision of privacy and comfort to the living area. Secondly, it provides a source of varied and novelty items for the farm diet, such as coffee, various shade-tolerant legumes, a wide assortment of fruits, and often bananas. This produce is harvested at periodic times throughout the year and lends variety that could not otherwise be afforded for the diet of the farm family. It may also serve as a small source of cash income throughout the year. Labor requirements are very low, with no power input and no chemical input. Productivity in terms of cash or usable energy is low. The homestead area is usually higher in fertility, however, because of the accumulation of nutrients from household or animal wastes caused by the net flow of nutrients into the area from surrounding fields.

Single-Crop Monoculture (6)

This type can be divided into two subtypes. On the friable soils we find monoculture of upland crops, while on the heavier soils with suitable water-holding capacity and/or suitable rainfall, the soil will be puddled for lowland rice. An essential requirement in this system, unless farm size is extremely small, is that power be available. Without power, other types of cropping patterns are more productive and are usually used. With lowland rice, monoculture can be practiced on a somewhat larger farm size, without power, than can the growing of upland crops. The requirements in terms of energy input for upland crops are: moderate labor investment, high power requirement, and a low chemical input, giving low-to-moderate cash and energy returns. For lowland rice the labor requirement is somewhat higher, but the power requirement is moderate. Usually the chemical input to lowland rice is moderate. Productivity of the single crop is usually higher under lowland than under upland conditions, and classified as high.

Multicrop Sequences (7)

In multicrop sequences the human energy input where field crops are used is still moderate, but the power requirement soars and is classified as very high. The chemical requirement is also high. Productivity in terms of cash and usable energy is high to very high. This is an extremely efficient system, but suited only to areas where power is readily available. It is especially suited to small power units. If large power is used the growing season must be longer, allowing for ample time between crops because of scheduling problems of the larger power units. With a relatively short growing season of five to six months, if multicrop sequences are used, the power source must be small enough to service economically a relatively small area of 1 to 3 or 4 hectares so that it is readily available when needed. The multicrop sequence also has a high power requirement for weed control purposes. Large tractors, unless chemical weed control is utilized, are as yet not suitable for mechanical weed control under high rainfall conditions on the heavy, sticky soil types characterizing most of the humid tropics. Weed control also has a strict time requirement if done mechanically.

The multicrop sequences are extremely productive in terms of energy. They are one of the key study areas for the IRRI multiple cropping research work. Included in the data are complete energy requirement profiles over time, agronomic characteristics, pest management practices, and the integration of various types of sequences into the total farm system. An example of an energy balance in a four-crop-per-year system is shown in Table IV. Less intensive patterns use far less chemical energy and are generally more efficient, although also less productive. The variable inputs are chemicals and power, with the ratio being 3:1. These data agree with those of Francis and Heichel (2) and Black (3).

Table IV. Relative Energy Balance for Three Power Sources in an Intensive Year-Round Cropping Pattern,[a] IRRI, 1973

	Energy balance (Mcal/ha)		
	Hand labor	Hand labor + carabao	Hand labor + hand tractor
Power source	845	2,783	2,012
Other variable inputs (mostly chemical)	6,035	6,035	6,035
Total energy used	6,880	8,815	8,047
Marketable energy	56,395	55,089	50,290
Marketable energy per Mcal used	8.20	6.25	6.25

[a]Assumed energy equivalents: Human labor—0.175 Mcal/h; animal power—2.4 Mcal/h; fuel—8.45 Mcal/1; heat of combustion of dry matter—3.700 Mcal/kg; value of goods and services—2.59 Mcal/P.

Intensive Vegetable Production (Sometimes with Intercropping) (8)

The intensive growing of vegetables is the next stage in intensification as farm size decreases, the labor density increasing as markets become available. Our research separates out two types of vegetable production. First are the field vegetables, grown on relatively large areas, that is, up to 1/2 hectare per field of a single species of vegetable. The other type is intensive intercropping, either on trellises or in the ditch-and-dyke system, or intercropping within longer-duration crops. We are accumulating descriptive data of an economic, social, and agronomic nature to describe these systems and their place in agricultural development. Intensive vegetable production, regardless of the method used, has a very high labor input, with low power and very high chemical inputs. Productivity in terms of cash return is very high, but the energy output is moderate to high. Except in certain well-defined cases, the multicrop sequence generally blends over time into vegetable production, with small areas of vegetables being planted in one or more of the crop seasons. This area usually increases as the farmer has a more available market, or as his cash requirements become higher. As his family size increases and more labor is available, vegetable production is also encouraged. The economic stability of vegetable crops is considerably lower, however, because of high fluctuation in market prices. In most cases, if farm size is about 1/2 hectare, the question is not whether a farmer should grow vegetables, but what portion of his total system should go into the vegetable enterprise.

Improved Complex Intercropping of Field Crops (9)

With friable soils, either at high or at lower levels of fertility, if the farmer has no power source available, the most efficient use of his resources is usually through intensive intercropping of field crops. This system is adapted to a wide range of market availability and environmental conditions. The critical determining factor as to whether the farmer intercrops with field crops or chooses the more intensive crop sequencing is his power availability. If he has no power, sequencing of crops as described above is not efficient or feasible. With no power the farmer cannot completely till his soil for seedbed preparation more than once a year. This single tillage is usually done during the dry season.

The advantage of the intensive intercrop sequence of field crops is the long effective growth duration of the pattern. This makes labor use more efficient during peak labor demand periods (4). The crops are usually planted at staggered intervals with the beginning of the rains. In this manner the farmer takes advantage of the early natural "flush" of nutrients with the first rainfall. The system is characterized by mixtures of species of different relative growth rates. The early-maturing crops may be tall in stature but are planted at low populations so that they are harvested before the later-maturing crops reach their reproductive stage.

A typical example would be the very popular corn/rice/cassava interplanting of Indonesia. The corn is harvested before the rice heads. The next crop to be harvested is rice, which is harvested before the cassava begins to spread and completely cover the soil. The cassava is harvested after 9 or 10 months. This system permits a single major tillage of the soil once a year during the harvest of cassava in the dry season. During the long rainy season lasting 6 to 7 months, the farmer simply practices the required low level of weed control. The nature of the crop mixtures and the canopy orientation keep the soil covered throughout the long growing season, minimizing the need for weed control. This system, however, begins to go out of balance as fertility declines in the soil. With diminishing fertility, the crop canopy becomes more sparse and the farmer adjusts to lower plant populations. The crop–weed balance is shifted in favor of the weeds.

Normally, with a lack of cash inputs such as fertilizer, the system will gradually change toward more and more tree crops. This intensive intercropping system is extremely flexible, and the species composition of the mixture depends on environmental conditions. With poor soils the mixture will be dominated by cassava; with very uncertain rainfall and poor soils, the predominance of trees in the system will be more evident. The system will also be varied according to the labor availability in the farm family. If the children in the family are young and not able to do heavy work, the system will often by characterized by very complex mixtures requiring little heavy labor. These require a "tending" that is easily done by small children or women. As the children grow older and the labor picture changes to one where there is potential for heavier manual labor, the system will be altered to involve more tillage with fewer plant species in the mixture. This is probably our most fascinating cropping system to study in terms of resource utilization because of its flexibility.

THE POTENTIAL FOR MODIFIED "TRADITIONAL" SYSTEMS IN A HIGH-MANAGEMENT AGRICULTURE

The IRRI research so far has looked at the simpler mixtures because of the difficulty in researching complex ones. Our data on this intercropping system involved physiology studies, plant population and timing trials, and weed control and fertility studies. The data begin to show the broad adaptability of this system in terms of different physical and socioeconomic resources.

The short-season intercrop combinations, such as corn–mung bean or corn–peanut, or corn–soybeans, sometimes show a productivity advantage over monoculture, but their biological stability seems to be a major factor in their use. The

Table V. Comparison of Corn Borer Infestation on Corn with or without Peanut Intercrop in Two Cropping Densities at 56 Days after Planting (IRRI, 1972 Wet Season)

Corn population (plants/ha)	Peanut intercrop	Borer-infested plants (%)	Borers (number/plant)	Feeding or exit holes (number/plant)	Feeding tunnels (number/plant)
40,000	yes	30	0.4	0.5	0.4
40,000	no	86	2.6	3.1	2.7
20,000	yes	21	0.4	0.5	0.5
20,000	no	60	2.0	2.1	2.0

wide corn row spacing in the corn–soybean intercropping system of Indonesia reduces downy mildew and corn borer infestation, the two most severe problems in growing corn. An example of the effect on insect infestation is shown in Table V (5). Corn borers are far less numerous in intercropped combinations. The effect on weed–crop balance is equally dramatic (Table VI) (6,7). Intercrop combinations generally compete better with weeds and require less input for weed control.

Surprisingly, when modern varieties are used in such a system, it may respond to high levels of management, even though the system evolved under conditions of low management. Corn and rice intercrop combinations show better response to nitrogen than do their monoculture checks (Tables VII, VIII). The intercrop combination shown in Table IX was more efficient in its uptake of

Table VI. Gross Return for Corn, Mung, and Corn and Mung Intercrop Averaged Over Corn Populations and Nitrogen Levels (IRRI, 1973 Dry Season)

Crop	Gross return ($/ha)		Increase (%)
	No weed control	Weed control[a]	
Corn[b] alone	194	366	88
Mung[c] alone	371	438	18
Corn and mung	504	586	16

[a]Butachlor at 1.5 kg/ha active ingredient.
[b]$0.12/kg.
[c]$0.34/kg.

Table VII. Corn (Early Thai Composite, 85-Day Maturity) and Rice (IR442-2-58, 120-Day Maturity) Intercropped at Varying Levels of Nitrogen Farmer's Field, Laguna, 1973, Wet Season (Average of 4 Replications)

Crop	Yield (t/ha) Rice	Yield (t/ha) Corn	Total value ($/ha)[a]
60 kg/ha N			
Corn	–	3.9	583
Rice	4.2	–	493
Rice and corn	1.5	2.9	611
120 kg/ha N			
Corn	–	4.0	597
Rice	4.4	–	515
Rice and corn	2.2	2.8	687
180 kg/ha N			
Corn	–	4.3	642
Rice	3.9	–	463
Rice and corn	2.2	4.0	865
240 Kg/ha N			
Corn	–	4.4	656
Rice	3.0	–	358
Rice and corn	2.0	3.4	732

[a]$120/ton of rice; $149/ton of corn.

Table VIII. Dollar Return per Dollar of Added N in Corn–Rice Intercropping (Average of 4 Replications) Farmer's Field, Laguna, 1973 Wet Season

N increment (kg/ha)	Dollar return/dollar of added nitrogen: Rice alone	Corn alone	Intercrop
60–120	2.2	1.1	5.6
120–180	–4.4	3.3	13.3
180–240	–7.8	1.1	–10.0

Table IX. Total Nitrogen Uptake in Aboveground Plant Parts at Maturity of Corn, Rice, and a Corn–Rice Intercrop under Various Nitrogen Levels, Farmer's Field, Laguna, 1973, Rain-Fed

	Nitrogen content (kg/ha)		
Crop combination	Corn	Rice	Corn + rice
60 kg/ha N			
Corn	104	–	
Rice	–	95	
Corn + rice	52	61	113
120 kg/ha N			
Corn	81	–	
Rice	–	62	
Corn + rice	47	54	101
180 kg/ha N			
Corn	95	–	
Rice	–	68	
Corn + rice	85	56	141
240 kg/ha N			
Corn	99	–	
Rice	–	91	
Rice + corn	73	67	140

nitrogen. The response of traditional intercropping systems to high levels of management has been reported by others (8).

Few research data are available on tree intercrop systems, but initial results show equally favorable trends in productivity and biological stability under resource-limiting situations. The socioeconomic advantages of such systems have been discussed.

THE FARMER'S CHOICE OF CROPPING PATTERNS

In the great majority of cases we find that farmers choose, not just one cropping pattern representing a single type of farm enterprise, but several different kinds of cropping and animal systems that can be viewed as different but interrelated enterprises. A farmer will include in his system a portion of his farm devoted to intensive sequential cropping, a portion to field vegetables, and perhaps a portion to tree-fruit crops. He may have one or more animal enterprises. When viewed as a whole, these combinations tend to make more efficient use of his labor, power, and cash resources, and give him far greater diversity and quality in his diet than he would experience were he to grow a single staple crop, or even a single cash crop, which would force him to buy his entire food supply. This general principle was shown to hold for "optimal" systems through programmed models for Thailand (9). We must remember, however, that this model pertains to the "small" farmer whose limited resources preclude his entering a power-based, capital-intensive, service-oriented economy.

THE DEVELOPMENT OF "APPROPRIATE" TECHNOLOGY FOR SMALL FARMERS IN THE LOWLAND TROPICS

Realizing that regardless of the degree and extent of infrastructure development possible, constraints on production will always exist, and we should realistically appraise goals for farmers experiencing these limitations.

The most effective long-range plan for developing an effective and appropriate cropping systems technology to reach these masses of tropical farmers will then have a twofold approach:

First must come a conceptualization of the needs and resources available to meet these needs for the small tropical farmer. Second, we must provide improved cropping systems of a wide range of types, designed to fit potentially available resources and to meet farmer needs. If we are to be successful in this endeavor, we must not slacken efforts in traditional crop improvement programs (plant breeding and physiology, for example). But we must erase from our minds the picture of wheat, corn, or rice stretching unbroken from horizon to horizon as a solution to the problems of small farmer agriculture in the humid tropics. Interdisciplinary "systems-oriented" teams must give new direction to the development of technology to reach disadvantaged farmers. This technology can be more efficient than our present cash and power-intensive type, but it applies, in most cases, to resource-limiting situations. Ultimate systems will involve intensive crop sequences, intercrops of annuals, annuals and trees, and tree mixtures. We must learn where each system is best adapated and how it works. This, in itself, requires considerably more knowledge about the complex biological and sociological interactions of tropical crops than we now possess.

REFERENCES

1. Ruthenberg, H., 1971, *Farming systems in the tropics,* Clarendon Press, Oxford.
2. Francis, C. A., and Heichel, G. H., 1973, Efficiency of energy production in maize–bean and other mixed cropping systems, Paper presented at the SAS 1973 meetings, Las Vegas, Nevada. *Agronomy Abstracts,* 1973 Annual Meetings.
3. Black, J. N., 1971, Energy relations in crop production—a preliminary survey, *Ann. Appl. Biol.* **67:** 272–278.
4. Norman, D. W., 1968, Why practice multiple cropping, *Samaru Agric. Newsl.* **10** (6): 107–116.

5. International Rice Research Institute, 1974, Annual Report for 1973, Los Baños, Philippines.
6. Bantilan, R. T., Palada, M. C., and Harwood, R. R., 1974, Integrated weed management: I. Key factors affecting crop-weed balance, *Philippine Weed Sci. Bull.* 1(2): 14.
7. Harwood, R. R., and Bantilan, R. T., 1974, Integrated weed management: II. Shifts in composition of the weed community in intensive cropping systems, *Philippine Weed Sci. Bull.* 1(2): 37.
8. Enyi, B. A. C., 1973, Effects of intercropping maize or sorghum with cowpeas, pigeon peas or beans, *Exp. Agric.* 9: 83–90.
9. Grimble, R. J., 1973, The central highlands of Thailand. A study of farming systems, Overseas Development Administration Special Report, Wye College, University of London.

COMMENT

Fabio Higuita · *Instituto Colombiano Agropecuario, Bogotá, Colombia.*

Although multiple cropping is a very old practice, there is little written on its economic aspects. It is the best way to increase food production in tropical countries with a high population density. Most less developed countries are in the tropical zone, where year-round temperatures are favorable and solar radiation is greatest. The more developed countries do not possess as favorable climatic conditions, yet they have abundant food supplies. An analysis of the intercropping system of cultivation as practiced in Asia shows that it is possible to have three, four, or even five crops per year, with greatly increased total production. China has largely solved its employment–population problem by intensive systems for soil management that require much hand labor.

While multiple and intercropping have been used in Colombia for over 300 years, scientific techniques have been applied only for 70 years, and have been improved only recently by experimental results shared by IRRI. Double crops are frequent in Colombia, and combined exploitation of coffee and cocoa crops has been practiced for several centuries. On some plantations, three or four crops are already common. The Experimental Center of Tibaitatá in Bogotá has shown that three successive crops are feasible. For example, rotation of corn/cabbage/onions does very well in the high, cool regions of Colombia. Agricultural authorities are confident that multiple cropping will increase both the quantity of food crops and employment in the densely populated areas of the country.

Multiple cropping is based on the efficient use of physical resources—climate and soil—and social resources—human and economic—in order to obtain as much yield from as many crops as possible in the smallest amount of time on a given acreage. It requires the efficient integration of all of the resources of the farm or agricultural enterprise. The physical and economic resources of the small farmer must be enhanced by this technique to obtain increased agricultural production. Without increase in food production to match population growth, catastrophe will ensue. It is exceedingly fortunate that conditions of climate and soil, and the characteristics of the population in most Latin American countries offer exceptional opportunities to implement the technique of multiple cropping, because the populations of Latin America are accelerating rapidly.

38

Genetics of Food Crop Improvement

Dale D. Harpstead and M. W. Adams

Department of Crop and Soil Sciences
Michigan State University
East Lansing, Michigan

Man's food-procuring habits underwent a change about ten thousand years ago when he began to select plants for food. He thus initiated the engineering of his food supply and laid the foundation for crop cultivation. His dependence on wild plants and hunted animals decreased as cultivated plants became a more dependable source of food. Through the cultivation of crops more people could live together in mutual support. The interdependent community was formed. Man had invented civilization.

Only the instruments of trial, error, and observation were available to guide early man in his food selection. These instruments allowed him to become dominant in his environment and to select plants to meet his food needs more satisfactorily. The first steps toward the improvement of crops must have been the rejection of those plants that produced adverse, or even toxic, reactions when consumed. We can only speculate on other plant characteristics eliminated through man's early evaluations.

Early in the selection process man must have chosen plants readily harvestable and easy to thresh. Seeds from these plants increased in frequency in the food collections. Likewise, the ability to store grain and still maintain its food qualities was of vital importance. It was this capability that freed man from his roving existence and gave him moments of leisure from food acquisition so he could confront second-echelon problems in his environment.

Several millennia may have passed before man became aware that, through selection, he had the power to change the characteristics of the plants he cultivated. With this newly discovered power, man could do such profound things as adjusting the cycle of crop growth to fit the patterns of his environment.

The time eventually came when man perceived his needs to be more than those of simple survival, and the esthetic qualities of plants became important. This must have led to the preservation and propagation of fruits with special shapes, colors, odors, or flavors. By any measure we apply today, early man's efforts in plant selection were a phenomenal success. The evidence of his handicraft still exists in the crops we grow. Man had wrestled with the gods and won.

GENETIC CONSEQUENCES OF SELECTION

It would be difficult to credit early man with actions that went beyond plant selection based on phenotypic expression. Naturally occurring variation and natural hybrids among variant types formed the genotypic basis for his success as we understand it today. By being alert to the occurrence of useful new plant types, man selected and preserved variant forms in nature that would have expired but for human intervention. Maize, wheat, and most edible beans are prime examples of man's role in preserving useful variation.

"Fitness," as described by the evolutionist, does not necessarily equal "yield" in an agronomic sense. A plant that can persist in nature can be described as "fit" and yet be of little or no value as a producer of food. Examples of this are the wild, grassy relatives of modern wheat and barley. These species remain untended in their environments, while selected crop plants persist only through the intervention of man.

Just when man became a breeder of plants cannot be ascertained. However, we can be certain of his early role in the preservation of naturally occurring variations and in transporting plants from place to place. By bringing together plants of unlike characteristics he exposed them to the possibility of natural crossing and the formation of new genetic combinations. His transport activities also gave rise to the development of useful ecotypes adapted to specific environmental conditions. The favorable adaptive response in these plants served to meet the needs of man.

In retrospect, we can trace with reasonable accuracy the genetic consequences of man's early efforts at plant selection. The harvesting of selected plants and the continued replanting of his selections increased the frequency of desirable types within his harvested crops. Through cultivation man became the guardian of his crops and achieved the capability of preserving genetic variation that would not persist under natural selection. Finally, the selection of plants that provided him a harvest when others fell to disease or insects gave to him unique advantages in terms of a more stable food supply, enabling him to escape the specter of persistent or intermittent hunger (1).

The product of man's efforts was largely an accumulation of economically useful genetic traits that placed his crops on a path divergent from pathways directed by evolutionary forces. This remains today the hallmark of man's activity as a breeder of plants.

MANAGEMENT OF FOOD CROP GENE POOLS

Genetic research on a wide variety of organisms, from the classical studies of Mendel, Johannsen, and Morgan to the quantitative studies of Fisher, Wright, and Haldane, and on to the population studies of contemporary geneticists, have established a reasonably comprehensive theoretical basis for managing the gene pools of our major food crops. Throughout the earlier period, i.e., before 1900, plant breeding was more an art than a science, although important work was done in many applied directions, such as demonstration of hybrid vigor in variety crosses. Immediately following 1900, both pure-line or pedigree selection and work on inbreeding and hybridization were undertaken. Results in both the self-fertilizing and cross-fertilizing crop species have been substantial.

To a large extent the approach in the self-fertilizing cereal grains was directed at finding genetic resistance to a number of fungal, bacterial, and viral diseases. The primary method involved finding a source of resistance through the screening of thousands of lines in so-called world collections of germ plasm, and the incorporation of the resistant gene or genes into commercially acceptable varieties.

This is a task still going on, with some shift in emphasis from specific kinds of resistance (vertical resistance) in favor of building multiple types of resistance, or field tolerance toward a wide array of biological races of the parasite (horizontal resistance). This work is not limited to outcrosses with rare genotypes discovered through a screening process. It also includes extremely wide crosses (interracial, interspecies, and intergeneric), and even mutations are used in the continuing campaigns waged by breeders against the dominant plant pathogens.

Fortunately, most of these campaigns have eventually been won by the teams of breeder/pathologists/agronomists engaged in these vital tasks. But many contests are still undecided. These research teams are constantly exploring new strategies of disease and pest control. One approach is the multiline variety, a composite of lines each carrying resistance to a different biological race of the pathogen, the makeup of the composite being changed as new pathogenic races increase or older races decline in relative abundance in the areas of production.

Breeding strategies to increase yield, once largely neglected except in hybrid crops, are being reemphasized. Mass selection for yield, once passed over by breeders because of a low level of progress, has now been shown to be an effective method when practiced in bulk gene pools tested under conditions where the effects of the microenvironment are accounted for. The initial failure of this method is now known to have resulted from a strong genotype created by environmental interactions and the confounding effects of environmental gradients in the field. Even a trait of low heritability, such as tiller number, may respond to mass selection with appropriate selection procedures (2).

Plant breeding theory stipulates that selection progress is proportional to the available genetic variance. Although this principle has often been ignored in the past, there is a reawakening to its general validity. This is apparent in several modern programs, where emphasis is being given to such operational techniques as creating bulk hybrid populations, interposing generations of random mating in a selfing series, recrossing selected lines as parents before they reach homozygosity, and the incorporation of a gene for male sterility in a bulk population to promote outcrossing (T. Ramage, personal communication, 1974).

Another strategy of great promise is that of focusing upon new objectives and problem areas heretofore thought unattainable. Examples include breeding for tolerance to soil salinity by searching for genes of specific effects, and by resorting to interspecific crosses to wild, weedy relatives of domesticated species (J. E. Grafius, personal communication, 1974).

Genetic–cytoplasmic male-sterility systems are being exploited to produce hybrid cereals such as wheat. In barley, a unique system involving trisomy is being developed to produce the true hybrid. The impact of these techniques on commercial production of grain has not yet been felt.

In crop species where controlled hybridization is commercially feasible, the choice of breeding strategy for quantitative traits, including yield, depends to a large extent upon the magnitudes and proportion of variances attributable to genes that act additively, with some degree of dominance, or that show pronounced genic interaction (epistasis).

In maize, sorghum, and several other predominantly cross-pollinated crops, controlled hybridization has been practiced for many years, with results well known to food producers. The use of hybrid maize, involving a considerable seed production technology, has unfortunately not spread into all maize-producing regions. Synthetic varieties of maize, superior to local, unimproved varieties but not requiring the elaborate seed production of true hybrids, show great promise in those regions where hybrid maize is impracticable. The genetic basis of synthetic varieties consists essentially of genes showing additivity and, to a lesser extent, dominance.

Where an appreciable proportion of the genetic variance for yield is attributable to genes showing *overdominance,* i.e., the single locus heterozygote superior to either homozygote, then production of the true hybrids is definitely indicated, and clearly defined methods exist for their development (3).

If considerable genetic interaction (epistasis) prevails for yield, in addition to additivity and dominance, hybridization is indicated and the best method of detecting the unique paired combination of lines that are superior appears to be the cyclic single-cross-selection procedure (4) (5).

The genetic model that the breeding team must deal with in improving performance is a function of the particular genetic population at hand, its previous selection history, and the array of simple and complex traits to be improved. Over against the genetic model is the environment, both physical and biological, and the shifting patterns of interactions between genetic and environmental effects. Crop improvement research is dedicated to the understanding of these effects and to the identification and quantification of the biological principles or laws that function. Crop breeding as an engineering discipline is directed at building superior populations using these principles.

Yield

Yield is the economically useful portion of the total dry weight produced by a crop. In the cereals and grain legumes yield refers to the weight of seed produced per unit of land. In other species it is the useful fruit, the clean fiber, the tonnage of roots or tubers, the dry weight of leaves, etc., per unit area of land.

Although much is known about the external manifestations of yield in our basic food plants, the processes leading to yield are still only partially understood. It is too simplistic to treat yield as a "character" with specific genes governing its expression. Absolute yield, as distinguished from yield differences, is a complex phenomenon, involving in its development most of the physiological and morphological processes of the plant's growth, and a major share of its genetic endowment.

Genetics of Yield

Because individual plants or plant progenies in the segregating generations of a cross between differently yielding parents differ almost imperceptibly in yielding ability across the range from low to high, and because a fraction of such yield differences can be shown to be heritable, geneticists have considered yield to be a *quantitative* trait. They have attributed the yield differences in such populations to genes that are numerous, of approximately equal effects, randomly distributed among chromosomes, and additive in their effects. The term used to designate such genes is *polygene,* and the variation determined by polygenic differences is designated as additive genetic variance. However, when polygenes interact among themselves, nonadditive variation results. The more sophisticated genetic analyses of yield per se in cereals and grain legumes generally suggest that both additive and nonadditive genetic effects are operative.

When genes affecting yield and/or vigor of growth interact almost exclusively in a nonadditive way, the outcome is heterosis (hybrid vigor). The effects of heterosis are utilized in true hybrid crops, such as maize and a few other highly cross-pollinated species, augmenting yield by 15–20%.

While the findings from statistical genetics give some guidance to breeders in the choice of breeding and selection schemes, they are of little direct aid in the problem of unraveling the complex developmental–physiological network that leads to yield in crop plants.

A start at this problem has been made in three broad research areas: (1) the study of yield components, their interactions, and genetic control; (2) the architecture of the plant; and (3) the study of the physiology of yield.

Components of Yield

Yield is expressible in terms of the number and sizes (weights) of the economic product. These components are identifiable in cereal grains, for example, as number of spikes (or panicles) per plant or per unit area, number of seeds per spike, and seed weight (6). In grain legumes the corresponding yield components are number of pods, number of seeds per pod, and seed weight. Generally these components are genetically independent, and determined by genes that show a low level of interaction (or none). However, the components of yield are usually negatively associated with each other; i.e., large numbers are associated with small size, and vice versa. This component compensation is probably caused by intraplant competition for limited metabolic resources during the processes of sequential development (7).

Yield analysis based on the immediate morphological components of yield has provided further insight into the basis of yield differences among genetic strains, and is now leading crop scientists to examine more critically the complete architecture of a plant in relation to its yield potential.

Plant Architecture

Architecture in the context of plant yield refers to both internal and external structure, that is, to number, size, and arrangement or display of those organs and tissues of a plant that in some way relate to, or affect, yielding ability.

A great deal of attention was focused on plant architecture as a result of the successes of the semidwarf cereals (8). Let us note that while we speak of architecture and physiological processes separately, functionally there is a high degree of correlation between them. Semidwarfism in cereals, for example, renders such plants more efficient in utilization of nitrogen.

Leaf number, leaf size, leaf angle, and leaf position have all been studied relative to their effect on yield. Plant height, number of branches, number of racemes, length of internodes, ovule abortion frequency, percent blossom drop, and harvest index are other components that, in some species, affect yielding potential.

The particular combinations of architectural characteristics that would tend to maximize yields have not yet been determined for many crops, though this is an objective of plant breeders. It must be emphasized that the cultural conditions under which a crop is grown plays a major role in the choice of the optimum combination of characteristics making up an ideal plant type.

One may logically raise the question, "Why is plant architecture important to yield?" The common dry edible bean provides some of the answers. Yield in beans is most closely dependent upon number of pods per plant (or per unit area of land). Pods are borne in clusters (racemes) which occur only at the nodes or joints of stems. Plants with many nodes–an architectural feature–will have more opportunities to form pods than plants with few nodes. Plants with many nodes can be either tall plants, or short but excessively branching. Plants with many nodes will also have more leaves than those with few nodes. The leaves, being more numerous, may intercept more sunlight and thus be beneficial, or so numerous that they cause mutual shading, not favorable to increased yield. Thus plant architecture plays its role.

Having mentioned light interception, we bridge the gap between architecture and physiology and comment briefly upon some of the vital metabolic processes in plants related to yielding potential.

Yield Physiology

Complete understanding of the physiology of yield has not been achieved. A number of component physiological processes have been identified, however, as contributory to, or determinants of, yield.

Some of these processes, such as basic rates of photosynthesis and rates of dark- and of photo-respiration, although gene-dependent, may be so solidly built into the fundamental character of each species that there is little immediate promise of being able to influence yield by breeding for more favorable levels of these processes. It is now clear, for example, that our major food plants fall into two distinct categories with respect to their rate of CO_2 uptake per unit of leaf area. (A third category exists, the photosynthetic system of the *Crassulacea,* called Crassulacean acid metabolism; because none of our major food crops are characterized by this mechanism of CO_2 fixation, it is not further discussed here.)

The distinction is based upon whether the initial fixation of CO_2 in chloroplasts is catalyzed by the enzyme ribulose diphosphate carboxylase, or by the enzyme phosphoenolpyruvate carboxylase, and whether the initial fixation product is a 3-carbon atom sugar phosphate (the C3 pathway) or a 4-carbon atom dicarboxylic acid (the C4 pathway), catalyzed by two different enzyme systems, respectively. Some of the CO_2 fixed via the C3 pathway is almost immediately released from an early intermediate compound by another enzyme system in a process known as photorespiration, thus leading to an overall lowered rate of net CO_2 fixation in C3 plants as compared to C4 plants. Furthermore, there are significant differences in leaf anatomy between C3 and C4 plants that enable C4 plants to be more efficient in net CO_2 fixation (9). Crop plants are identified as belonging to either the C3 or the C4 group.

Maize, sorghum, and sugarcane are representative of C4 species; the other cereal grains and grain legumes belong to the C3 species. Transformation of a C3 plant into a C4 plant by traditional breeding (including mutation) methods does not appear promising (10). Nor have the considerable efforts to find low photorespirers among C3 plants been successful up to the present. Rewards from the more imaginative methods, such as directed gene transfers and somatic cell genetics, while provocative and highly challenging, lie in the future.

Factors that lead to apparent increases in photosynthetic rates, such as stomate and mesophyll resistance to CO_2 movement, rate of translocation of fixed carbon out of the leaf, size of the storage organ (sink) to which photosynthate is translocated, and/or the availability of alternative sinks, may be more amenable to genetic change through breeding than the basic photosynthetic process itself (11, 12). Selection for increased sink size, that is, size of the ear or ear number in maize, head size or number in cereal grains, etc., may be the most effective way of changing genetic composition to achieve maximum utilization of photosynthetic capacity.

The ability of a crop to respond to mineral fertilizer and supplemental irrigation has been invaluable in the cereal grains for the production of high yields. Capacities for differential uptake and utilization of many different mineral nutrient elements are under genetic control in both cereals and grain legumes (13, 14, 15), and some genetic regulation probably exists in all the basic food plants. There has been, however, little deliberate exploitation by breeders of these capacities other than the systematic use of high fertilizer levels in the breeding and testing of new varieties.

With shortages of fertilizers, particularly nitrogen, increased attention is being paid to the detection and use of genotypes that prove efficient in N uptake or utilization. In the food legumes, efficiency of biological N_2-fixation is being given high research and development priority. Biological engineers of the near future may become involved in the technology of developing bacterial or mycorrhizal strains capable of fixing nitrogen in the root environment of maize, wheat, and rice, and incorporation of N_2-fixing organelles from certain algae into cells of higher plants.

There is some interest in breeding plants that yield well at low input levels of mineral nutrients. To the extent that a more efficient uptake and utilization of mineral nutrients results, such efforts would be worthwhile. However, the really high yields necessary in food crop production demand soils well supplied with nutrient minerals, and no amount of genetic amelioration will overcome the basic needs of the crop for plant foods.

The other side of the coin is that of sensitivity to mineral toxicities, such as from saline soils, or soils high in available aluminum or manganese. There is hope from work currently underway in some species that salt tolerance can be increased. This would be a very significant achievement if accomplished in any of the basic food crops, for it would enable the exploitation of desert lands not now deemed arable because of their salinity.

NUTRITIONAL QUALITIES

In 1896, a maize selection experiment was initiated in the Agricultural Experiment Station at the University of Illinois to produce high- and low-protein maize varieties. A stated objective was to increase nutritional quality via high-protein selection (16). This initial work used a locally adapted maize variety from which individual ears were analyzed for percent of protein. The ears with the highest and lowest protein values gave rise to lines in a divergent selection scheme. It is of scientific interest to know that this experiment is still in progress and has proceeded through more than 75 generations of selection. Results after 50 generations are shown in Figure 1 (17). The success in selecting for increased

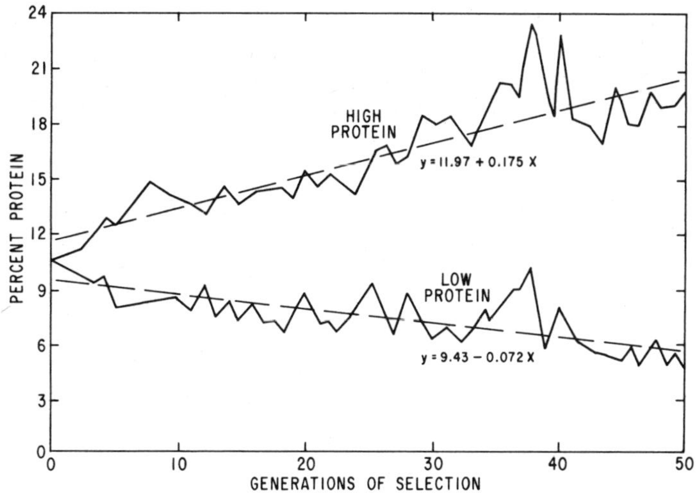

FIG. 1. Effect of 50 generations of selection for high and low oil protein content of corn. **Solid lines indicate actual data, broken lines indicate trend (reference 17).**

protein content was spectacular; however, the practical results were disappointing.

Systematic animal feeding trials using these maize selections were reported in 1922 (18). As the total protein in the kernel increased, the nutritive value of the protein decreased largely because of an increase in the zein fraction. By 1924 the monumental works of Osborne on the fractionation and evaluation of plant proteins had been widely disseminated (19). More systematic selection attempts were made to modify maize protein content without significant success. In these experiments, as the protein content was increased, the zein or alcohol-soluble fraction increased at an even more rapid rate (20). This observed relationship in maize served to curtail extensive additional plant breeding research on the nutritional quality of cereal grains.

A second relationship observed in chemical composition of cereal grain that impeded progress in the quest for higher nutritional quality was the negative correlation between grain yield and protein content. This relationship was so constant that existence of a "universal nitrogen constant" was postulated in 1949 (21). This declared, in effect, that the maximum amount of nitrogen absorbed by a crop species had an absolute ceiling, while yield, principally the accumulation of carbohydrates, was influenced both by genotype and environment (22). The validity of the "law" concept has been subsequently challenged in a series of studies that have shown the so-called barriers to be a product of the experimental model (23–25).

Only recently has significant progress been reported in the breeding of cultivars of wheat, oats, and rice, which indicates that the observed negative correlations between yield and protein content is not as great a barrier as originally thought (26, and B. O. Juliano, personal communication, 1974). While little success was achieved in initial plant breeding efforts to increase the protein content of feed grains, substantial success had been achieved in the production of higher protein wheat varieties. The key factor to be noted here is that this success was not measured in terms of the nutritional characteristic, but rather on the favorable milling and baking qualities associated with the higher protein cultivars.

Maize

Some of the earliest plant-breeding efforts aimed at the improvement of nutritional qualities of a food crop were in maize, and it is fitting that the first major breakthrough in nutritional quality came in that crop. The discoveries of the effects of the opaque-2 gene in 1964 and of a second gene, floury-2, in 1965 were major breakthroughs in the search for improved food crops (27, 28). The genes involved in these studies were previously known as a result of their phenotypic expressions in the maize endosperm. Each was recessive to a "normal" dominant gene and each was classically expressed through a soft, floury endosperm devoid of the "normal" vitreous starch fraction.

The most notable and beneficial effect of these modifying genes was the increase in the amino acid lysine in the endosperm protein from 1.6% in normal kernels to 3.7% in the opaque-2 stock and 3.3% in the floury-2 (29). However, perhaps equally significant was a parallel increase in the trytophan content with both genes and in methionine in the floury-2 stock. Both lysine and trytophan are limiting essential amino acids in maize endosperm protein, a fact that had been demonstrated many years earlier by Osborne and Mendel (30).

The increased lysine content of the modified kernels could be explained, in part, by a decrease in the synthesis of the zein fraction of endosperm protein. Zein had been shown to be nearly devoid of both lysine and trytophan in its molecular composition (19). Because the total protein content of the kernel had not been greatly affected by the presence of the mutant genes, the other protein fractions had increased at a rate proportional to the decrease in the zein fraction. In addition, the glutelin fraction in the mutant kernels was significantly higher in lysine than the same fraction in normal kernels (31).

The zein fraction in normal maize accounts for approximately 50% of the endosperm protein. Because this was reduced to less than half that amount in the kernels modified by the presence of the opaque-2 and floury-2 genes, a significant genetic control had been exercised over the nutritional characteristics of maize endosperm protein.

Extensive and early nutritional testing of the modified maize endosperm proteins has been reported by numerous authors (32–36). These early studies, confirmed by more recent nutritional research, established the superior nutritional quality of the protein synthesized when the recessive opaque-2 and floury-2 genes were present (37).

Other cereal grain food crops have protein contents closely resembling that of maize. Barley, wheat, sorghum, and millet all contain alcohol-soluble protein fractions similar to the zein in maize. Lysine is the first limiting essential amino acid in the protein, followed by either tryptophan or threonine as the second limiting amino acid. Rice and oats are exceptions to this pattern, as the alcohol-soluble protein fractions in these species are greatly reduced.

Barley

A direct outgrowth of the work that led to the production of a high-lysine maize was the systematic evaluation of the protein and lysine content of 1000 strains of barley in the World Collection. This work identified a single strain from Ethiopia with a higher lysine and a higher protein content than normally found in barley (38). This modified barley strain has been called *hiproly,* identifying these two properties.

A genetic analysis of crosses between the high-lysine barleys and the "normal" plants generally indicated that high lysine was a recessive characteristic and, in this regard, resembled the genetic situation in high-lysine maize. However, the effects of the gene in barley were of a much lower magnitude than the high lysine genes in maize. The reduction in the alcohol-soluble protein fraction was less, and the associated increase in lysine was proportionately reduced (39). Today, the development of a nutritionally superior barley has not gone beyond the experimental stage. Strains carrying the hiproly gene have generally been inferior agronomically largely because of shrunken kernel characteristics and low fertility (seed set) associated with the mutant gene. Whether these are pleiotropic effects or closely linked genetic effects remains to be established.

Sorghum

Sorghum endosperm protein is among the poorest in the cereal grains in terms of nutritional quality. Lysine is the first limiting amino acid, with a strong negative correlation between lysine and total protein content (40). The initial efforts directed toward genetic modification of this protein source met with disappointment. Extensive testing of materials out of the World Collection of sorghums failed to locate a clear-cut genetic system that would function in a pattern similar to the known genes in maize or barley. Large differences in total protein were observed, and it was postulated that the increased protein per se, coupled with the relatively small increases in lysine observed, would be a valuable addition to making sorghum a food source (41).

More recently a major breakthrough has occurred in sorghum research with the discovery, in two Ethiopian varieties, of a simple recessive genetic trait conditioning protein synthesis and lysine content. The chemical analyses of these high-lysine types closely parallel the analyses of the high-lysine maize selections. Nutritional evaluation based on rat feeding trials gave weight gains four times greater after 28 days than was obtained when normal sorghum was fed (42). This discovery appears to represent a most significant step forward in the improvement of the nutritional quality of grain sorghum.

Wheat

Wheat is used primarily as a human food and is a relatively abundant producer of protein. Nevertheless, the biological value of wheat protein is low and tends to be only slightly superior to the protein of maize. It is clearly deficient in lysine (43).

More than 15,000 lines from the World Wheat Collection have been analyzed in the search for high lysine genes (44). This work has failed to uncover heritable genetic systems similar to those in maize and barley. The range of protein and lysine content among various strains from the world collection was large. This appears to offer some hope that cultivars high in protein, with reasonably high lysine content, can be produced through plant breeding.

Rice

Efforts to effect a nutritional improvement in rice have indicated a different approach to the breeding and genetics of the crop. The protein found in rice is of high nutritional quality when compared to most other cereal grains. The limiting qualities are closely associated with the low concentration of protein in the endosperm, usually less than 7% in polished grain. This low concentration becomes a problem when rice is the principal food source, unsupplemented by more concentrated protein sources. Various high-protein cultivars (12 to 13% as compared to 6.5 to 7% in normal rice) have been isolated and tested.

Many of the strains that resulted from the initial work proved to be highly influenced by environmental conditions, and also reflected a negative correlation between protein content and quality (45). One line of rice has been identified with an available protein content of approximately 10%; it is not greatly influenced by environmental conditions and can be incorporated into commercial rice varieties (B. O. Juliano, personal communication, 1974)

Other Cereals

During the past decade there has been increasing public interest in a new man-formed cereal grain, triticale. This is a stable hybrid between durum wheat and rye, produced through the doubling of the hybrid chromosome complement. This cereal not only possesses many of the desirable agronomic qualities from both of its parental ancestors, but it also enjoys some of the nutritional superiority of rye (46). The techniques used to produce triticale hold the promise that more complicated genetic engineering feats can be accomplished, permitting selective hybridization with specific nutritional goals as objectives.

Legumes

So far, the discussion of nutritional quality has been limited to the cereals. However, seed legumes are vitally important components of an adequate diet. Their importance as a food crop lies in their protein content being two to four times as concentrated as the proteins in cereals. Secondly, the protein of legume seeds complements the cereal proteins by having an abundant supply of the amino acid lysine, although they too may be limiting in sulfur-bearing amino acids, especially methionine. The chief limiting factor associated with the use of legumes as food is in the level of toxic or antimetabolic components they contain. These factors may limit the intake of these foods and/or require drastic heat treatment to inactivate their deleterious effects.

Among commonly eaten legume species, little progress has been made in the reduction or modification of the undesirable nutritional factors through genetic selection. An exception, however, may be seen in soybeans, where one of the four known trypsin inhibitors in that species has been shown to be under genetic control and can be associated with specific varieties (47, 48).

Other Crops

Root crops also contain examples of superior and inferior nutritional qualities. The protein content of the potato may vary between 1 and 4% and is closely associated with specific genetic backgrounds. Toxic alkaloids have also been shown to be under genetic control in the potato and may, unless selected against, become a problem in food production.

Cassava, a widely consumed root crop, normally contains toxic levels of hydrocyanic acid (HCN) in wild or unimproved species. Selection against this factor has been effective in isolating "sweet" varieties as compared to the "bitter," or high HCN, wild types.

NEW FRONTIERS

Each day more people become dependent on a single plant staple for most of their diet. Such dependence greatly increases the vulnerability of a population to inadequate diets when even minor fluctuations occur in total crop production.

Production Efficiency

Several morphological and physiological components that are contributory to food production have been noted. There is evidence that most, if not all, of them are under some degree of genetic control, thus implying that through plant breeding techniques, strains possessing favorable gene combinations for all the components could be developed. Such strains should indeed be truly superior in yielding potential.

Two very pragmatic considerations cannot be overlooked.

1. It has been difficult to show, for example, that increasing photosynthetic efficiency, per se, results in a corresponding yield increase, or that making maize leaves more erect to intercept more sunlight increases yield. Why, one might ask, should breeders try to select for a component that is not directly correlated with yield? The answer is that yield is both sum and product of many different components, and that subefficient levels of two or more components in a

genotype may render that particular genotype low yielding and generally incapable of responding to selection for only a single component. Simultaneous selection for several components, both architectural and physiological, is required in order to minimize bottlenecks in the plant's ability to produce a superior yield.

2. Hand-in-hand with selection for multiple criteria must go the task of fitting the genetic patterns into the environmental network. That is, optimum output from the genetic constitution of a plant is only feasible in a favoring environment of physical, biological, and management factors. The breeder must be both geneticist and agronomist.

In spite of the major advances that have been made in the understanding of gene action and the new insights made in the physiological functioning of the plant, it does not appear likely that these developments, standing alone, will add startling new increments to our crop-yielding capacities. The greater yielding efficiency of modern F_1 hybrids and semidwarf cereal varieties grown in highly favorable environments has underscored the importance of matching genotype and environment in achieving maximum productivity. Most of the progress that will be achieved in increasing the yield of staple food crops during the next decade will come as a result of the further application of these principles. Major changes in the basic physiology of crop plants that would lead to higher crop yields still are not clearly in focus in published research results. If new discoveries were to be revealed today it is unlikely that they could be incorporated into newly developed crop varieties in less than a decade.

Nutritional Factors

Breeding basic food crop plants to produce a more nutritious product still remains one of the great challenges for plant breeders. The use of known modifier genes in maize, barley, and sorghum offers a ray of hope for millions of persons living on subsistence diets. To date, only limited success has been achieved in the incorporation of these genes into useful varieties. The lack of success has been largely caused by the unfavorable agronomic qualities associated with these genes in their initial form. The breaking of linkages with deleterious genes and the incorporation of favorable genetic modifiers have greatly increased the likelihood of success in the pursuit of more nutritious varieties.

Second generation high-lysine maize varieties recently developed in the CIMMYT programs have gone a long way toward recovering flinty endosperm types that closely resemble the kernel qualities of "normal" varieties. These newer varieties are the product of genetic plant-breeding programs designed to incorporate useful modifier genes together with the original high-lysine gene.

Only recently have plant-breeding programs been initiated that are designed to select genotypes with higher nutritive values not directly related to known amino acid balance or protein content. Preliminary results indicate that it is possible to select for increased biological efficiency of protein utilization in triticale. It is too early to predict how generally applicable these results may be (F. C. Elliott, personal communication, 1974).

It is tempting to believe that we now have available all that is necessary to capitalize on "crash" programs to upgrade both yield and quality in our basic food crops. While large new investments of both time and money would result in substantial progress in many areas, fundamental work on key plant-breeding problems cannot be abandoned. New tools are needed to evaluate the heritable variances in the determination of yield and nutritional quality. When quality is a factor we are poorly prepared to detect nutritional alteration of lesser magnitude than a major change in the product. Nor are we able to screen the large numbers of genotypes that would have to be screened if the desired gene were rare or if the desired effect were determined by as few as five recessive genes, each one exerting a partial effect on the whole. We are not yet prepared to play the numbers game. We must rely largely on chemical procedures and hope they will reflect the true nutritional quality in the product when it is used as food.

It is gratifying to witness the progress that has been made in yield, adaptation, disease and insect resistance, nutritional quality, and efficiency of production in our basic food crops. Time alone will tell whether or not we will be successful in meeting our total food needs and, at the same time, provide an adequately nutritious diet when only one crop or a very few food crops are available. The success we achieve during the rest of this century will be the product of highly integrated research programs that bring to bear the forces of chemistry, genetics, physiology, agronomy, and nutrition, each complementing the other in the quest for superior plant production. The stakes are very high in this game—it is one we dare not lose.

REFERENCES

1. Allard, R. W., 1960, *Principles of plant breeding,* John Wiley & Sons, New York, 485 pp.
2. Redden, R. J., and Jensen, N. F., 1974, Mass selection and mating systems in cereals, *Crop Sci.* **14:** 345–355.
3. Comstock, R. E., Robinson, H. F., and Harvey, P. H., 1949, A breeding procedure designed to make maximum use of both general and specific combining ability, *Agron. J.* **41:** 360–367.
4. Hallauer, A. R., 1967, Development of single-cross hybrids from two-eared maize populations, *Crop Sci.* **7:** 192–195.
5. Ehdaie, B., and Cress, C. E., 1973, Simulation of cyclic single cross section, *Theor. Appl. Genet.* **43:** 374.
6. Grafius, J. E., 1965, A geometry of plant breeding, *Res. Bull.* No. 7, Mich. A.E.S.

7. Adams, M. W., 1967, Basis of yield component compensation in crop plants with special reference to the field bean, *Phaseolus vulgaris, Crop. Sci.* **7:** 505–510.
8. Adams, M. W., 1973, Potentials of field beans and other food legumes in Latin America, Proceedings of a seminar sponsored by CIAT, Cali, Colombia, pp. 266–278.
9. Black, C. C., Jr., 1973, Photosynthetic carbon fixation in relation to net CO_2 uptake, *Annu. Rev. Plant Physiol.* **24:** 253–286.
10. Kreidemann, P. E., 1971, Crop energetics and horticulture, *Hortic. Sci.* **6:** 432–438.
11. Evans, L. T., 1972, Storage Capacity as a Limitation on Grain Yield, International Rice Research Institute, Rice Breeding Annual Report, pp. 499–511.
12. Ogren, W. L., 1974, Paper prepared for FAO/TAC working group seminar on grain legumes, ICRISAT, Hyderabad, India.
13. Gorsline, G. W., Thomas, W. I., and Baker, D. E., 1964, Inheritance of P, K, Mg., Cu, B, Zn, Mn, Al and Fe concentrations by corn (*Zea mays* L.) leaves and grain, *Crop Sci.* **4:** 207–210.
14. Foot, B. D., and Howell, R. W., 1964, Phosphorus tolerance and sensitivity of soybeans as related to uptake and translocation, *Plant Physiol.* **39:** 610–613.
15. Polson, D. E., 1968, Physiological–Genetic Investigations of the Differential Response of Navy Beans (*Phaseolus vulgaris* L.) to Low and High Zinc, Library, Michigan State University, East Lansing, Mich.
16. Hopkins, C. G., 1899, Improvement in the chemical composition of the corn kernel, *Ill. Exp. Sta. Bull.* **55:** 205–240.
17. Woodworth, C. M., Leng, E. R., and Jugenheimer, R. W., 1952, Fifty generations of selection for protein and oil in corn, *Agron. J.* **44:** 60–65.
18. Showalter, M. F., and Carr, R. H., 1922, Characteristic proteins in high- and low-protein corn, *J. Am. Chem. Soc.* **44:** 2019–2023.
19. Osborne, T. B., 1924, *The vegetable proteins,* Longmans, Green and Co., New York.
20. Frey, K. J., 1951, The interrelationships of proteins and amino acids in corn, *Cereal Chem.* **28:** 123–132.
21. Willcox, O. W., 1949, Keys to abundance, *Better Crops Plant Food* **33** (4): 9–15 and 46–48.
22. Willcox, O. W., 1954, Quantitative agrobiology: I. The inverse yield law, *Agron. J.* **46:** 315–320.
23. Black, C. A., and Kempthorne, O., 1954, Willcox's agrobiology: I. Theory of nitrogen constant 318, *Agron. J.* **46:** 303–307.
24. Black, C. A., and Kempthorne, O., 1954, Willcox's agrobiology: II. Application of the nitrogen constant 318, *Agron. J.* **46:** 307–310.
25. White, W. C., and Black, C. A., 1954, Willcox's agrobiology: III. The inverse yield-nitrogen law, *Agron. J.* **46:** 310–315.
26. Frey, K. J., 1973, Improvement of Quantity and Quality of Cereal Grain Protein; Alternate Sources of Protein for Animal Production, National Academy of Sciences, pp. 9–41.
27. Mertz, E. T., Bates, L. S., and Nelson, O. E., 1964, Mutant gene that changes protein composition and increases lysine content of maize endosperm, *Science* **145:** 279–280.
28. Nelson, O. E., Mertz, E. T., and Bates, L. S., 1965, Second mutant gene affecting the amino acid pattern of maize endosperm proteins, *Science* **150:** 1469–1470.
29. Nelson, O. E., 1969, Genetic modification of protein quality in plants, *Adv. Agron.* **21:** 171–194.
30. Osborne, T. B., and Mendel, L. B., 1964, Nutritive properties of proteins of the maize kernel, *J. Biol. Chem.* **18:** 1–16.

31. Jimenez, J. R., 1966, Protein fractionation studies of high lysine corn, *in: Proceedings of the High Lysine Corn Conference,* June 21–22, Purdue University, Lafayette, Indiana (1966), E. T. Mertz and O. E. Nelson (eds.), Corn Industries Research Foundation; A division of Corn Refiners Association, Inc., 1001 Connecticut Avenue, N.W., Washington, D.C., pp. 74–79.
32. Mertz, E. T., Vernon, O. A., Bates, L. S., and Nelson, O. E., 1965, Growth of rats fed on opaque-2 maize, *Science* **148:** 1741–1742.
33. Pickett, R. A., 1966, Opaque-2 corn in swine nutrition, *in: Proceedings of the High Lysine Corn Conference,* June 21–22, Purdue University, Lafayette, Indiana (1966), E. T. Mertz and O. E. Nelson (eds.), Corn Industries Research Foundation; A division of Corn Refiners Association, Inc., 1001 Connecticut Avenue, N.W., Washington, D.C., pp. 19–22.
34. Bressani, R., 1966, Protein quality of opaque-2 maize in children, *in: Proceedings of the High Lysine Corn Conference,* June 21–22, Purdue University, Lafayette, Indiana (1966), E. T. Mertz and O. E. Nelson (eds.), Corn Industries Research Foundation; A division of Corn Refiners Association, Inc., 1001 Connecticut Avenue, N.W., Washington, D.C., pp. 34–39.
35. Pradilla, A., Harpstead, D. D., Linares, F., Sarria, D., and Tripathy, K., 1969, Ensayos analiticos y biologicas de la proteina del maiz modificado por el gene opaco-2, *Antioquia Med.* **19** (3): 201–211.
36. Harpstead, D. D., 1971, High-lysine corn, *Sci. Am.* **225** (2): 34–42.
37. Bressani, R., Braham, J. E., and Behar, M., 1972, (eds.), *Nutritional improvement of maize,* Proceedings of an International Conference held at the Institute of Nutrition of Central America and Panama (INCAP), Guatemala City, March 6–8 (1972), Audiovisual Aids Section of INCAP, Guatemala City, Guatemala, C.A., 317 pp.
38. Hagberg, A., and Karlsson, K. E., 1969, New approaches to breeding for improved plant protein, International Atomic Energy Agency, Vienna, Austria, pp. 17–21.
39. Munck, L., 1972, Improvement of nutritional value in cereals, *Hereditas* **72:** 1–128.
40. Collins, F. C., and Pickett, R. C., 1972, Combining ability for grain yield, percent protein, and g Lysine/100 g protein in a nine-parent diallel of sorghum bicolor (L.) Moench, *Crop. Sci.* **12:** 423–425.
41. Verupaksha, T. K., and Sastry, L. V. S., 1968, Studies on the protein content and amino acid composition of some varieties of grain sorghum, *Agric. Food Chem.* **16:** 199–203.
42. Singh, R., and Axtell, J. D., 1973, High lysine mutant gene (hl) that improves protein quality and biological value of grain sorghum, *Crop. Sci.* **13:** 535–539.
43. Hegsted, D. M., Trulson, M. F., and Stare, F. J., 1954, Role of wheat and wheat products in human nutrition, *Physiol. Rev.* **34:** 221–258.
44. Johnson, V. A., Mattern, P. J., and Schmidt, J. W., 1972, *in: Symposium: Seed proteins,* G. E. Inglett (ed.), Avi Publishing Co., Westport, Connecticut, pp. 126–135.
45. Juliano, B. O., 1972, *in: Symposium: Seed proteins,* G. E. Inglett (ed.), Avi Publishing Co., Westport Connecticut, pp. 114–125.
46. Hulse, J., and Laing, E. M., 1974, *Nutritive value of triticale protein,* International Development Research Center, Ottawa, Canada, 184 pp.
47. Single, L., Wilson, C. M., and Hadley, H. H., 1969, Genetic differences in soybean trypsin inhibitors separated by disc electrophoresis, *Crop. Sci.* **9:** 489–491.
48. Clark, R. W., Mies, D. W., and Hymowitz, T., 1970, Distribution of a trypsin inhibitor variant in seed proteins of soybean varieties, *Crop. Sci.* **10:** 486–487.

COMMENT

Federico R. Poey · *Semillas Poey, S.A., Mèxico, D.F.*

Although genetic principles are universal, their application to plant breeding in tropical latitudes must be adapted to the local agronomic conditions and objectives, which are different from those in temperate regions. Generally, there is either no, or very limited, mechanization available in the tropics, and the methods for marketing and using the products are primitive. The kinds of breeding program used are determined mainly by the type of farmer who will benefit from them. In the tropics there are two principal types of farming: One is mechanized in an attempt to imitate the modern U.S. farmer, while the other is the small or subsistence farm, owned and operated by a man who has a totally different cultural attitude and motivation. Present breeding programs have so far been of direct benefit only to the former, while the subsistence farmer has received little or no benefit. The need to direct efforts toward both types of farmers complicates the objectives of tropical breeding programs.

Genetic–Environmental Interaction

Genetic–environmental interaction is basic to the concept of plant breeding, but it has been underestimated in most tropical programs. The generally optimum agronomic conditions of the experimental fields offer an environment that contrasts with the inadequate conditions of the average farm. To this interaction with the selected genotypes must be added that due to the wide variation in soil and agricultural practices, all of which minimize the expected gain in yield of the improved varieties based on evaluations from experimental fields only. These interactions also affect the nutritional value of the crops.

The traditional way the farmers utilize their crops should also be considered. In many instances these are different from those considered in the experimental field. For example, farmers may desire to utilize their corn crop as forage rather than for grain alone.

The genetic–environmental interaction can be measured through statistical regression techniques utilizing yield and environmental indices from the locations for which the improved variety is to be recommended (1,2). In most tropical countries, yield evaluations are conducted in various locations on an annual basis, with some varieties consistently repeated. Interpretation of these data and the ecological identification of environments could "regionalize" areas of adaptation for specific genotypes. This is a new field of research for which existing information can be considered as an excellent starting point.

The International Maize and Wheat Improvement Center (CIMMYT) use stability parameters in its wheat-breeding programs, with excellent results. The improved wheat varieties from CIMMYT are adapted to a wide range of environmental conditions and have gained great popularity in different countries on different continents. The stability concept, however, should not be overemphasized to the point of expecting universal varieties for staple food crops. Local improvement programs should always produce better varieties that would interact positively with local conditions, resulting in higher yields than those obtained with stable varieties adapated to a wide range of environments. In addition, the extensive use of a few varieties implies a risk of devastating losses by insects and disease.

Uniformity versus Variability

In temperate climates, typified by the United States, uniformity in a crop is considered almost as important as yield per se. However, in tropical countries a certain genetic variability within a crop is desirable in order to improve its adaptation. That variability can contribute to toleration of the usually highly erratic natural environmental conditions, as well as local agricultural practices. On self-pollinated crops such as wheat, multilineal varieties offer the proper mechanism to maintain the recommended variation. On cross-pollinated crops such as corn, desirable variation exists in most tropical commercial hybrids and in improved varieties created by mass selection or synthetic combination of lines. In the case of tropical hybrids, certain variability is present as a consequence of the limited selfing commonly practiced in inbred lines. This limitation is necessary to prevent an excessive loss of vigor that results from too much inbreeding of tropical materials.

It is important to recall that some important staple food crops have had their centers of origin in Latin America, for example, corn, beans, and potatoes. It is known that in such centers great species variability is present–an asset for the breeding programs using these crops. Variability is carefully preserved in germ plasm banks in Mexico, Honduras, Colombia, and Peru. Recently, these collections have been subjected to systematic field evaluations by local and international institutions, to establish their yield and nutritive potential. However, present breeding programs have not taken full advantage of these germ plasm banks. For corn in Mexico and Central America, for example, only the Tuxpeño and Caribe varieties have been utilized. For the higher plateaus of Mexico, only the Chalqueño, Cónico, and Celaya strains have been used. Enough variability may still be found in these strains to continue genetic progress, but a greater knowledge of the available potential would be useful.

Simultaneous Improvement of Yield and Protein

It is generally accepted that simultaneous progress may be difficult if two characteristics are negatively correlated. This simplistic conclusion must be reconsidered. Harpstead and Adams mentioned progress in the simultaneous selection for high yield and protein content in wheat, barley, and rice in spite of the negative correlation reported for these two variables.

Both characteristics–yield and protein content–depend on many genes. When only one component is selected, e.g., protein, progress results in an accumulation of favorable genes for increasing protein content. At the same time, the other factor, yield, which depends on many different genes, tends to stay at the same level in the absence of selection, as theoretically no genetic change in gene frequency takes place for this characteristic. Selections for high protein content would not change the yield potential, nor would selection for yield potential alone change protein content. When these modified populations are included in a correlation analysis, the independence of the magnitude of the expression of the two selected variables is emphasized.

Another explanation for the negative correlation found in these variables has to do with the selection criterion used. Protein is commonly measured in percent, so that the apparent increase in protein content obtained by selection can be a consequence of the indirect selection toward low carbohydrate content. Because carbohydrates account for the largest proportion of the dry weight in cereal kernels, the total weight of the kernel is reduced when the carbohydrate portion is reduced, allowing a negative correlation between yield and protein content.

Another way of measuring protein in cereals can be in absolute weight produced by the plant, which could have advantages during the selection process if protein were processed separately from carbohydrates. But, when the consumer, whether person or animal, ingests the cereal directly, the percentage of protein is important as a criterion of nutritive quality. One way to reconcile these criteria in selection programs can be by limiting the minimum kernel size or weight per plant, followed by selection for percentage of protein. We have some evidence in Mexico, for corn populations that were not previously selected for yield or protein, that shows a very low correlation between grain weight and protein content. This evidence suggests that the negative correlation generally observed is not a natural phenomenon, but one that is induced indirectly as a consequence of selecting toward only one of the two variables.

Harpstead and Adams mentioned that progress in selection is proportional to the existing genetic variance. In this sense, it has been repeatedly demonstrated that a wide variability exists in protein and amino acid values in cereals. In corn, for example, this variability persists in opaque-2 even at its higher concentrations of lysine and tryptophan. Also, great variability is found in the germ–endosperm relationship in corn. The germ, with its higher quality and relative amount of protein, represents another source of available genetic variability for the nutritional improvement of corn.

There are two main obstacles to the simultaneous selection for yield and protein: (1) the lack of simple, rapid, nondestructive, and economic methodology to identify the protein in a large number of samples, preferably in individual kernels; and (2) separating environmental from genetic effects in the expression of protein values.

In conclusion, it is biologically, statistically, and logically possible to improve protein and yield simultaneously in staple food crops. The biological support for this is that protein synthesis utilizes, basically, metabolic pathways different from those for carbohydrates and depends on different genetic mechanisms. The statistical explanation is that, even with low frequency of optimum gene combinations, and despite significant environmental effects, adequate sampling and proper experimental designs can be used to separate genetic from environmental effects. This means reducing one component–carbohydrates–in favor of the other–protein–while the yield factors can be selected for independently.

References

1. Eberhart, S. A., and Russell, W. A., 1966, Stability parameters for comparing varieties, *Crop Sci.* **6**: 36–40.
2. Márquez Sánchez, F., 1974, El Problema de la Interacción Genético-Ambiental en Genotecnia Vegetal, Patena, A.C., Chapingo, México.

39

Genetic Improvement of Cereal Proteins

Edwin T. Mertz

Department of Biochemistry
Purdue University
Lafayette, Indiana

Cereal proteins are inferior nutritionally to the proteins in milk, meat, and eggs because of inadequate levels of the amino acid lysine. With the discovery in 1963 by Mertz, Bates, and Nelson (1) that the maize mutant opaque-2 had nearly twice as much lysine as ordinary maize has, scientists realized that cereal grain proteins could be improved in quality by genetic manipulation. The recent discovery of high-lysine mutants of barley (2) and sorghum (3) raises the hope that all cereals can be improved in protein quality.

Agricultural scientists agree that more efficient use of the earth's land resources is required if world food production is to keep pace with world population. One way to use land more efficiently is to replace present cereal grains with grains of higher protein quality. The use of a high-quality protein cereal such as opaque-2 maize in the diet of humans provides a quality of protein previously available only from a good mixture of normal cereals and legumes, or from meat, milk, and eggs. The latter three require much larger areas of land per calorie of food, and legumes are usually lower yielding than the cereal grains.

If we assume that the FAO pattern of 5.2% lysine (4) is ideal for the infant, it is possible to compare the lysine content of common cereals and selected high-lysine mutants. This comparison is shown in Table I, based on data that we obtained in our laboratory. The protein levels of the various cereals are shown in column 2, the lysine levels based on protein, in column 3, and the percent of the ideal FAO level is given in column 4. On the basis of these data, the best of the cereal grains, oats, has about 73% of the ideal level, and the poorest of the grains, sorghum and millet, 36% of the ideal level. The sample of high-lysine

Table I. Lysine Content of Cereals and Selected High-Lysine Mutants

Cereal grain	Protein (%)	Lysine (g/100 g protein)	Percent of ideal level
Maize 4858[a]	10.5	2.7	52
Maize 4855,[a] high lysine	10.9	4.5	87
Maize 4856,[a] high lysine	10.1	4.7	90
Sorghum, normal[b]	13.1	1.8	35
Sorghum, high lysine[b]	18.5	3.3	63
Barley, normal[c]	19.8	3.3	63
Barley, high lysine[c]	19.4	5.6	108
Rice BB, normal[d]	6.9	3.7	71
Rice BP1761, high protein[d]	15.4	3.4	65
Wheat, Genesee, normal[e]	12.1	3.0	58
Wheat, Purdue 4930, high protein[e]	17.3	2.9	56
Oats, Noble, normal[f]	18.9	3.8	73
Millet[g]	14.5	1.9	36

[a]4858:CIMMYT normal yellow flint synthetic. 4855:CIMMYT yellow hard endosperm opaque-2 synthetic. 4856:CIMMYT yellow soft endosperm opaque-2 synthetic. From CIMMYT, Mexico City.
[b]Normal sorghum kernels: high-lysine sorghum. High lysine (hl hl hl) kernels from F_2 segregating heads derived from crosses between "normal" (low lysine) plants and the high-lysine sorghum line IS 11758.
[c]Normal barley: Bomi barley variety. High-lysine mutant: mutant 1058 from Risø, Denmark.
[d]Normal rice: Blue Bonnet variety. High protein rice:BP1 761 from IRRI.
[e]Normal wheat: Genesee, variety of New York soft wheat. High-protein wheat: Purdue 4930-A6-28-2-1.
[f]Normal oats: Noble, a Wisconsin variety.
[g]Millet: Finger millet, variety from Uganda supplied by Dr. S.A. Eberhart, Iowa State University, Ames.

barley that we analyzed contained 5.6% lysine, which is an excellent level. The double mutant of opaque-2 and brittle-2 also has an ideal level of 5.3% (Table II). Normal maize contains 52%, whereas opaque-2 maize, as currently produced in Mexico, contains 87–90% of the ideal level. Sorghum contains only 35% of the ideal level, but high-lysine sorghum has nearly double this amount (63% of the ideal level). The data in Table I indicate that wheat contains about 57% and current varieties of rice 71% of the ideal level of lysine.

It is obvious from the data in Table I that the plant breeder, by appropriate manipulation of the gene pools, can increase the lysine content of several cereals to a level approaching that found in meat, milk, and eggs.

The cereal chemist is especially interested in knowing more about the chemical changes that occur in the proteins to bring about these increases in lysine. In order to learn more about the nature of these changes, we fractionated the endosperm proteins in the various cereal samples by the Landry-Moureaux method (5). This method is outlined in Table III. Table IV shows the results of

Table II. Nitrogen Distribution in Endosperm of Double Combination Mutants of Maize[a]

Fraction	Endosperm genotype					
	su_1o_2	sh_1o_2	sh_2o_2	sh_4o_2	bt_1o_2	bt_2o_2
I	22.7	39.9	25.3	43.3	23.3	22.3
II	3.0	1.8	1.2	6.5	2.7	2.9
III	9.0	1.6	1.1	3.9	2.5	5.5
IV	14.2	16.4	26.1	8.7	13.1	12.2
V	45.3	32.2	35.4	26.8	50.2	48.0
Total N extracted	94.2	91.9	89.1	89.2	91.8	90.9
Lysine (% of total protein)	3.9	4.8	4.2	4.0	4.8	5.3
Tryptophan (% of total protein)	0.8	1.2	1.2	1.2	1.4	1.3

[a]Percent of total nitrogen.

fractionating the endosperm proteins in the isogenic mutants opaque-2, floury-2, the double mutant of opaque-2 and floury-2, brittle-2, and the double mutant of opaque-2 and brittle-2, in the Ohio background (6). Results are also shown for the fractionation of the high lysine mutant opaque-7 in the W22 background (6). These data show that the introduction of the opaque-2, floury-2, brittle-2, or

Table III. Landry-Moureaux Fractionation Sequence D

Fraction	Solvent[a]		Time of agitation (min)	Protein fractions
I	NaCl 0.5 M	(4°C)	60	Albumins
			30	Globulins
			30	
	Water		15	
			15	
II	Isopropanol 70% (v/v)	(20°C)	30	
			30	Zein
			30	
III	Isopropanol 70% (v/v)		30	
	+ 2-ME 0.6% (v/v)	(20°C)	30	Zein-like
IV	Borate buffer pH 10		60	
	+ 2-ME 0.6% (v/v)	(20°C)	30	Glutelin-like
V	Borate buffer pH 10		60	
	+ 2-ME 0.6% (v/v)		30	Glutelin
	+ SDS 0.5% (w/v)		15	Residue

[a]2-ME: 2-mercaptoethanol. Borate buffer: borate, NaOH, NaCl μ 0.5. SDS: sodium dodecylsulphate.

Table IV. Nitrogen Distribution in Maize Endosperms[a]

Fraction	Oh43						W22		
	Inbred genotype								
	+	o_2	fl_2	fl_2o_2	bt_2	bt_2o_2	+	o_7	o_7o_2
I (saline)	5.8	13.6	9.2	17.0	12.1	22.3	6.9	16.6	17.6
II (zein)	59.0	26.9	49.1	25.0	26.1	2.9	40.6	20.3	8.7
III (zein-like)	5.8	8.4	9.0	15.2	15.4	5.5	15.3	12.0	15.1
IV (glutelin-like)	12.7	14.0	7.6	9.9	8.7	12.2	12.8	18.8	21.3
V (glutelin)	13.8	29.2	22.0	24.8	27.9	48.0	21.0	29.5	33.3
Total N extracted	97.1	92.1	96.7	91.9	90.2	90.9	96.6	97.2	96.0

[a]Percent of soluble nitrogen.

opaque-7 genes into a normal background increases the level of saline-soluble proteins, decreases the level of zein, and increases the level of glutelin (Fraction V).

Because the saline fraction (Fraction I) and Fraction V contain about 6 gm of lysine per 100 gm of protein, and Fraction II, zein, contains about 0.1% lysine, it is obvious that these changes will increase the lysine content of the mutant endosperms. It can also be noted that the double mutants, floury-2/opaque-2 and opaque-7/opaque-2, show changes that resemble those observed with opaque-2 without giving an effect higher than that observed with opaque-2 alone. In contrast, the double mutant brittle-2/opaque-2 shows substantially higher increases in saline-soluble and glutelin levels, and an almost complete disappearance of the zein fraction. Here one observes an additive effect of the opaque-2 and brittle-2 genes to give a product with much higher levels of lysine than are found in either opaque-2 or brittle-2 alone.

We have extended these studies to include sugary-1, shrunken-1, shrunken-2, shrunken-4, and brittle-1, and the double mutants of these single mutants with opaque-2. These data are shown in Tables II and V. The changes in fractions I, II, and V are similar to those observed with brittle-2 (Table V). However, the levels of lysine in the double mutants (Table II) are much higher than those observed in the single mutants, and resemble the levels found in the double mutant of opaque-2 and brittle-2.

Studies with the developing endosperms of the double mutant opaque-2/brittle-2 indicate that at no time during development, from 10 days postpollination on, is there any evidence that zein is being produced (Misra, Mertz, and Glover, in press). This has been confirmed with acrylamide gel electrophoresis, which shows the complete lack of the two normal components of the zein fraction.

Table V. Nitrogen Distribution in Opaque-2 and Several Nonfloury Endosperm Mutants[a]

Fraction	Endosperm genotype							
	+	o_2	su_1	sh_1	sh_2	sh_4	bt_1	bt_2
I	5.8	13.6	11.9	8.2	12.3	25.7	8.8	12.1
II	59.0	26.9	27.1	43.7	29.4	30.8	36.0	26.1
III	5.8	8.4	21.9	12.3	9.4	7.7	16.4	15.4
IV	12.7	14.0	9.1	14.4	15.0	8.3	8.3	8.7
V	13.8	29.2	22.8	16.3	23.6	23.6	27.4	27.9
Total N extracted	97.1	92.1	92.8	94.9	89.8	96.1	96.9	90.2
Lysine (% of total protein)	1.6	3.5	1.8	1.9	2.7	3.0	2.3	3.3
Tryptophan (% of total protein)	0.3	0.8	0.3	0.6	0.7	0.8	0.5	0.7

[a]Percent of that nitrogen in endosperm.

Table VI. Protein Distribution in High-Lysine Sorghum[a]

Type of sorghum	Fraction I	Fraction II	Fraction III	Fraction IV	Fraction V
Normal	15.3	26.4	26.5	4.3	22.5
High lysine	22.4	13.7	20.2	4.3	33.5

[a]High-lysine values average of assays from 5 segregating heads using high-lysine (hl hl hl) kernels from F_2 heads derived from crosses between normal plants and high-lysine sorghum line IS 11758. Lysine content of normal sorghum: 1.8 g/100 g protein; lysine content of high-lysine sorghum: 3.3 g/100 g protein.

Table VI shows the results of fractionating normal and high-lysine sorghum. Here again, one observes in the high-lysine sorghum an increase in Fraction I, a decrease in Fraction II, and an increase in Fraction V. Feeding tests with high-lysine sorghum demonstrate that it is much more nutritious than normal sorghum; weight gains in rats eating high-lysine sorghum were four times greater than in rats consuming the normal sorghum counterpart (3).

Table VII shows that the Landry-Moureaux fractionation of high-lysine mutant barley number 1508 also shows an increase in the glutelin fraction. It is obvious from these data that the maize, sorghum, and barley high-lysine selections all have shown similar changes in their protein patterns, and it is this rather than the development of any new proteins that is primarily responsible for the increase of the lysine content of the grain. One exception to these findings has been observed; namely, that the high-lysine mutant barley, hiproly, has been produced by a different set of genetic events. In this case, there is no drop in the level of prolamine, but there are marked increases in several high-lysine-containing proteins in the saline-soluble fraction (7).

In those high-lysine types where there is a marked reduction in prolamine, it has been observed that there is also a floury or soft type of endosperm. It is

Table VII. Protein Distribution in High-Lysine Barley[a]

	Albumin/globulin		Prolamine		Glutelin		Lysine g/100 g	
	Mutant	Normal	Mutant	Normal	Mutant	Normal	Mutant	Normal
Ingversen	46	27	9	29	39	39	7.0	4.7
Mertz	48	27	3	33	32	28	5.7	3.3

[a]Percent of total nitrogen in fractions. Purdue values based on Landry-Moureau fractions: albumin/globulin = Fraction I, prolamine = Fractions II and III, and glutelin = Fractions IV and V. Bomi barley (normal) and mutant 1508 kindly supplied by H. W. Ohm, Purdue University. The former contained 18.5% protein, the latter 19.8%. Ingversen's samples contained 10.2% and 10.1%, respectively.

possible, however, by selective breeding, to select for hard endosperm at the same time that one is selecting for high lysine content. A successful opaque-2 hard synthetic type has been developed by CIMMYT, and is represented by maize 4855 in Table I. The development of a hard endosperm type of maize in the United States has not progressed as far as that at CIMMYT. It is theoretically possible that one could also breed for hard endosperm types of high-lysine sorghum and high-lysine barley.

With the advent of hard endosperm types of high-lysine cereals, the cereal is difficult to distinguish, by physical means, from its normal counterpart. It therefore became necessary to develop a simple test to distinguish the hard endosperm type of high-lysine cereal from the normal cereal. We succeeded recently in developing a rapid test at Purdue based on the unusually high levels of free amino acids found in high-lysine mutants. The test is based on the use of ninhydrin (8), which gives a much stronger reaction with high-lysine maize, sorghum, and barley samples than with the normal counterparts. The ninhydrin screening test should be useful in the market place and in the research laboratory to identify high-lysine types of cereals.

It may not be necessary to achieve the FAO level of 5.2% lysine in all cereal grains used in animal and human foods. Nevertheless, this is a level to aim at, and there is no evidence at present to suggest that the plant breeder, by appropriate genetic manipulation of the gene pools, cannot attain this goal. However, the plant breeder must watch both the lysine level and the protein level. In rice, which has an unusually low protein level even for a cereal, the breeding for high protein has caused a reduction in the level of lysine in the protein (Table I). Theoretically, the introduction of high-lysine genes could restore the lysine level in the high-protein rice varieties, and perhaps bring them closer to the ideal of 5.2%.

FUTURE PROSPECTS

Breeding for improved nutritional value in cereals has a bright future. A search should be made for the opaque-2 type of mutant in all economically important cereal grains. There is a good possibility that such types exist in millets and that they could also exist in wheat. Another promising approach is the use of wide crosses between cereal grains to cross the high-lysine maize, barley, and sorghum types with cereal grains in which high-lysine types have not been found to date. For example, a wide cross between high-lysine barley and wheat would certainly improve the lysine content and raise it to a level intermediate between that of wheat (3%) and high-lysine barley (5%). It has been reported that such a wide cross has been achieved recently (9). A successful wide cross immediately available for exploitation is triticale, an artificial genus synthesized by combining the genomes of wheat (genus *Triticum*) and rye (genus

Secale). The lysine level per unit of protein in this wide cross is higher than that in wheat.

Another approach to improve nutritional value in cereals is to search for mutants that will overproduce the free amino acid lysine in the developing seed. If such overproduction is not lethal to the germination characteristics of the seed, this approach would be equivalent to lysine supplementation of cereals, and could improve all cereals that are limiting in lysine, as the search for high-lysine mutants accelerates. It is not too optimistic to hope that eventually all cereal species will carry substantially higher levels of lysine, thus closing the quality gap that now exists between cereal and animal proteins.

ACKNOWLEDGMENT

The author's research on maize has been supported by the Agency for International Development under contract *Inheritance and Improvement of Protein Quality and Content in Maize.*

REFERENCES

1. Mertz, E. T., Bates, L. S., and Nelson, O. E., 1964, Mutant gene that changes protein composition and increases lysine content of maize endosperm, *Science* **145:** 279.
2. Ingversen, J., Koie, B., and Holl, H., 1973, Induced seed protein mutant of barley, *Experientia* **29:** 1151.
3. Singh, R., and Axtell, J. D., 1973, High lysine mutant gene (hl) that improves protein quality and biological value of grain sorghum, *Crop Sci.* **13:** 535.
4. World Health Organization Technical Report Series No. 522, 1973, *Energy and protein requirements,* Report of a Joint FAO/WHO ad hoc Expert Committee, WHO, Geneva.
5. Landry, J., and Moureaux, T., 1970, Hétérogénéité des glutélines du grain de mais: Extraction sélective et composition en acides aminés des trois fractions isolées, *Bull. Soc. Chim. Biol.* **52:** 1021.
6. Misra, P. S., Mertz, E. T., and Glover, D. V., 1975, Studies on corn proteins VI. Endosperm protein changes in single and double endosperm mutants of maize, *Cereal Chem.* **52:** 161.
7. Munck, L., 1972, Improvement of nutritional value in cereals, *Hereditas* **72:** 1.
8. Mertz, E. T., Misra, P. S., and Jambunathan, R., 1974, Rapid ninhydrin color test for screening high-lysine mutants of maize, sorghum, barley, and other cereal grains, *Cereal Chem.* **51:** 304.
9. Bates, L. S., Campos, A. V., Rodriguez, R., and Anderson, R. G., 1974, Progress toward novel cereal grains, *Cereal Sci. Today* **19:** 283.

40

Production and Use of Protein Concentrates

Steven R. Tannenbaum

Department of Nutrition and Food Science
Massachusetts Institute of Technology
Cambridge, Massachusetts

The history of utilizing proteins in novel form dates back to gelatin manufacture from hides and bones. In this century the demand for new protein technologies and new sources of raw material first occurred in nonfood areas, such as paper and textile sizings, button manufacture, and even early attempts to make casein fabrics.

The demand for new sources of protein for use in foods is a much more recent phenomenon, dating back only to the 1950s, when the widespread prevalence of protein-calorie malnutrition began to be appreciated. Work at INCAP and other centers demonstrated that vegetable proteins could be blended to match the nutritive value of animal protein sources for human feeding. The demand for these nutritional developments might have been insufficient in itself to provide the impetus in research and development that began in the 1960s and has continued through to the present. A concomitant development in basic technology was also required, as well as an increased demand for technologically sophisticated protein products in nonnutritional applications.

The technological developments came from a variety of sources. For example, the plastics industry had already dealt with problems of fiber spinning and pellet extrusion on a very large scale. The use of extrusion technology for animal feeds was also well advanced. There were also significant technical developments in the manufacture of breakfast cereals and snack foods, and these developments could readily be transferred to protein products. It is probably no coincidence that the initial industrial ventures into textured protein products included some of the industrial leaders in breakfast cereals and animal feeds.

Table I. Per Caput Consumption of High Protein Foods[a]

Food	1972	1973	Change, %
Eggs	307 eggs	294 eggs	–5
Pork	67.4 lb.	61.6 lb.	–9
Beef	116.0 lb.	109.5 lb.	–6

[a]From: USDA, Economic Research Service, National Food Situation, May, 1974.

The final impetus for the unprecedented demand for protein concentrates in the last three years has come from the increased demand and prices for meat products, particularly in Europe and Japan. In the United States, per caput consumption of the more expensive high protein foods has actually decreased recently, as shown in Table I. This can probably be directly related to the enormous increases in the cost of all food (Table II), which has forced both families and institutions to substitute lower cost items into their budgets. In spite of the fact that the cost of protein in various protein concentrates has doubled in the past decade (equivalent to a rate of inflation of about 10% per year), the magnitude of the price differential between protein isolates and conventional high protein foods has continued, and possibly increased (Table III).

OILSEEDS

It has been estimated that there may be potentially 80 million tons of oilseed protein available per year for human and animal feeding by 1980 (1). The current rate of production is somewhat below this figure, being on the order of 58 million tons. The primary purpose for cultivation of oilseeds is to obtain edible oil for table purposes, or for use in manufacture of margarine or other shortening. The basic process for obtaining the oil is essentially the same for all oilseeds, and involves either pressing (primarily screwpress), solvent extraction,

Table II. Cost Increases of Various Foods

Food	Change in consumer price index, August 1972–August 1974
All food	+ 31%
Fruits and vegetables	+ 31%
Dairy products	+ 29%
Meats, poultry, and fish	+ 24%

Table III. Relative Cost of Protein

Source	Protein, ¢/lb. 1964	1974
Soy protein concentrate (70% protein)	24	48
Soy protein isolate (95% protein)	37	55
Torula yeast (50% protein)	30	60
Skim milk powder	37	180
Tuna (canned)	–	629
Bologna	–	973
Hamburger	–	530

or a combination of the two. The material remaining after removal of the oil contains fiber, carbohydrate, and protein. The protein can comprise up to 50% of this residue, depending upon the particular oilseed. This material is either discarded, used as fertilizer (a poor source because it decomposes too slowly), or used as a source of protein in animal feeds. Currently, only a small percentage is recovered in a form suitable for human foods.

The major factors limiting more extended food applications of these materials are the overly severe conditions under which most of them are handled to remove the oil, and their market image as fertilizer or animal feed. In addition, each of the oilseeds has specific, individual processing problems. In a general way, the oilseed proteins are the least expensive of all the potential new proteins in their simplest edible state, but additional refining to improve the properties to provide a more useful product invariably leads to cost increments that double or treble the price of the protein. There is no simple, consistent way to compare prices of a variety of new proteins, each of which may be suitable for different applications. It is also difficult and misleading to compare nutritive values of proteins, because their actual worth will depend upon a variety of external environmental factors, including the other components of the diet in which they are incorporated.

Soybeans

This is by far the most important of the oilseeds from a food standpoint, and has the most highly developed technology for its adaptation to food products. The entire technology, from treatment of the bean to production of protein concentrates, has recently been summarized (2,3). The oil is recovered primarily by solvent extraction, and the residue is approximately 50% protein. The defatted soy contains a number of undesirable factors that must be removed or inactivated. In particular, there are a number of physiologically active proteins, including one that inhibits the important digestive enzyme, trypsin, that must be inactivated by heat. Because the desirable proteins are also affected by heat in a manner that reduces their solubility and nutritive value, this process must be carried out with great care.

Other factors that limit the usefulness of soy protein are a bitter, beany off-flavor, and the presence of two soluble carbohydrates (raffinose and stachyose) that lead, in man, to gas production by intestinal flora, to distension of the gut, and to flatulence. Each of these factors is reduced in intensity by processes that purify the protein and lead to products of higher protein content.

The traditional Oriental use of the soybean follows three forms: a milklike aqueous extract (soy milk), produced by extraction of cooked beans at high temperature; a protein curd precipitated from soy milk, either by acidification or by addition of calcium salts (tofu); and a variety of hydrolyzed protein products made by fermentation processes (miso, shoyu).

The simplest method of purification used in Western countries involves immobilization of the protein and removal of extraneous materials. This is accomplished either by extraction with aqueous alcohol (70% ethanol or isopropanol), or by extraction with water at the isoelectric point of the proteins. For soy, the minimum solubility of the proteins is at pH 4 to 5. Either of these processes removes most of the undesirable soluble carbohydrates and some of the off-flavor, and gives a product that is approximately 70% protein. The product is called soy protein concentrate, and is suitable for addition to a variety of food products, or for the manufacture of texturized products.

An even more refined product is made by carrying out a process that is actually the reverse of the one just described. Instead, the protein is solubilized by extraction at alkaline pH, the extract is separated from any insoluble residue, and the protein is precipitated by readjustment of the pH back to the region of minimum solubility. This cycle can be repeated a number of times to increase the purity of the protein. Products of this type are called soy protein isolates, and they are 90 to 99% protein. Almost all of the objectionable characteristics are removed, and the material can be incorporated into a large variety of food products. This material can be texturized by spinning into edible fibers, a process that will be more fully described later in the chapter.

Other Oilseeds

There are numerous other oilseeds of commercial importance that have unrealized prospects for production of protein concentrates. These include cottonseed, peanut, coconut, rapeseed, and sunflower. Each has its own peculiar problems of purification, but a more detailed discussion is outside the scope of this discussion (see references 4–6).

MARINE PROTEIN CONCENTRATES

Fish protein concentrate (FPC) can be broadly described as a product made from whole fish wherein the protein in the starting material is concentrated to produce a final product fit for human consumption. A comprehensive summary of developments in FPC production is contained in a recent book on the subject (7).

The basis for any FPC process is the removal of the two constituents that lead to rapid deterioration of fresh fish: water, which allows microbial spoilage; and lipid, which will allow deleterious oxidative changes. Although a variety of methods are available to achieve this end, the most common approach is to use solvent extraction for simultaneous removal of lipid and water. In the United States, two processes have been approved by the Food and Drug Administration—one using isopropyl alcohol (Nabisco-Astra Corp. and U.S. Bureau of Commercial Fisheries), and one using a two-step extraction with ethylene dichloride followed by isopropyl alcohol (Viobin Corporation).

The major advantage of FPC is the high biological value of its protein, which approximates that of animal proteins. Because of this, only small amounts added to cereals lead to relatively high increments in nutritive value. FPC also faces a myriad of problems, including high cost and poor functional properties in foods. The true cost of FPC will only be known when plants have been in operation long enough to determine actual operating costs. The cost is, however, strongly tied to that of the raw material, fish. Therefore, the process can be economical only where fish is in excess and inexpensive, and probably where an FPC process can be integrated directly into an existing fishing industry. Recent increases in the price of solvents will have a significant impact on the cost of solvent-produced FPCs.

The poor physical properties of FPC present a problem similar to that initially faced by soy protein. On the basis of work done on solubilization by chemicals and enzymes, there is good reason to expect that these problems can eventually be solved. These types of processes will obviously involve increased costs, but if the case is similar to soy, the added utility of the product may compensate for the increased price.

A major problem faced by FPC is the availability of raw material. The fisheries biologists greatly overestimated the available catch in the 1960s, and overfishing and the vagaries of nature have created scarcity where there once was surplus. For this reason, more attention is being paid to sources of raw material that were previously neglected. One example is the Atlantic squid, which has possibilities for conversion into a high-quality protein concentrate (8). Another is the Antarctic krill, which is supposedly available in millions of tons per year and is being actively exploited by the Soviet Union.

Special consideration should be given to the type of multiple-use schemes developed for the Chilean fish resource (9), because of the great efficiency of coupling protein concentrate production directly to a marketable food product.

SINGLE-CELL PROTEIN

SCP has become, by definition, a generic term for crude or refined sources of protein whose origin is unicellular or simple multicellular organisms, i.e., bacteria, yeast, fungi, and algae. The production of SCP is a more complex process than that used for FPC and is shown schematically in Figure 1, which is self-explanatory. Each step in the overall operation is denoted by a separate block, and either some, or all, of these steps would be required in an individual process. Most processes for SCP are basically similar, except for the type of organism and carbon substrate used. One of the major attractions of SCP is that it is a protein resource that can be produced without resort to an agricultural base. In contrast to FPC, SCP will probably prove most economical in very large

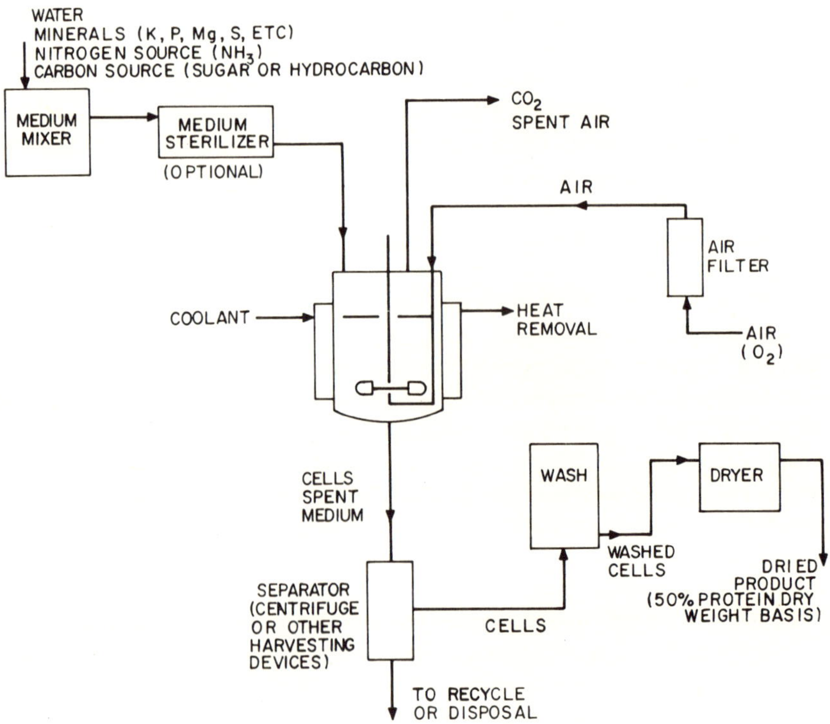

FIG. 1. Simplified flowsheet of production of single-cell protein.

plants producing hundreds of thousands of tons of material annually. The technological, economic, and nutritive aspects of SCP have recently been summarized (10).

In terms of world interest, most attention is being paid to processes that utilize hydrocarbons or derivatives as the sole energy source for growth of the microorganism. This would include gas oil, refined petroleum fractions, or alcohols. Other raw materials of interest include molasses, starch, sulfite waste liquor from paper manufacture, cheese whey, and cellulose. The particular raw material of choice depends on locale. Thus, natural gas or methane would be of great interest in areas such as the Middle East or the North Sea, where it is available in abundance.

Methane has notable advantages and disadvantages. It is very cheap and leaves no residue in the final product. However, it requires a sophisticated fermentation system to prevent formation of hazardous gas mixtures, it is limited to growth of bacteria, it requires large quantities of oxygen, and produces more heat.

Although gas oil has been used extensively in Europe for animal feed products, a product made from this petroleum fraction would not be permitted in food without costly purification to exclude potentially harmful residues. Most work has centered on use of highly purified paraffinic hydrocarbons that, in themselves, would be safe in a food. Sulfite waste liquor and whey are of interest in locales where they are now discarded, and, along with starch and molasses, may be used to produce cells by conventional fermentation technology. Another carbohydrate, ubiquitous in nature and of potential future interest, is cellulose. The main problem is the conversion of cellulose to metabolizable sugar in a manner that would be economically competitive with more readily available fermentable carbohydrate.

Bacteria, yeasts, fungi, and algae are all in active consideration for pilot or commercial scale processes. Algae represent a distinctly separate group because they utilize carbon dioxide as their carbon source. *Spirulina maxima,* a type of blue-green alga, has been used since ancient times by peoples near Lake Chad in Africa, and was probably also used by the Aztecs in ancient Mexico. The primary limitation on this and other types of algae is economic. Some types of algae also have problems of flavor and protein digestibility. The most popular organisms appear to be yeasts, which somehow seem more familiar to human experience. They have been used in foods as vitamin additives and flavoring agents, have protein contents on the order of 50% of dry weight, and are easier to recover from fermentation broths than bacteria are. The species of interest are mainly *Saccharomyces* and *Candida.* Bacteria could ultimately possess a number of advantages over other organisms. They have higher growth rates and higher protein contents, but are less well known in human nutritional experience.

It is now generally agreed that SCP can, and should, play a significant role in providing an alternative to oilseeds to meet future world protein needs. Undoubtedly the initial major role will be in animal feeds, but gradually contributions to direct human food use will also increase. SCP has been considered as one of the possible feed inputs for a computerized model of projected protein requirements of the European Economic Communities, United Kingdom, and Japan (1). Assuming that the use of SCP in these countries in 1980 would not be more than one-half the technically feasible maximum level, the projections suggest that consumption of SCP might be about 1.4 million tons in 1980. This would be equivalent to about 2 million tons of oilseed cake on an equal protein basis. Factors that could moderate these estimates include the current energy crisis, the overall shortage of capital for new plant investment, and strong negative consumer or governmental reaction to the concept of proteins produced using petroleum-based sources. There are currently under construction plants with about 3×10^5 tons per annum capacity, based upon hydrocarbon fermentation technology, with plans for producing about an equal amount in planning stages. However, most recent attention has been given to utilization of alcohols as a substrate, particularly methanol, and by 1980 this technology may well provide plant capacity equal to, or greater than, fermentation of n-paraffins.

The future extent of direct SCP use in foods is more certain than it is in animal feeds. There are currently two industrial projects directed toward this end, including one on torula yeast grown on ethanol (Standard Oil of Indiana), and another on fungi grown on carbohydrates (Ranks Hovis Macdougall, Ltd., and Du Pont, Inc.). The extent of direct usage by 1980 will depend, to a great extent, upon the resolution of safety factors, such as the problem of dietary nucleic acid tolerance, and upon the adaptability of the organisms to food fabrication requirements.

USE OF PROTEIN CONCENTRATES IN FOOD PRODUCTS

Because the most widely used protein concentrate is from soy, it would be well to look first at current uses for these products. The various types of soy products currently being marketed in the United States are listed in Table IV, and the types of food products that incorporate these proteins are listed in Table V. Of all the food products listed in Table V, the greatest recent growth has come in the meat product area because of the economic factors mentioned earlier, and these applications demand the most sophisticated soy technology.

The development of products from protein concentrates that simulate meat, fish, and shellfish from a textural point of view has led to wide acceptance of substitute foods. There are a number of technological approaches to this end that have been reviewed in depth elsewhere (11,12), and will be briefly described here. The potential benefits offered by these products include lower cost,

Table IV. Types of Soy Products Currently Marketed in the United States

Product
Canned soybeans
Flour and grits
Concentrates
Isolates
Enzyme-modified products
Milks
Whey–soy blends
Texturized
Cheeses
Extruded
Spun

controlled nutrient composition, and the possibility of restructuring lower cost cuts of meat to reduce waste and economic loss.

The simplest approach to texturization is the fabrication of "chewy" granules that simulate ground meat. The basis for this approach is the use of isolated gluten at concentrations in the formulation high enough to produce stiff doughs. These doughs, containing suitable flavor and color, are extruded, sliced, and dried. When rehydrated they may be used directly in casseroles.

Another approach employs thermal denaturation of systems containing high concentrations of dissolved protein to form "chewy gels" (Figure 2). This process can be made more or less continuous through the use of the same type of cooker-extruders used in the fabrication of snack products or in the preparation of full-fat soy flours. The products are based mainly on soy proteins, and preparations containing as low as 70% protein can be utilized. The texture of the final product can be varied over a wide range, from tough to tender. As in the case of granules, these products are mainly intended for use in stews and casseroles, and as ground meat extenders.

Table V. Types of Foods Containing Soy Products

Bakery products
Dairy products:
beverages; desserts; cheeses; toppings
Meat products:
meat patties and loaves; sausage products; bacon substitutes; meat granules
Infant formulations
Special dietary foods

The most sophisticated process, and also the most expensive, utilizes oriented protein fibers (Figure 3). The fibers are made primarily from soy protein preparations of greater than 70% protein content (usually 90% or more) and 95% soluble at alkaline pH. The protein is solubilized in alkali at pH 12 at a concentration of 12 to 14% to give a viscous dope. This is then extruded through spinnerettes into a coagulating bath of acid and salt to set the fibers. There are approximately 16,000 fibers in a single tow and fiber diameters vary from 0.001 to 0.030 inch. The tow is taken up from the bath onto a series of reels that stretch the fibers and allow excess salt and acid to be washed away.

The final products are prepared by blending washed fibers with fat, flavors, coloring, supplemental nutrients, stabilizers, and protein binders. The binder protein is usually egg albumin, which is used because of its thermosetting properties. The cost of this expensive ingredient contributes significantly to the ultimate cost of the product. The blended fibers are then transferred to a blender-cooker and are finally converted into slices, cubes, bits, or granules. The entire process, beginning with extraction of soy protein to final fabricated food, can be carried out on a continuous basis. The composition of these products is

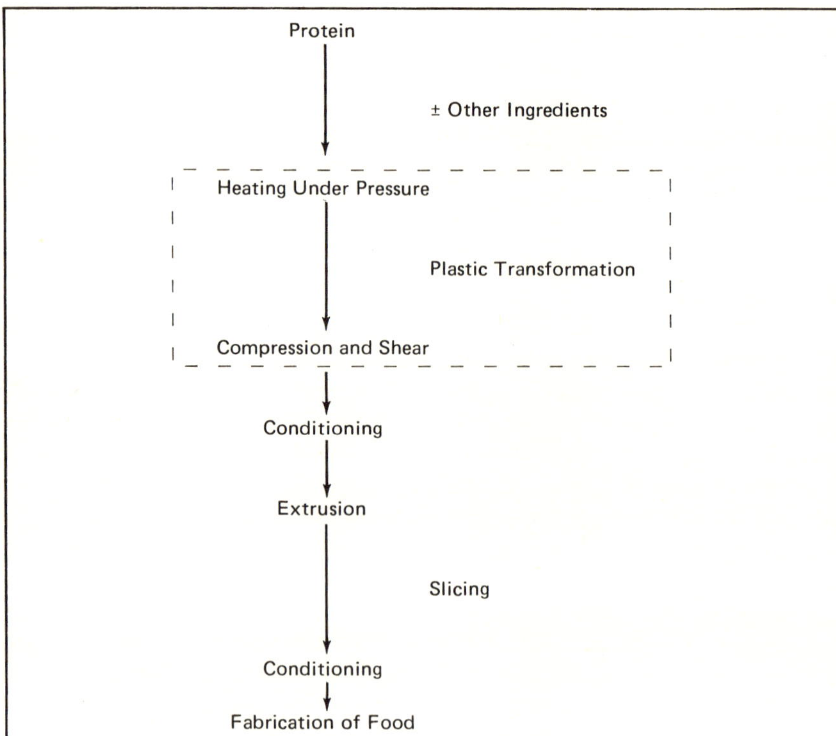

FIG. 2. Extrusion technology.

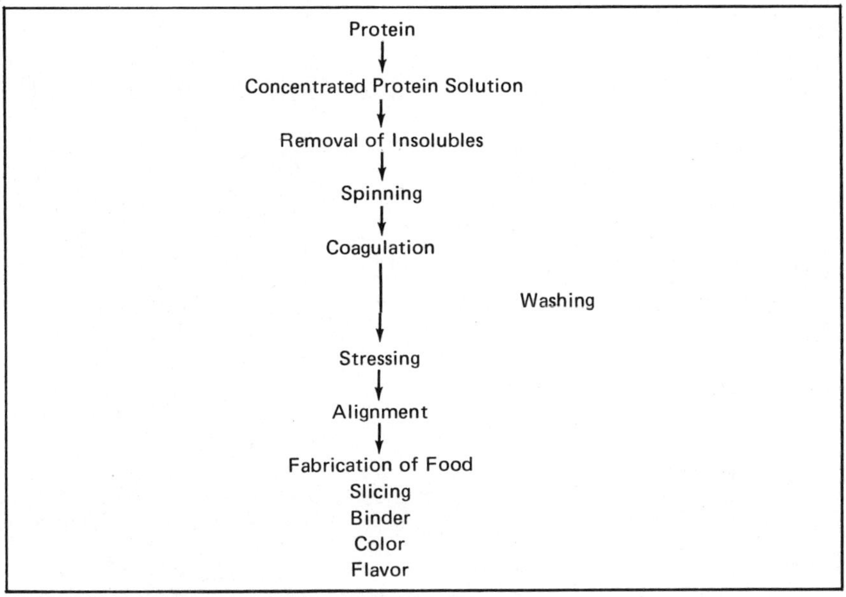

FIG. 3. Fiber-spinning technology.

such that they are approximately 40% soy fiber; the remainder is composed of varying quantities of the other ingredients. It is possible that the optional ingredients include lower cost cuts of meat that could contribute flavor and color.

CONCLUSIONS

Because of simple economic factors, protein concentrates may be expected to play an ever-increasing role in protein food products. As of this moment soy completely dominates the marketplace and a sophisticated technology for texturization of soy has been developed. An added advantage for soy is that only a small fraction of the crop is used directly for food; most goes to animal feed. In addition to soy, there are large potential reserves of other oilseeds, and increasing amounts of a variety of SCPs are likely to begin to appear between now and 1980.

To what extent will these alternate proteins serve as resources for protein concentrates directly utilizable in foods? This will depend in large part upon the qualities, characteristics, and costs of any new protein concentrate. It is my guess that soy will not be supplanted for some time to come, if ever, but that multiprotein blends, engineered for specific product applications, will be the next stage in our still-developing protein technology.

REFERENCES

1. Food and Agriculture Organization, 1971, *U.N. agricultural commodity projections,* Rome, pp. 1970–1980.
2. Smith, A. K., and Circle, S. J., 1952, *Soybeans: Chemistry and technology,* Vol. 1, Avi Publishing Co., Westport, Connecticut.
3. Wolf, W. J., 1971, Soybeans as a food source, *Crit. Rev. Food Technol.* **2** (1): 81.
4. Martinez, W. H., Bernardi, C. C., and Goldblatt, L. A., 1971, Potential of cottonseed: Products, composition, and use, *in: SOS/70, Proc. Third Intl. Congr. Food Sci. Tech.,* Washington, D.C., p. 248.
5. Hagenmaier, R., Cater, C. M., and Mattil, K. F., 1973, Aqueous processing of fresh coconuts for recovery of oil and coconut skim milk, *J. Food Sci.* **38** (3): 516.
6. Sosulski, F. W., Sabir, M. A., and Fleming, S. E., 1973, Continuous diffusion of chlorogenic acid from sunflower kernels, *J. Food Sci.* **38** (3): 468.
7. Tannenbaum, S. R., Stillings, B. R., and Scrimshaw, N. S. (eds.), 1974, *Economics, marketing, and technology of fish protein concentrate,* M.I.T. Press, Cambridge, Massachusetts, 500 pp.
8. Kahn, L. N., Berk, Z., Pariser, E. R., Goldblith, S. A., and Flink, J. M., 1974, Squid protein isolate: Effect of processing conditions on recovery yields, *J. Food Sci.* **39** (3): 592.
9. Rutman, M., and Heimlich, W., 1974, The fish protein hydrolyzate (FPH) process. A target design approach, *in: Economics, marketing, and technology of fish protein concentrate,* S. R. Tannenbaum, B. R. Stillings, and N. S. Scrimshaw (eds.), M.I.T. Press, Cambridge, Massachusetts, pp. 135–161.
10. S. R. Tannenbaum, and D. I. C. Wang (eds.), 1975, *Single-cell protein–II,* M.I.T. Press, Cambridge, Massachusetts, 707 pp.
11. Glicksman, M., 1971, Fabricated foods, *Crit. Rev. Food Tech.* **2** (1): 21.
12. Gutcho, M., 1973, *Textured foods and allied products,* Noyes Data Corp., Park Ridge, New Jersey.

COMMENT

Arthur D. Odell · *Industrial Grain Products, Montreal, Canada.*

In his overview of the production, fabrication, and utility aspects of protein concentrates, Tannenbaum has rightly stressed some of the major practical constraints associated with the more novel members of this group of materials. I concur with his analyses and predictions of the role of these materials for the short-term future.

Vegetable Proteins

For the near, and indeed, the longer term, soy may be expected to play a major role in the noncereal vegetable inputs for human dietary support and supplementation. Certainly, in the broad spectrum of vegetable proteins, soy products are impressive. From defatted flours upward through concentrates to isolates, protein densities rise from 50% to better than 90%, while protein efficiency ratios for the same categories trend toward the reverse direction, from 90% of that in casein to approximately 65%. Purification, then, imposes nutritional sacrifice, somewhat compensated for by the elimination of some undesirable components, by gain in protein density, and by enhancement of functionality for food fabrication.

There are sound reasons to regard single component soy products as "first generation" food components that can, and should, team up with synergistic companion proteins from other sources. Such second, third, or fourth generation mixed products can be much more cost-effective through more intense nutritional impact. Multiprotein blends are almost mandatory for future vegetable-based protein foods–a trend started by Incaparina and since followed by wheat/soy blend (WSB) and corn/soy milk (CSM).

It can be predicted that the major spur to the commercial achievement for fabricated protein foods based on synergistic mixtures will come from the beneficial economic impact on the grocery bills of affluent societies. There will be commercial opportunities for products that, when used for extension or replacement, will have the approximate nutritional equivalence to expensive natural meats. Such nutritional equivalence is of increasing importance in the research and development expenditures by commercial firms. Common sense urges an equivalency approach, and regulatory agencies in affluent societies are increasingly insistent that it can be achieved. In such a regulatory climate, synergistic protein blends or fortification with limiting essential amino acids are the only alternatives. For example, blends of wheat gluten and soy protein in the correct ratio to combine individual PER values of 1.0 and 2.0 can give a product equal to casein in nutritional merit.

The number of man-years of effort and the funds expended to bring soy protein technology to where it stands today are awesome. Fortunately, as new sources of vegetable protein become available at the commodity level, most of this expertise will be directly applicable to new materials. In Canada, we are looking very intently at the possibilities inherent in rapeseed, sunflower, faba beans, field peas, and others. Canada will soon have available a federally assisted, but industry-run and financed, Pilot Plant Corporation facility ready to assist anyone, anywhere, in developing new technologies for proteins, oils, and starches.

Marine Protein Concentrates

Marine protein concentrates have serious problems to face. Their cause has not been helped by overoptimistic assessment of the seas as a source of conventional fish, but the most serious problem is that of cost: cost of solvents, costs of harvesting, and most prohibitive of all, price competition for fish and edible fish wastes by the fish meal industry for use as animal feed products. While much criticism has been leveled at FPC because of almost total absence of physical functionality, it is almost axiomatic that if raw material costs, reliability of supply, and process costs were comparable to those that apply to vegetable products, then the incentive would be present to create these desirable attributes. At this time, however, accurate, full-scale process costs are unknown, and raw material costs fluctuate wildly, always trending upward.

Single-Cell Proteins

From a rather daring and somewhat dubious concept of a few years ago, single or simple multicells have recently made tremendous gains in stature and practicality in their current stance as sources of animal feeds. This development can at least relieve pressure on human food supplies. For direct human use, the greatest successes to date have been with yeasts, which are hardly new. SCP is here to stay, however, and many of the processing problems that still remain in this technology will yield to concentrated engineering effort. Perhaps more troublesome may be the need to reduce nucleic acid contents and the carry-over of undesirable substrate components into the final product. The recent rises in energy costs have not only dealt severe blows to the cost of conventional foods, but may well require an agonized reappraisal of the cost components for new foods such as SCP.

Subject Index

Index of Countries and Geographical Areas